COVID-19 Impacts on Child Health

COVID-19 Impacts of Child Health

Jessica L. Peck
Editor

COVID-19 Impacts on Child Health

A Holistic Framework for Pediatric
Supportive Care

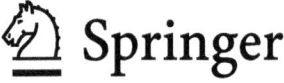 Springer

Editor
Jessica L. Peck
Clinical Professor, Louise Herrington
School of Nursing
Baylor University
Dallas, TX, USA

ISBN 978-3-031-80368-0   ISBN 978-3-031-80369-7   (eBook)
https://doi.org/10.1007/978-3-031-80369-7

This Springer imprint is published by the registered company Springer Nature Switzerland AG
The registered company address is: Gewerbestrasse 11, 6330 Cham, Switzerland

If disposing of this product, please recycle the paper.

Introduction

A joyful heart is good medicine, but a crushed spirit dries up the bones.
—Proverbs 17:22

During the first week of March in 2020, I was at the state capitol building in Austin, Texas for a nurse practitioner event. As I was sitting in the auditorium, I felt a tap on my shoulder. Behind me was the Director of Government Affairs, whispering there was a news crew in the lobby, asking if I'd mind giving a quick interview. I was no stranger to media engagements and it was not uncommon for local media to cover health events occurring in the legislature. Without any hesitation or angst, I casually strolled out of the auditorium and crossed the cavernous atrium without a care in the world while admiring the majesty of soaring columns carved from pink Texas granite. I was in no rush while getting fitted with a microphone and internally formulating a few responses to routine questions I anticipated on nurse practitioner care. Little did I know as I looked up and into the camera lens, I would suddenly become like Alice in Wonderland, falling down an unexpected rabbit hole into a world gone mad, where things became curiouser and curiouser by the moment. The news reporter's first question to me inquired about my reaction as a nurse to the COVID-19 virus. It is an indescribable understatement to say I was caught off guard. I stumbled. I mumbled. I wondered internally why she was asking me about an obscure virus that was at this point seemingly nowhere near Texas and irrelevant to pediatrics in the moment. Media rumblings were dismissed as fear mongering by seasoned health professionals who remembered previous outbreaks like the Severe Acute Respiratory Syndrome (SARS) outbreak of 2003. SARS was first reported in China but had resulted in around 8000 cases globally and only a handful of cases in the United States. I walked away from the interview confused and disconcerted, but shook it off as a one-off and resumed what was a very typical legislative day under a cheerfully blue Texas sky.

I left straight from the capitol to vacation with my family in San Francisco for Spring break. As we arrived, news of the Princess cruise ship stranded off the California coast floated over the airwaves as my husband and I exchanged quizzical expressions over the heads of our young children, struggling to interpret how this should direct our actions. We arrived at Oracle Park to tour the home of the San Francisco Giants, where we were met by employees who were unsure what to do with us. After much whispering and back-and-forth walks to the manager's office, we were simply told the stadium was closed to tours for the day with no further explanation than a shoulder shrug. At the Walt Disney Family Museum, we found a notice explaining they were closed for the day to clean but not to worry; they planned to reopen the next day. On a boat ride to Alcatraz, we were surrounded by public chatter with growing concern and curiosity. Little could we appreciate the foreshadowing looming that day in the literal shadows of the world's most infamous prison. We decided it was wisest to go home and as we arrived at the airport, we were greeted by sirens, lights, and caution tape accompanying a news crew covering a singular COVID-19 case of an infected airline worker. Palpable panic was rapidly rising in the gathered crowds hovering at each gate, anxious to get out of there. As we waited for our flight, my phone began to ping ominously with news from home that the Houston Livestock Show and Rodeo had been cancelled. An event revered in Space City since 1932, the reverberations of cancellation felt catastrophic, as we knew only the most severe circumstances would halt an event that welcomes millions of guests each year raising millions of dollars for scholarships. After our flight arrived in Houston late that evening, I had a primal parental urge I couldn't really explain to immediately go buy food and supplies. As I entered the grocery store near the midnight hour with my teenaged daughter, I was shocked to see a line waiting with staff controlling timed entry. The shelves looked barer than before Houston hurricane preparation, which left me with a feeling of fear and dread as I bought an off-brand, random assortment of food and household items I often had to climb or crawl to reach on the shelves. I saw public shaming of carts piled high and experienced moral distress as I struggled between buying enough for my family while considering needs of the other families around me.

The next morning, I was scheduled to practice at a primary care clinic in suburban Houston, where I was employed at the time. I went with trepidation but found the morning to start off somewhat routinely with newborn visits and well child care showing up as scheduled. That temporary reassurance abruptly ended with a visit from the local health department, who shoved a handful of COVID-19 testing swabs at me with little explanation and left. Then the phones started ringing… and ringing… and ringing. The first was a family who had just returned from New York City. Their toddler was symptomatic for COVID-19 and had a presumptive exposure. What should they do, they asked me. I distinctly remember where I was standing with the phone in my hand, looking around at my clinic full of staff and waiting room full of families, all looking to me to tell them what to do. Time stood still and all sound stopped. I remember looking down in what felt like slow motion at the casual, comfortable dress I was wearing, typical for me on clinic days in professional attire but comfy enough to play with kids. I stared at my ballet flats with shiny buttons on the toes and I suddenly felt completely and utterly ridiculous. I realized this was war. I needed sneakers. I needed scrubs. I needed a pony tail. I needed personal protective equipment (PPE), but this was a small, independent, brand-new clinic. We didn't have a stockpile of masks or gowns—why in the world would we have needed them? I ended up *sharing* a *used* N-95 mask with another nurse at the clinic, whose husband had found it in the garage after previously wearing it to paint something. We passed it back and forth, sanitizing it as best we could while trying not to poison ourselves. I turned the back alley of the clinic into a drive-through clinic and testing site. I shut down the waiting room. I created emergency protocols. I swabbed snotty noses while kids coughed in my face as I wondered internally if I was endangering my family or if I'd even be able to go home. And life as we knew it died that day. The world would never be the same.

This is my story. There are literally millions of other healthcare providers with their own story, many, if not most, more tragic than mine. I have never been more proud to stand shoulder to shoulder with other direct care providers. I want the public to know that there are many brave individuals who did their very, very best and sacrificed much to do it. Some even sacrificed their own lives. Thank you is not enough.

It's easy to look back with 20/20 hindsight, but it's *impossible* to overemphasize the complete and utter blindside that came to healthcare professionals in March of 2020. The overall sentiment was being completely stunned... stunned at the lack of preparation, lack of warning, lack of coordination in response, lack of PPE, lack of credible information, lack of support... and the list goes on and on. I watched as physicians and advanced practice clinicians desperately made social media pages documenting the details of their clinical encounters daily in an attempt to connect with others who were watching people die in droves. I watched as nurses were expected to show up to work in the face of a deadly virus while carrying their reused PPE in paper bags for weeks on end, even creating repair kits to make a one-use disposable mask stretch for weeks if not months. I watched as emails came through from my local health system, requiring me to take online classes on ventilator management and be prepared to be called to intensive care service. (This was way out of my scope of practice and I had no practical experience managing a ventilator at all). I watched as my nurse practitioner students set up temporary hospitals barracks-style in New York City, cared for an outbreak on an aircraft carrier in Guam, sat with dying patients while their families watched helplessly on video, helped birthing mothers bring new life into the world without a single support person present, told parents of children in the neonatal intensive care unit they had to choose only one person to be a designated visitor, and tried to comfort hospitalized children who were not permitted to have a caregiver present. There emerged an immeasurable trove of trauma I still have not recovered from to this day. I asked my students in what ways I could support them during these early days of the outbreak. Below are representations of some of those requests, but I warn you. Proceed reading with caution. Take care of your heart and get a tissue.

> It has been a stressful last month but I also have been working the last 10 days, testing anywhere from 100 to 150 COVID tests myself daily, so it has been chaotic. I sadly had an elderly patient who I had seen as his provider in the last week, with positive results who committed suicide so he wouldn't infect his wife who was traveling to care for their children at the time. So that has been very tough to process.

I just learned that a dear friend of mine and co-worker died today from COVID-19. It is very unexpected as my unit has decided to not take any patients diagnosed with COVID-19 and has put in place a lot of measures to keep our unit safe. I was told she was only symptomatic for 4 days before she passed.

I called my work and learned half of our patients now have COVID-19. They are not doing well because they are immunocompromised. I work with acute neurological patients. They moved all of our positive patients to one end of the hall with makeshift plastic shower curtains to separate. We do not have N95 or other necessities. We are reusing masks.

Please pray for our patients, families, and bedside nursing staff as we navigate through changes in visitation policies caused by an upswing of COVID-19 cases. We are overwhelmed struggling with staffing full and overflow units and our patients are dying alone. This week has been the most difficult I have experienced in my career.

The moral distress of patients dying alone in itself is difficult for the entire team and something I would never have imagined. I've been living in a trailer self-isolating and haven't seen my family in a month.

During this time, I was serving as president of the National Association of Pediatric Nurse Practitioners, a 3-year term to which I had been elected in March of 2019. The weight of responsibility was crushing. Not only was I worried about my own family, my students in graduate nursing education, and my patients and their families in clinical practice, I had the responsibility of leading my colleagues through what was certainly the darkest time in my professional experience existing over a span of nearly 30 years. I remember sitting in a hotel parking lot in San Francisco during my "vacation" on an emergency executive board meeting conference call (this was unimaginably before videoconferencing was the norm). We discussed cancelling our annual conference scheduled to occur the next week, an event nearly half a century in tradition in which we expected more than 2000 nurse practitioners to gather as experts in pediatrics and advocates for children. This was a multi-million dollar decision for the organization and I imagined the impact of all the participants who had already paid for travel. As we came to a voice vote, I was called upon first and felt like my vote of "aye" to cancel was in the deepest, most slow-motion voice you can imagine. Little did we know, this would soon be the least of our concerns as greater tragedies awaited. I led this 9000 member organization from the 8 × 10 confines of my home office and desk computer, which granted me a tiny window into the world of my colleagues. I made high-stakes decisions with precious little information and even less time as I fully realized the magnitude and weight of my words. Life was literally in the balance. I started a podcast before professional organization podcasts were common, simply recording them on my laptop and sending them out as an urgent message to rally the troops in the trenches. I learned with the rest of the world how to go live on social media as I feverishly tried to give much-needed information to our members. I hosted the first-ever virtual conference from my desk at home, trying to foster connections in a profession crushed by the weight of the pandemic.

As the historical weight of this moment sunk in, I realized I had a responsibility to objectively measure the impact of the pandemic on our profession. Along with my colleague Dr. Jennifer Sonney, we designed and delivered the first-ever survey of advanced practice pediatric nursing professionals. The results were devastating.

Measured in March of 2021, 34% of our colleagues indicated moderate or extreme concern for burnout, while 25% felt nervous or anxious and 15% felt depressed or hopeless (Peck & Sonney, 2021). One year later, we reissued the survey and found the spirit of our colleagues to be much more distressed with 87% of our colleagues now reporting professional burnout. Additionally, concern over worsening pediatric mental health outcomes increased from 74% to 94%, with nearly 60% reporting extreme concern. Close to half of respondents reported increased concern for child abuse. Almost 90% reported responding to misinformation as the primary barrier faced in clinical practice (Sonney & Peck, 2023). The impacts were widespread, not only impacting clinical arenas, but also delayed critical pediatric research efforts and significantly impacted student progression and clinical training with severely limited clinical experiences. There were more than 200 pages of open comments submitted in this survey that took several days and several boxes of tissues to get through. It will take years if not decades for the pediatric care continuum to recover. It is my hope every nurse reading this will take time to read the articles Dr. Sonney and I published to illuminate the experiences of our colleagues.

Although there was much reporting on the impact of COVID-19 on health professionals in general and with particular emphasis on emergency or intensive care providers, there was little attention paid to pediatrics as a discipline. I watched as the collective public narrative emerged that COVID-19 was not a threat to children. And while it was true that the pandemic (thankfully) spared children from a similar burden of morbidity and mortality experienced in the adult population, I watched as their world crumbled around them.

Consider these generational milestones:

- *Where were you on VE Day?*
- *Where were you when JFK was assassinated?*
- *Where were you when the Challenger exploded?*
- *Where were you on 9/11?*

This generation of youth will now ask, *"Where were you when quarantine started?"* It's a sobering thought. In past generations, the aforementioned events all had something in common. They sparked a sense of unity and a desire to serve the collective good. These tragedies and trials brought people together. COVID-19 was distinctly different in that it tore the world apart. Children watched as partisan politics created angry accusations and divisions. Children watched as their schools closed, along with every social outlet and safety net. Children watched as their parents lost their jobs or struggled to work from home while managing homeschooling and coping with no childcare. Other children watched as their parents left every day to risk their lives in frontline service capacities, coming home and removing their clothing in the garage before running to the shower. Estimates tell us that more than 10 million children in the world experienced the death of their parent or caregiver. Children watched the faces of their smartphones and other screens, desperate for human interaction as waves of loneliness and anxiety crashed relentlessly. Children watched adult faces disappear behind masks, with eyes full of worry and fear visible. Children learned words like social distancing and personal protective equipment. The world watched as two children sat on the concrete of a Taco Bell parking lot, trying to get internet access for schoolwork. The world watched as the National Center for Missing and Exploited Children raised alarms about skyrocketing reports of child predators abusing children through social media messaging amid unfathomable demand for child sexual abuse materials.

The truth is, COVID-19 created a catastrophic social, emotional, and psychological injury to the heart and soul of children that will be generations-long in the processing and healing. As adult stewards of their future, we must do better. The COVID-19 pandemic crushed the collective spirit of the world, but a joyful heart is good medicine. The question is, where can we find joy in the midst of such great suffering? I believe the answer to that question lies in the pages of this book. Here you will find brilliant voices of innovators, leaders, scientists, clinicians, and researchers who collectively pursue a mission of stewarding well the future of the world's children. These brave souls find audacious optimism in the face of utter pessimism. They have learned to find peace in chaos, joy in sorrow, and comfort in pain. They have raised their voices in a collective clarion call to the future. They have humbly shared their mistakes and gratefully shared their victories. It should be noted this work is far from complete and discerning readers will note omissions of additional considerations or reflect with their own updated experience or data. This is not meant to be a complete record but simply a starting place with a historical lens for future vision. It would be remiss of me to not share with you the great personal cost it took for some of these writers to relive and share their experiences. The word of the year for 2020 was "unprecedented" and it couldn't be more reflective of the realities faced by the healthcare community. I ask that you extend grace as you read, recognizing the rapid evolving that is occurring and will continue to occur. This historical account represents a snapshot in time, with recognition that language, knowledge, practice guidelines, and other information will continue to change as we continue to learn. You are invited to step into a vast array of clinical environments and listen to the stories of witnesses who have lived to share their stories here in the pages of this book. There will be another global pandemic or other disaster that inevitably threatens child health, but you can learn from their lessons, glean from their wisdom, and benefit from their experience. It will take our collective courage and shared strengths to build a better world for tomorrow, but I believe that it is possible by stewarding these lessons of the past to build a bridge of hope to the future.

To all the healthcare professionals who bravely fought on the front lines of the COVID-19 pandemic, we owe you a debt of gratitude. This disaster befell a healthcare system long fractured and vulnerable, exposing what we as healthcare providers have seen behind the scenes for decades. People deserve better and I believe we are capable of creating better. May future readers of this work honor your legacy by carrying forward the good work started here.

https://www.jpedhc.org/article/S0891-5245(23)00214-6/fulltext
https://www.jpedhc.org/article/S0891-5245(21)00094-8/fulltext

Clinical Professor   Jessica Peck
Louise Herrington School of Nursing
Baylor University
Dallas, TX, USA
jessica_peck@baylor.edu

References

Peck, J. L., & Sonney, J. (2021). Exhausted and burned out: COVID-19 emerging impacts threaten the health of the pediatric advanced practice nursing workforce. *Journal of Pediatric Health Care, 35*(4), 414–424. https://doi.org/10.1016/j.pedhc.2021.04.012

Sonney, J. T., & Peck J. L. (2023). The cost of caring during COVID 19: A clarion call to action to support the pediatric advanced practice nursing workforce. *Journal of Pediatric Health Care, 37*(6), 658–672. https://doi.org/10.1016/j.pedhc.2023.08.003

Contents

Acute Care Implications: Principles of Inpatient Management

Amanda Johnson

When written in Chinese, the word crisis is composed of two characters.
One represents danger and the other represents opportunity.

—John F. Kennedy

Introduction and Background

In the beginning of 2020, the coronavirus disease 19 (COVID-19) pandemic changed how pediatric hospitals in the United States and around the world cared for patients. Pediatric healthcare professionals (HCPs) prepared for the worst and waited. Scheduled surgeries halted, pediatric emergency departments had limited patients, and parental fear of hospital care was prevalent. Children sheltered in place at home and did not go to school. While adult-focused providers were overwhelmed with patients and makeshift triage centers were constructed to provide care, pediatric hospitals were nearly empty and quiet. This emptiness allowed for opportunity to assist pandemic response efforts by transforming pediatric intensive care units (PICUs) into adult intensive care units (ICUs) and/or having pediatric HCPs work in adult COVID-19 units in other parts of an adult-based hospital. Ethically, it was distressing for pediatric HCPs to see empty beds and available resources when adult care providers and units were in dire straits. Although providers were willing, the challenge was how to do it safely, effectively, within the scope of certification and licensure while not leaving vulnerable children without care. In some instances, PICUs were split into hybrid units in which most beds were designated for adults in COVID-19 specific units with a reserved remainder for children.

A. Johnson (✉)
Rush University, Chicago, IL, USA

University of Chicago, Chicago, IL, USA
e-mail: amanda_johnson@rush.edu

J. L. Peck (ed.), *COVID-19 Impacts on Child Health*,
https://doi.org/10.1007/978-3-031-80369-7_1

1

The unknown epidemiology and clinical course for COVID-19 in pediatrics caused HCPs to extrapolate information from case reports, professional social networks, and weekly government updates. The first reports of the effects of COVID-19 in pediatrics came from China in early 2020, with most children experiencing mild symptoms; however, about 6% of children had more severe symptoms requiring escalated respiratory support (Dong et al., 2020). Five percent (672) of children in the United States with a positive diagnosis of COVID-19 between April and October 2020 required hospitalization and 4% (38) of these children required respiratory mechanical ventilation (Parcha et al., 2021). Healthcare professionals did their best to translate the information that was known into best practice, often shifting strategies week-to-week in response to rapidly evolving information.

Emerging variants of COVID-19, particularly the Delta variant, caused an acceleration of positive pediatric cases in the United States in mid-2021. Mandates on masking and social distancing were lifting, and schools were reverting to in-person learning, factors which promoted viral transmission. COVID-19 vaccinations were not yet approved for children under the age of 12 years, leaving them vulnerable to infection. PICU admissions related to COVID-19 increased during July–September 2021. Approximately 10% of these admissions required respiratory mechanical ventilation, but overall hospital admissions for children remained low in comparison to adults with the Delta variant (Bahl et al., 2023). The Omicron variant became prominent in fall of 2021, and although more contagious with shorter incubation period, it did not increase PICU admissions (Bahl et al., 2023).

As the general population continued to resume pre-pandemic norms, pediatric hospitals were overwhelmed in 2022 with a so-called tripledemic. Many PICUs were over capacity as respiratory coinfections were prevalent. The tripledemic, consisting of concurrent outbreaks of respiratory syncytial virus (RSV), influenza, and COVID-19 (in addition to rhinovirus and enterovirus) caused a surge of children requiring respiratory support, mechanical ventilation, and cardiovascular support. The tripledemic strained pediatric hospitals unprepared for the influx in patients. Makeshift triage centers once used for adult COVID-19 patients were now being used for care of viral coinfections in pediatric patients. This surge was not isolated to COVID-19, but it is prudent to discuss the repercussions of isolation recommendations and the subsequent unseasonal resurgence of common respiratory infections that had been very low in the pediatric population over the previous 2 years. Pediatric hospitals continue to seek balance of a new era of care as the pandemic transitions into an endemic phase.

Points of Care

Framework of Transforming PICUs for Adult Care

In early 2020, adult ICUs globally were overwhelmed at capacity for admissions, causing distress among HCPs. In the United States, daily debriefs were broadcasted in certain states to discuss COVID-19 deaths, hospital bed allotments, and ventilator availability in the state. There was a need to be resourceful with cancellation of elective surgical cases and further discussions within each institution about how to allocate bedspace. Across the world and in the United States, adult ICUs or entire floors were transformed to care for patients with COVID-19. The COVID-19 units were converted into negative pressure areas or fitted with HEPA filtration to cohort patients and prevent viral spread. Special considerations were taken when transforming these units to limit staff from exposure, such as having intravenous infusions outside the room to be programmed or changed by the nurse, and computer workstations outside of the room with capability to view the patient through a window into the room to minimize HCP exposure and usage of personal protective equipment (PPE) (Halpern et al., 2020).

Pediatric patients had less severe physical symptoms from COVID-19 in the beginning; however, adults, especially adults with comorbidities such as hypertension, type 2 diabetes mellitus, chronic obstructive pulmonary disease, and cardiovascular disease, presented 5–7 days after onset of illness in acute respiratory failure complicated by shock, acute kidney failure (AKI), acute respiratory distress syndrome (ARDS), and arrythmias requiring intensive care therapies that could only be provided in ICUs with HCPs who are trained to manage these complications (Remy et al., 2020). In the United States during this time in 2020, there were approximately 68,000 adult intensive care beds being filled and approximately 5000 PICU beds available (Remy et al., 2020). Pediatric intensivists are trained to manage respiratory failure and complications of shock, AKI, and arrythmias. However, questions arose how governmental bodies, professional associations, and institutions should or even could support care delivery of the adult patient in the PICU.

Accreditation and licensure are factors that need to be addressed prior to changing care delivery policies because in most cases approval to provide care is dependent on federal and state laws and regulations governing the jurisdiction of the institution (Halpern et al., 2020; Remy et al., 2020). In March 2020, the United States federal government signed into law the "Coronavirus Aid, Relief, and Economic Security Act" (CARES Act) to include Good Samaritan protection for HCPs. Individual state governors made executive orders to allow HCPs to expand their scope of practice. Retired HCPs were allowed to return to work during the public health emergency. The National Association of Pediatric Nurse Practitioners (NAPNAP) amended their position statement on age parameters, previously updated in 2019, to protect pediatric nurse practitioners who were faced with the challenge of caring for adults. NAPNAP's position was to support adult care by pediatric HCPs if it was done safely, within the boundaries of their state's nurse practice act, and if they could hand-off care to an adult provider when able (Worsely, 2019). There was an expansion on HCP ability to perform telehealth in more locations with more diverse delivery modalities. Also, HCPs were able to quickly obtain out-of-state licenses to allow help in different states with the ongoing crisis. These changes gave protection to pediatric HCPs and allowed PICUs to care for adult patients.

Major metropolitan areas and defined geographical areas developed central command centers to communicate hospital capacities and supplies to triage and facilitate transfers as needed (Christian et al., 2014; Halpern et al., 2020). This communication allowed Massachusetts General Hospital, a children's hospital, to transfer their remaining pediatric patients in their PICU to other freestanding children's hospitals in Boston to allow their PICU to be transformed into an adult ICU (Yager et al., 2020). Globally, similar triage centers and transformations of PICUs were occurring. In France, one hospital chose to transform the PICU into an adult ICU and makeshift a PICU as part of the emergency department (Chomton et al., 2021). Other institutions divided the PICU into both adult ICU care and PICU care.

There had to be preparation of the PICU space to occupy adult patients. Pediatric patients' small size with relation to pediatric equipment would not be satisfactory for adult care. Considerations for endotracheal tube size, laryngoscopes, central and peripheral vascular access, dialysis catheters, urinary catheters, extracorporeal membrane oxygenation (ECMO) cannulas, temporary transvenous pacing catheters, adult defibrillators, adult crash carts, and suction catheters all had to be stocked and distributed to the PICU (Chomton et al., 2021; Halpern et al., 2020; Remy et al., 2020). Each room was transformed if not already negative pressure, HEPA filters were installed to create isolation rooms, cardiorespiratory monitors were reconfigured to adult parameters from pediatric parameters, adult hospital beds replaced cribs, intravenous pumps were reconfigured for adult programming, and if possible, space was configured outside of the room to allow the patient to be visualized without entering the room (Halpern et al., 2020; Remy et al., 2020; Wasserman et al., 2021). If a shared pediatric/adult space was created, special care to keep pediatric supplies separated from adult supplies was considered. If able, the unit had two different supply areas and a physical barrier erected between the two sides of the unit to avoid cross contamination (Halpern et al., 2020).

As the physical space was prepared, staff were educated in days (not weeks or months) to care for adult patients. Part of the rapid education for pediatric nurses included orientation in an adult ICU paired with an adult nurse for a few shifts. The focus of this orientation was to learn non-weight-based medication dosing, adult inotropic medications, ventilator management, and documentation (Wasserman et al., 2021). This orientation allowed the newly trained pediatric nurse to orientate other pediatric nurses to the care of the adult patient with COVID-19.

Policies and protocols were also written in days, not months, as had been the norm. Policies for PPE were distributed and reviewed by pediatric nurses, although each institution had a different evaluation process. Quick references for protocols regarding COVID-19 intubation, sedation, suctioning, prone positioning, and ECMO in adults were printed and kept in several locations on the unit for review. Pharmacists created medication dosing cards and provided education on medications specific to COVID-19 treatment strategies, such as antivirals (Halpern et al., 2020). Some institutions used their simulation centers to help pediatric HCPs practice these new protocols (Yager et al., 2020). Emerging evidence on the care for COVID-19 caused policies and protocols to continually change; these changes were disseminated during daily rounds, emails, and ongoing staff education.

Consideration was taken when deploying staff into newly formed adult ICUs. A tiered strategy was incorporated when divvying up staff to allow the most experienced critical care staff be the point of direct care (Halpern et al., 2020). In some institutions, adult critical care professionals had a consultation role, overseeing the newly created adult ICUs while hospitalists, pediatric intensivists, subspecialities, and anesthesiologists provided direct patient care in the ICUs (Remy et al., 2020). Other institutions had adult critical care professionals round daily either virtually or in person with the "new" adult HCP to discuss points of care and to provide education on adult-specific processes and myocardial infarctions (Wasserman et al., 2021). Teams were created with specialists to perform intubations, central venous access, and ECMO cannulation. Nurses were also redeployed from surgical areas, general pediatric floors, and pediatric emergency departments. Their ICU experience was factored for acuity of direct patient care; nurses without ICU experience were used at times to assist patient care, turning, bathing, disinfecting, and obtaining supplies (Chomton et al., 2021; Remy et al., 2020). Part of the treatment of COVID-19 with ARDS was turning the patients prone. Assistance available to help turn large adult patients provided ergonomic protection and allowed for both staff and patients to remain safe during repositioning. The complement of staff helped nurse-to-patient ratios remain low, given the high acuity.

Special considerations including sedation preference, alcohol withdrawal, pressure ulcers, and other adult comorbidities should be included in education if PICUs are transformed again to care for adult patients (Chomton et al., 2021; Remy et al., 2020). In adult ICUs, patients are typically sedated with propofol, a medication not commonly used in pediatrics because of the concern for propofol infusion syndrome. Pediatric HCPs might not feel comfortable titrating propofol to a higher dosing that is acceptable in adult care. About 20% of adult ICU patients are at risk for developing alcohol withdrawal syndrome, and signs of alcohol withdrawal should be reviewed with pediatric HCPs (Remy et al., 2020). A withdrawal assessment scale should be included in documentation education when transforming a PICU to an adult ICU. Pediatric patients do develop pressure ulcers; however, adult patients are more severely affected because of their body habitus, poor perfusion with illness, and peripheral vascular disease. Pediatric HCPs should be conscious of using skin barriers proactively and use a skin assessment scale when caring for critically ill adults.

Rapid transformation of PICUs into adult ICUs was successful during the beginning of the COVID-19 pandemic. Most of the care focused on cardiopulmonary physiology and multiple system organ failure, for which pediatric HCPs are comfortable providing care (Wasserman et al., 2021). The COVID-19 pandemic demonstrated that pediatric HCPs are resilient in a crisis. However, there is remaining concern for long-term ramifications of the pandemic causing burnout and HCPs leaving the bedside.

Management of COVID-19

In the beginning of 2020, pediatric patients admitted to the PICU for management of COVID-19 represented between 2% and 4% of all pediatric patients with COVID-19 in the United States, with the mortality rate reported between 1% and

4% (Kache et al., 2020; Parcha et al., 2021). Because of the limited number of pediatric patients seeking health care, the International COVID-19 PICU Collaborative was formed in March 2020 to help provide real-time information across the world with virtual meetings every week (Shekerdemian et al., 2020). Globally, low- and middle-income countries had a higher mortality rate for pediatric patients with COVID-19 compared to high-income countries, which could be reflective of the overall healthcare system capacity in these countries (Kitano et al., 2021). Pediatric patients under the age of 1 year had the greatest risk of requiring hospitalization and mortality, non-distinguishable by country income (Kache et al., 2020; Kitano et al., 2021). The treatment strategies described in this section were translated into practice for pediatric patients who presented throughout the pandemic with the novel COVID-19 and Delta and Omicron variants.

Signs and symptoms of COVID-19 observed in pediatric patients were like adult patients' symptoms but without, in most cases, onset of hypoxemia. Pediatric patients had gastrointestinal symptoms with vomiting and diarrhea more frequently than adults but generally did not warrant PICU admission. Other common symptoms included fever, cough, sore throat, rhinorrhea, headache, and shortness of breath (Kache et al., 2020). Multisystem inflammatory syndrome in children (MIS-C) was seen in pediatric patients presenting with mild-to-severe multiorgan involvement and will be discussed in detail under complications (Kache et al., 2020).

Respiratory symptoms associated with COVID-19 prompted the most PICU admissions during the pandemic (Shekerdemian et al., 2020). If children presented with mild distress without hypoxemia or increased work of breathing, they were discharged home to be monitored by the caregiver. If the child had moderate-to-severe respiratory distress with hypoxemia, it warranted admission to the PICU or general unit for oxygen supplementation. Non-invasive oxygen supplementation included low flow nasal cannula and if needed, escalated to high flow nasal cannula (HFNC), continuous positive airway pressure, or bilevel positive airway pressure, depending on the response to the treatment (Kache et al., 2020). Most children were discharged home about 7 days after weaning oxygen support (Chao et al., 2020). There was a low percentage of pediatric patients requiring escalation to invasive mechanical ventilation with concern for ARDS (Chao et al., 2020; Kache et al., 2020). If mechanical ventilation was required because of concern for airborne infection, the most skilled provider or intubation team was recommended to perform the procedure with video laryngoscopy, if available, to increase the distance between the HCP and patient (Chao et al., 2020; Kache et al., 2020). A cuffed endotracheal tube was recommended with inflation of the cuff once position was confirmed to help decrease airborne pathogen contamination. Mechanical ventilation management strategies for pediatric patients with ARDS secondary to COVID-19 were treated as any pediatric patient with ARDS. There was a paucity of information in the beginning of the pandemic regarding pediatric patients with COVID-19 and ARDS, resulting in treatment strategy selection based on published pediatric case reports and extrapolating information from adults with COVID-19 and ARDS. Prone positioning, escalation of positive end expiratory pressure (PEEP), escalation to high frequency oscillatory ventilation, nitric oxide, and ECMO were all considerations to individualize patient care without significant evidence of changes in the outcome (Kache et al., 2020).

Healthcare professionals provided hemodynamic monitoring in pediatric patients with COVID-19 in the PICU and included observation for signs of shock: tachycardia and hypotension. Compensated and uncompensated shocks were treated using best practice national guidelines, the 2020 Surviving Sepsis Campaign for treating shock at the time. Epinephrine or norepinephrine was recommended as first-line inotropic support. It was also recommended to obtain cardiac biomarkers, echocardiography, and electrocardiogram with any present concern for myocarditis and hyperinflammatory process (Kache et al., 2020). If able, the HCP placed an arterial pressure line to monitor mean arterial pressures with adjunctive therapies for the treatment of sepsis. If escalation to ECMO was required for hemodynamic stability, it was not contraindicated; however, there were limited patients requiring escalation.

Therapeutic medication treatment strategies for care of symptoms evolved throughout the pandemic and at times changed day-by-day depending on the most recent evidence in adult clinical trials. Acetaminophen was recommended in the beginning for treatment of febrile state and myalgia because there was concern of nonsteroidal anti-inflammatory drugs (NSAIDs) to worsen COVID-19 symptoms (Kache et al., 2020). In pediatric patients with severe respiratory illness, dexamethasone was recommended as there was improvement in mortality of adult patients when it was used with patients already requiring oxygen support or mechanical ventilation (Younis et al., 2021). Dexamethasone was not found to improve outcomes in adults if administered in individuals without a respiratory support requirement. The pediatric clinical outcome information regarding use of dexamethasone was extrapolated from adult clinical trials, and discussion of use in pediatrics was case-by-case, dependent on severity of illness of the individual. There were also several pediatric patients who received azithromycin with concern for co-infection of pneumonia with COVID-19 with moderate-to-severe respiratory distress (Shekerdemian et al., 2020).

During the pandemic, the Food and Drug Administration (FDA) under the Coronavirus Treatment Acceleration Program expedited new medical products for use in patients suffering with symptoms related to COVID-19 and hoped to lessen the mortality rate that was growing exponentially daily in adults. Clinical trials were performed as soon and as safely as possible to assist in development of treatment options. These clinical trials included investigating use of antivirals already established for care of other illnesses. The antivirals that were used as treatment in clinical trials in adults included: chloroquine/hydroxychloroquine, ivermectin, lopinavir/ritonavir, remdesivir, and tocilizumab, which were given to adult patients who were gravely ill without improvement in symptoms with other treatment strategies (Younis et al., 2021). The results extrapolated from these expedited adult clinical trials were then reviewed in light of the identified concern and considered for use in pediatrics. In late Spring 2020, chloroquine/ hydroxychloroquine was authorized for emergency use by the FDA in hospitalized patients weighing greater than 50 kilograms with severe symptoms of COVID-19, but authorization for emergency use was later revoked in June 2020 with little-to-no improvement found and increased risk of side effects noted in patients receiving this medication. There were pediatric patients with severe respiratory symptoms who received hydroxychloroquine during the emergency authorization (Chao et al., 2020; Shekerdemian et al., 2020). Tocilizumab was administered as a single agent and in combination with hydroxychloroquine during PICU admissions in Spring 2020 in five children who were severely ill in the United States (Shekerdemian et al., 2020). In late Fall 2020, the FDA approved use of remdesivir in adult and pediatric patients 12 years of age and older and weighing at least 40 kilograms with emergency use authorization for pediatric patients weighing at least 3.5 kg hospitalized with confirmed COVID-19 (U.S. Food & Drug Administration, 2020). The recommendation was for the pediatric HCP to monitor laboratory values including complete blood count (CBC), complete metabolic panel (CMP), and and international normalization ratio (INR) as a baseline and intermittently while receiving remdesivir therapy (U.S. Food & Drug Administration, 2020).

There were several pediatric institutions in the beginning of the pandemic that did not experience any children with COVID-19 or only provided care to a single case or two. Pediatric consortiums were most important during the pandemic to help disseminate best practice strategies with a limited number of pediatric patients becoming severely ill from COVID-19. Pediatric professionals in infectious disease were invaluable during the pandemic to support the constantly evolving and changing practice over the first year of the pandemic prior to vaccine availability.

Risk Factors for Pediatric Patients

Adult patients with comorbidities had a higher morbidity and mortality rate when infected with COVID-19. There were also common themes in underlying medical conditions noted in pediatric patients with COVID-19 which required escalation of intensive care. Obesity was an underlying condition that caused both adult and pediatric patients to more likely require ICU care with increased support (Chao et al., 2020; Shekerdemian et al., 2020; Wanga et al., 2021). Obese children were twice as likely to require admission to the PICU than non-obese children. Younger children and adolescents were found to have a higher risk for requiring PICU admission (Esposito et al., 2021). Pediatric patients with underlying chromosomal abnormalities, neurological, developmental, or metabolic disease were also associated with a higher admission rate to the PICU with more severe symptoms (Schroeder et al., 2023; Wanga et al., 2021). Another comorbidity in pediatric patients was asthma, which caused a longer length in PICU stay, longer requirement of respiratory support, development of pneumonia, and more likely need for inotropic support when compared to pediatric patients without asthma (Schroeder et al., 2023). Diabetes mellitus types 1 and 2 and hypoglycemia were chronic endocrine conditions which required higher level of care in a PICU (Banull et al., 2022). There was concern that poorly controlled glycemia caused higher inflammatory response to COVID-19. An underlying diagnosis of adrenal insufficiency was treated with stress corticosteroid dosing in the presence of COVID-19 as is common with other acute illnesses. The more comorbidities a pediatric patient had, the more severe symptoms with COVID-19 and higher rates of admission to the PICU (Schroeder et al., 2023).

Consideration of socioeconomic status should also be factored into the risk profile of a pediatric patient with COVID-19 who required admission to the PICU. Lower socioeconomic status impacts healthcare across the continuum, and patients with COVID-19 were not immune to this impact. Poor overall access to health increases risk of comorbidities described in this section and by in turn increased risk of a PICU admission.

Multisystem Inflammatory Syndrome in Children (MIS-C) a Complication of COVID-19

Beginning in April 2020, pediatric patients were evaluated for a hyperinflammatory state with symptoms that were concerning for Kawasaki disease or toxic shock syndrome; however, the symptoms did not quite fit perfectly into either of these known diagnoses. The Centers for Disease Control and Prevention (CDC) announced a health advisory for a multisystem hyperinflammatory state in pediatrics (MIS-C) with a clinical presentation about 2–6 weeks after having COVID-19 or suspected of having COVID-19. The presentation criterion for MIS-C at this time were defined as (1) being less than 21 years of age with fever, (2) elevated inflammation serum markers, (3) hospitalization for severe illness with multisystem organ involvement, (4) no other possible diagnoses, and (5) tested positive for COVID-19 or have recent COVID-19 infection or exposure (Kache et al., 2020). Pediatric HCPs were put on high alert of the severity of MIS-C with concern for septic shock, myocarditis, cardiopulmonary arrest, and pediatric death with recent COVID-19 infection. When MIS-C was first recognized, it affected school age children 5–11 years old more than other ages; however, with the Omicron variant children age less than 5 years presented in higher frequency with MIS-C (Campbell et al., 2022). Black, Hispanic, and Asian children were more likely to experience MIS-C compared to White children.

Recommended laboratory evaluation for pediatric patients with concern for MIS-C includes C-reactive protein (CRP), erythrocyte sedimentation rate, fibrinogen, procalcitonin, D-dimer, ferritin, brain natriuretic peptide (BNP), and lactic acid dehydrogenase serum levels; if elevated, the HCP started treatment. Cardiorespiratory function was reviewed with echocardiography, electrocardiogram, chest radiograph, and/or chest computed topography scan. If the child presented with mucocutaneous lesions, conjunctival injections, and elevated serum BNP, there was a higher incidence of coronary artery abnormalities (Kalyanaraman & Anderson, 2022). There was a higher prevalence of pleural effusions and bilateral pulmonary consolidations with concern for pneumonia noted on chest radiograph in pediatric patients with MIS-C compared to children with just COVID-19 (Kalyanaraman & Anderson, 2022). Consultation with cardiology, rheumatology, and infectious disease provided an interprofessional approach to treatment strategies for MIS-C as treatment evolved with more cases seen. Each organ system affected was treated with appropriate strategies for shock, AKI, and myocarditis. Fluid resuscitation, milrinone, and epinephrine were found effective in the treatment of shock with MIS-C (Abrams et al., 2022). The first patients affected by MIS-C were prescribed intravenous immunoglobulin (IVIG), steroids, and at times infliximab or anakinra because of the anti-inflammatory effects; patients were noted to have good results with this combination (Abrams et al., 2022). In June 2020, the American College of Rheumatology published guidelines for first-line treatment of MIS-C which included IVIG and baby aspirin, and glucocorticoids for patients in shock or organ failure (Abrams et al., 2022). If the patient was refractory to this treatment, then the HCP was recommended to prescribe high-dose glucocorticoids or anakinra (Abrams et al., 2022). Empiric antibiotics were prescribed to all patients with concern for severe MIS-C until cultures were negative.

Outcomes and the number of MIS-C cases improved with each new variant of COVID-19. In the United States, the highest number of cases were reported during November 2020 through February 2021. At the height of this wave, there were over 250 cases in a week (Campbell et al., 2022). In comparison, during the Omicron wave occurring December 2021 through March 2022, the height of cases in the United States was reported at less than 150 a week (Campbell et al., 2022).

There was opportunity to review the MIS-C cases and better define criteria for HCPs to use to help diagnosis MIS-C. For example, it was observed that MIS-C patients have higher CRP levels when compared to patients with Kawasaki disease and toxic shock syndrome. The higher CRP level is more useful when differentiating these diagnoses in comparison to reviewing ferritin and fibrinogen levels. At the time of writing this chapter, the CDC current criteria for MIS-C include (1) fever greater than or equal to 38 °C, 2) severity of illness requires hospitalization, (3) CRP greater than or equal to 3.0 mg/dL, AND (4) at least two of the following: shock, mucocutaneous involvement, gastrointestinal (abdominal pain, vomiting, or diarrhea), cardiac (left ventricular ejection fraction less than 55%, elevated troponin, or coronary artery dilatation), hematology (platelets less than 150,000), OR COVID-19 status (positive COVID-19 antigen 60 days prior or detection of antibody with current illness, or close contact with confirmed COVID-19 case 60 days prior) (Banull et al., 2022). When pediatric patients started receiving the COVID-19 vaccine, the prevalence of MIS-C patients continued to decrease and most importantly, there was a significant decrease in mortality related to MIS-C. An updated case definition was constructed in 2023 to revise the 2020 criterion with an overarching aim to increase specificity and decrease misclassification.

The neurocognitive long-term effects of MIS-C are still being reviewed. At the time of writing this chapter, there was limited data available. There is some concern for decreased executive functions and lasting emotional and behavioral problems causing a disruption in learning and social interaction related to MIS-C (Otten et al., 2023). Continued research is needed to assess the complications of MIS-C over the next several years.

Viral Coinfections

Viral coinfections (such as occurred in the tripledemic) in pediatrics increase morbidity and mortality with longer length of stays and increased ventilatory requirements with admission to the PICU. During the pandemic hospital admission, rates for pediatric patients with RSV decreased significantly related to sheltering in place and limited interactions (Bozzola et al., 2022). In 2022, children were being re-introduced to in-person learning, mask mandates were dependent on each state requirement, and adults had the opportunity to vaccinate, resulting in fewer hospitalizations. These changes caused children to be exposed to common viral illnesses that they had less exposure to over the last 2 years of the pandemic. It is common to observe ebbs and flows year-to-year with the severity of common viral illnesses that require hospitalization, but the unprecedented influx of acutely ill pediatric patients during the tripledemic in 2022 is worth discussion. It is important for HCPs to understand the impact of "re-opening" a country after restrictions enacted by a pandemic and consider implications for PICU care.

Bronchiolitis secondary to RSV, influenza, rhinovirus, enterovirus, and COVID-19 coinfections caused a surge in PICU admissions, not only for children less than 1 year of age but it also affected toddlers at a significantly higher rate than in previous viral seasons before the pandemic (Bozzola et al., 2022). This higher rate of admission in older children is speculated to be related to lack of exposure and immunity to these viruses during the pandemic. Some pediatric patients with coinfections required admission to the PICU for both non-invasive and invasive respiratory support. Supportive care of symptoms of a viral illness continued to be the only treatment strategy. A subset of these patients required escalated cardiovascular support with inotropes and ECMO. The length of stay in the PICU increased for patients who presented with coinfections. There were several states with limited PICU availability during this surge, which caused some children to be transferred to adjacent states, sometimes several hundred miles away from their home.

Barriers and Breakthroughs

Caregiver Presence

Visitor restrictions were applied across all healthcare settings to limit exposure to COVID-19 and conserve the amount of PPE that was available at the start of the pandemic. Adult healthcare settings enacted a strict no visitor policy in March 2020. If an adult patient sought care, they would be dropped off at the hospital, and if admitted, the rest of the care would be discussed by phone or video call to their family members. There were countless hospitalized adult patients who died without family at their bedside during the pandemic because of the great risk for potential exposure to COVID-19. Children's hospitals throughout the United States and globally also adjusted their visiting policies. Family-centered care, once a core tenant in children's hospitals, now became a barrier and introduced more distress on caregivers and children.

Most children's hospitals initiated a screening policy for all visitors and limited visitors to one caregiver at the bedside (Bloxham et al., 2023; Hart & Taylor, 2021; McBride, 2021). The screening policy asked about recent symptoms that could be related to COVID-19 and often included a temperature screen when entering the building. The caregiver who was allowed to be at the bedside most of the time had to be someone who lived with the patient. Once admitted to the hospital and depending on the hospital policy, the caregiver was limited to the patient's room for the entire hospital stay and another caregiver was not allowed to come and relieve them. Other hospitals did allow for an exchange of caregivers after an extended period. There were some hospitals that required the caregiver to be tested for COVID-19 prior to being allowed to stay. The caregiver at the bedside was required to wear PPE, which could include a mask, gown, gloves, and eye protection dependent on the individual hospital policy. At the very least, a mask was always worn with compliance to national guidelines and recommendations. No siblings were allowed to visit during this time. In some institutions, their policy was already written to include no sibling visitation during winter months in the United States, particularly when viral illnesses were more prevalent, and this was a way to help decrease transmission (McBride, 2021).

The barrier of limited caregiver presence during the pandemic impacted communication, patient and caregiver's mental health with social isolation, and potentially impacted external burdens such as care for other children and work status. Post-traumatic stress symptoms were described by both patients and caregivers after being hospitalized during the pandemic in the PICU (Lessa et al., 2022). Restrictions in caregiver presence also impacted end-of-life care conversations.

Caregiver's communication with HCPs was limited and segmented. Prior to the pandemic, many children's hospitals invited the caregiver to participate in daily rounds with the interprofessional team. This allowed the caregiver to listen to the plan of care and ask questions. During the pandemic, caregivers were often not included on daily rounds to help decrease the risk of transmission. If the caregiver was included on daily rounds, often the HCPs stood at least 6 ft. apart with some professionals on video calls to limit the number of members of the team. This in turn caused limited communication for the caregiver, potentially decreased the opportunity to hear everything that was discussed, and limited ability to see nonverbal cues. The caregiver at the bedside was left to decipher the plan and notify other family members. Healthcare professionals did their best to provide updates to family members not at the bedside by relying on technology to have video meetings; however, there are known limitations in this means of communication compared to face-to-face interactions (Lessa et al., 2022; McBride, 2021).

Children were restricted to their room during the pandemic and only interacted with the caregiver at bedside and HCPs who entered the room when required. The restriction of visitors caused children to feel lonely and miss their other family members. Phone calls and video chats helped the child feel less lonely; however, this was not the same as personal contact. Prior to the pandemic, children's hospitals would rely on the child life department to help provide social interaction and distraction for the hospitalized patient; however, during the pandemic, child life accessibility was very limited because of the patient's inability to leave the hospital room. This loneliness was also noted in the caregiver at the bedside who might not be able to leave for fear or not being able to return and stay with the child in the hospital.

External burdens that had the potential to be impacted by the visitor limitation included the caregiver's job status and strain on home life. If the caregiver did not have the option for remote working, there was concern that being unable to leave the hospital would cause them to lose their job. The caregiver at the bedside also could not retreat home to care for other children or maintain daily household needs. The caregiver might have to ask other family member or friends to help care for their other children. In a time when everyone was sheltering in place, these external burdens could potentially cause an increased anxiety and worry because of visitation policies in place (Hart & Taylor, 2021).

Healthcare professionals did their best to navigate a hospital during a time when there was an inability to provide family-centered care. There were valid reasons at the time for limiting the visitation, and HCPs pivoted to support the family the best they could with supplying updates in person when able and via phone and video calls. As the recent pandemic comes to an end, it is important for HCPs to focus on rebuilding family-centered care, carefully evaluate unintended impacts of well-intentioned policies, and plan for the future.

Learner Training

The pandemic impacted learner training for all HCPs. Each group developed strategies to mitigate limited interactions with patients and certain diagnoses to still graduate competent and proficient HCPs. There was concern for reduced clinical experiences, limited exposure to clinical team structure, and benefits of exposure to telehealth and simulation. As this chapter is being written, the healthcare system is observing graduates of a pandemic at work and there is no data published on if there has been a change in care from this impact.

In March 2020 when hospitals were restructuring their workforce, many medical students and nursing students were removed from clinical experiences completely. Other HCP students were given limited clinical experiences when safely able. The Graduate Medical Education made recommendations for residents and fellows to be divided into different teams to limit exposure to direct patient care, limit use of PPE, and preserve providers to be able to provide care if there was an exposure or infection (Blankenburg et al., 2022). This divided team approach had residents and fellows working remotely either from home or housed in another part of the hospital away from direct patient care. These individuals would still participate in patient care by listening to daily rounds and performing chart reviews. Their counterparts were then present for the direct patient care. Patient exams were often performed by only one member of the team to limit the exposure risk to the rest of the team. The residents and fellows reviewing charts from afar were able to become competent and efficient at gathering data and reviewing differential diagnoses.

There was concern over the limited number of diagnoses trainees were being exposed to in pediatrics. Elective surgeries had halted, pediatric viral illnesses were decreased, and overall, there were limited number of pediatric patients hospitalized. The limited diagnoses also limited interaction between service lines. There was little education being discussed in virtual daily rounds, and subspeciality services were not visible for what used to be routine daily discussions. Collaborative patient care was challenging during segmented discussions among HCPs. Simulation training was used to augment teaching on certain diagnoses and complex medical care that might need special attention given the limited number of patients observed during the pandemic (Blankenburg et al., 2022).

There were, however, breakthroughs to enhance learning with the pandemic besides the use of simulation; learners were given options to engage via telehealth and virtual meetings. Trainees were able to participate in telehealth appointments with pediatric subspeciality teams. These appointments offered the trainee the opportunity to practice gathering histories and learn how to ask questions to elicit information instead of performing a hands-on exam. The trainee could simulate a real in-person experience by meeting with the patient and caregiver first and then having the supervising HCP join the appointment to discuss potential differentials and next steps in the plan of care. This allowed the trainee to receive some education and learn alongside supervising HCPs how to complete a telehealth appointment. Virtual meetings and conferences were another breakthrough for education. For example, prior to the pandemic, weekly grand rounds, morning report, and patient specific conferences for education were completed in person. During the pandemic, these meetings became virtual, and now after the pandemic, most of these meetings have stayed in a hybrid format. This now allows more flexibility in the participant's schedule to attend these meetings, allowing for better attendance and at times better dialogue and education. National conferences also went virtual, allowing for continuing education from experts at all levels of learning.

There is continued opportunity for trainees to have different learning opportunities without direct patient care. Technology is continuing to evolve, and future use of virtual reality or gaming services might continue to enhance the trainee's education. These opportunities might not have been explored if it weren't for the pandemic, which allowed HCPs to entertain new ways to augment direct patient care.

Surgical Pediatric Subspecialty Care

When elective surgeries were stopped in March 2020, pediatric surgical subspeciality were left to wait and see what the next steps would be. It was unclear how long elective surgeries would be stopped, unclear how COVID-19 would impact pediatric care, and unclear how children were going to be kept safe during the start of the pandemic. Pediatric otolaryngology, neurosurgery, orthopedics, plastics, general surgery, and urology were all affected during the pandemic with both a decrease in case volumes and referrals. Pediatric patients were not seeking routine healthcare during the pandemic and concerns found on a routine exam that usually prompted a referral to a subspecialist did not happen. For example, pediatric otolaryngology had a significant decrease in surgical cases sustained for a prolong period related to social distancing, mask mandates, and decrease in viral illnesses affecting routine surgical cases such as tonsillectomy and tympanostomy tube placement (Jones et al., 2021).

There were children who presented to the emergency room with semi-urgent, urgent, and emergent surgical requirements. There were strategies to ensure these cases were done safely for both the child and the healthcare staff. All children who required a surgical procedure had to have a COVID-19 test completed prior to proceeding to the surgical suite. If the patient was COVID-19 positive, a conversation occurred among the surgical team, anesthesia, and surgical staff to either delay or to proceed with the case, dependent on the urgency of the case and severity of COVID-19 symptoms. There was an additional risk to provide anesthesia to a patient with COVID-19. If the patient was not stable enough to wait for the results of the COVID-19 test, then they were emergently taken to the surgical suite with precautions taken as if the patient was positive for COVID-19. These precautions included performing surgery in a negative pressure operating room, having only the anesthesiologist in the room for intubation to not expose other members of the team, limiting the number of members of the team to those mandatory to do the surgical case, and everyone in the room using requisite PPE. There were limited resources in some hospitals and surgical cases impacted resources available, such as postoperative care with mechanical ventilation and expected length of stay within the PICU or general pediatric floor. It was imperative for active communication among the interprofessional team with each case to discuss resources available during each wave of the pandemic.

As the pandemic continued, adult surgical subspecialities applied a medically necessary time sensitive (MeNTS) risk-stratification score to allow for a method to triage surgical cases to weigh the need for surgical intervention (Slidell et al., 2020). This scoring system was adapted and changed to reflect pediatric care such as chronic conditions and congenital anomalies not considered in the adult score. This allowed for better risk-stratification scores to be discussed among the team and complete pediatric surgical cases that were needed (Slidell et al., 2020). The risk-stratification score was flexed dependent on the needs of the individual institution. The creation and use of a risk-stratification score let pediatric patients undergo needed surgeries, but also started conversation on the outcome and means to conservative management. The pandemic drove surgical subspecialities to pause and have a conversation regarding next potential steps in care (e.g., conservative management of appendicitis with antibiotic therapy and observation versus surgical removal). These pauses and inabilities to rush to surgery during the pandemic prompted a breakthrough to consider nonoperative strategies when able.

Lessons Learned

Pediatric Trauma

During the pandemic, children were sheltering in place and not attending school, which brought a change in the type of trauma HCPs witnessed in the hospital. There was a sharp decrease in the number of orthopedic traumas from decreased travel, fewer motor vehicle crashes, and decreased participation in sport activities. However, in 2020, firearm-related injuries became the leading cause of death in pediatrics. There was almost a 40% increase in the number of firearm-related deaths from 2019 to 2020, and a significant increase was related to self-inflicted injuries (McGough et al., 2022). The severity of these traumas added tension to an already strained healthcare system in both the use of limited resources and mental health of HCPs. The increase in firearm mortality has caused HCPs to call for increased education on gun safety in the home and reinforces the need to continue interprofessional conversation regarding federal and state laws.

There was concern for increased abusive trauma during the pandemic. Children were not going to school or day care with mandated reporters and were sheltering in place with their caregivers, who had several reasons to be stressed related to socioeconomics and overall heightened concern of the pandemic itself. There are mixed data on if there were an increase or decrease in the number of abusive traumas during the pandemic; however, patients who presented with injuries related to abusive trauma presented more severely and required acute care interventions (Klover et al., 2021; Sanford et al., 2021). The variable reports of abusive trauma during the pandemic should cause a pause to ponder if abusive trauma decreased or if it was underreported because the patient never came to the hospital and was not in the care of anyone besides the abuser. There is concern for underreporting because abusive trauma that was evaluated was more severe, which might mean less severe abusive trauma did not seek medical attention. If there is another pandemic, pediatric HCPs should continue to be diligent to ensure the safety of children who remain vulnerable to abuse during stressful times.

Mental Health and Suicide

Mental health is described in more detail later in chapter "Mental Health: Assessment of Risk, Clinical Manifestations, and Access to Care" and elsewhere in this book, but it would be remiss if it was not briefly discussed as a lesson learned in the acute care setting. During COVID-19, suicide rates in 2021 in children were the highest in over 50 years. Not all suicide attempts are completed, and pediatric HCPs in the acute care setting treated children who attempted suicide by self-inflicted gunshot wounds, hanging, and ingestion. The pandemic caused loneliness, post-traumatic stress from COVID-19, anxiety, depression, stress in the household, and reliance on social media, which can contribute to suicide thoughts and actions (Barteck et al., 2021). Pediatric HCPs had to be prepared during the pandemic and even now to face challenges of caring for children in acute liver failure from acetaminophen overdose, severe hypoxic injury from hanging with neurological sequelae, and neurological devastation from self-inflicted gunshot wounds. Pediatric HCPs have the training to help care for this patient population, but there needs to be mindfulness on the emotional toll on HCPs when they care for these patients at an alarming rate. It is also important to note the limited number of mental health hospitals or wards for pediatric patients to continue to get care after they are medically ready for discharge. The increased number of suicide attempts has strained the healthcare system without enough access to provide continued care outside of the acute care setting. There was no prediction for the increase in the rate of suicide attempts in children during the pandemic. It is imperative to develop better integration of mental health screening and care into everyday health care to potentially provide support to stop suicide thoughts and attempts.

Intracranial Infections

Another diagnosis that impacted pediatric acute care during the pandemic was the increased incidence of bacterial intracranial infections secondary to otitis media and sinusitis with recent COVID-19 infection or co-infection at the time of diagnosis (Khuon et al., 2022). It is unclear if there is a direct relationship between the increase in intracranial infections with COVID-19, or an indirect relationship with children not being evaluated by primary care provider to treat otitis media or sinusitis completely, or a combination of both. Pediatric patients with intracranial infections can present with mild persistent symptoms such as headaches, orbital edema, forehead edema, and mastoid pain; however, they can also present obtunded, with seizure activity, and stroke-like symptoms which warranted PICU admission for treatment. These patients required interprofessional collaboration with infectious disease, neurosurgery, otolaryngology, neurology, at times hematology, and intensive care. The acute care setting did not predict an influx in this patient population, which potentially put a strain on resources in the PICU. Patients with intracranial infections require an extended length of stay for coordination of care with either continued rehabilitation or home health for long-term antibiotic therapy. There is also the lesson learned to encourage patients with symptoms with concern for otitis media and sinusitis to have close re-evaluation for potential requirement of antibiotic therapy.

Fragility of the Health Care System

Another lesson learned; the United States healthcare system was fragile during the pandemic and continues to attempt to recover while this book is being written. Free standing pediatric hospitals are still financially impacted by lost revenue during the pandemic. There was increased demand for adult acute care; however, in pediatric free standing hospitals children stopped getting routine care, did not have elective surgeries that financially support hospital revenue, and employees were furloughed, and/or employee benefits were potentially augmented (Blumenthal et al., 2020). A number of primary care offices could not keep their doors open and closed permanently, leaving an already vulnerable population more vulnerable without availability to care. There were also many caregivers laid-off or unemployed during the pandemic. This high rate of unemployment potentially caused some children to be uninsured and unable to seek healthcare with concern for high cost to the caregiver. There must be consideration moving forward on the implications of having a healthcare system based on fee-for-service for financial security and how another pandemic might impact pediatric hospitals with already precarious financial security. There also must be conversations moving forward on how to best support HCPs and prevent them from leaving the bedside with a continued shortage of all workers in the healthcare system.

The other area of impact that revealed fragility of the healthcare system in the acute care setting was the number of supply chain issues during the pandemic (Goldschmidt & Stasko, 2022). Healthcare professionals were often asked to use the same PPE during the pandemic because of great concern of not having enough supplies. There were also many hospital supplies used for common practice that could not be distributed because of delays in transportation globally. These supply chain issues made HCPs change their policies and protocols for patient care. While these changes were necessary because of the lack of supplies, it does not make it the right answer for providing safe and ample care to patients. There needs to be consideration moving forward on how best to keep the healthcare system running with optimal supplies needed no matter if there is a pandemic or not.

Calls to Action
- Pediatric patients must continue to be able to receive healthcare during times of crisis and future pandemics. It is up to pediatric HCPs to have a voice to demand access to healthcare not be delayed or stopped.
- The healthcare system is fragile and unravelling with HCPs continuing to feel unsupported and leaving the workforce. There is a sense of urgency to focus on change before there is a complete collapse in the ability of the United States to adequately provide pediatric healthcare.
- There must be change in firearm safety education and legislation to protect children. Currently, penetrating injury from a firearm is the number one cause of pediatric death in the United States.

References

Abrams, J., Belay, E., Godfred-Cato, S., Campbell, A., Zambrano, L., Kunkel, A., Miller, A., et al. (2022). Trends and treatments for multisystem inflammatory syndrome in children (MIS-C), United States, February 2020-July 2021. *CID, XX*(XX), 1–9.

Bahl, A., Meilke, N., Johnson, S., Desai, A., & Qu, L. (2023). Severe COVID-19 outcomes in pediatrics: An observational cohort analysis comparing alpha, Delta, and omicron variants. *The Lancet Regional Health-Americas, 18*, 100405.

Banull, N., Reich, P., Anka, C., May, J., Wharton, K., Kallogjeri, D., Shimony, H., et al. (2022). Association between endocrine disorders and severe COVID-19 disease in pediatric patients. *Hormone Research in Pædiatrics, 95*, 331. https://doi.org/10.1159/000524595

Barteck, N., Peck, J., Garzon, D., & VanCleve, S. (2021). Addressing the clinical impact of COVID-19 on pediatric mental health. *Journal of Pediatric Health Care, 35*, 377–386.

Blankenburg, R., Gonzalez, J., Aylor, M., Frohna, J., McPhillips, H., Myers, R., & Waggoner-fountain, L. (2022). The impact of the COVID-19 pandemic on pediatric graduate medical education: Lessons learned and pathways forward. *Academic Medicine, 97*(3S), S35–S39.

Bloxham, J., Levett, P., Lee, J., Dvorak, C., Hodge, D., & Stewart, S. (2023). Identifying parent anxiety and family distress of critically ill children in response to changes in hospital visitation policies during the COVID-19 pandemic. *Journal of Pediatric Nursing, 68*, 87–92.

Blumenthal, D., Fowler, E., Abrams, M., & Collins, S. (2020). COVID-19—implications for the health care system. *The New England Journal of Medicine, 383*(15), 1483–1488.

Bozzola, E., Barni, S., & Villani, A. (2022). Respiratory syncytial virus pediatric hospitalization in the COVID-19 era. *International Journal of Environmental Research and Public Health, 19*(23), 15455. https://doi.org/10.3390/ijerph192315455

Campbell, A., Melgar, M., & Yousaf, A. (2022, December 8). *Updates on Multisystem Inflammatory Syndrome in Children (MIS-C): Epidemiology, case definition, and COVID-19 vaccination.* CDC. Webinar Communication.

Chao, J., Derespina, K., Herold, B., Goldman, D., Aldrich, M., Weingarten, J., et al. (2020). Clinical characteristics and outcomes of hospitalized and critically ill children and adolescents with coronavirus disease 2019 at a tertiary care medical center in New York City. *The Journal of Pediatrics, 223*, 14–19.

Chomton, M., Marsac, L., Deho, A., Maroni, A., Geslain, G., Frannais-Haverland, K., et al. (2021). Transforming a paediatric ICU to an adult ICU for severe Covid-19: Lessons learned. *European Journal of Pediatrics, 180*, 2319–2323.

Christian, M., Sprung, C., King, M., Ditcher, J., Kissoon, N., Devereaux, A., et al. (2014). Care of the critically ill and injured during pandemics and disasters: CHEST consensus statement. *Chest, 146*(4_Suppl), e61S–e74S.

Dong, Y., Mo, X., Hu, Y., Qi, X., Jiang, F., Jiang, Z., et al. (2020). Epidemiology of COVID-19 among children in China. *Pediatrics, 145*(6), e20200702.

Esposito, S., Caramelli, F., & Principi, N. (2021). What are the risk factors for admission to the pediatric intensive unit among pediatric patients with COVID-19. *Italian Journal of Pediatrics, 47*(103), 2–4.

Goldschmidt, K., & Stasko, K. (2022). The downstream effects of the COVID-19 pandemic: The supply chain failure, a wicked problem. *Journal of Pediatric Nursing, 65*, 29–32.

Halpern, N., Kaplan, L., Rausen, M., & Yang, J. (2020). *Configuring ICUs in the COVID-19 era.* Society of Critical Care Medicine. https://www.sccm.org/getattachment/03130f42-5350-4456-be9f-b9407194938d/Configuring-ICUs-in-the-COVID-19-Era-A-Collection

Hart, J., & Taylor, S. (2021). Family presence for critically ill patients during a pandemic. *Chest, 160*(2), 549–557.

Jones, J., D'Souza, J., Mantle, B., Jospeh, J., Arjmand, E., & McMurray, J. (2021). Comparison of pediatric otolaryngology clinical and operative case volume among surgical specialties in the COVID-19 pandemic. *International Journal of Pediatric Otorhinolaryngology, 147*, 1108806.

Kache, S., Chisti, M., Gumbo, F., Mupere, E., Zhi, X., Nallasamy, K., et al. (2020). COVID-19 PICU guidelines: For high-and limited-resource settings. *Pediatric Research, 88*, 705–716.

Kalyanaraman, M., & Anderson, M. (2022). COVID-19 in children. *Pediatric Clinics of North America, 69*, 547–571.

Khuon, D., Ogrin, S., Engels, J., Aldrich, A., & Olivero, R. (2022). Increase in pediatric intracranial infections during the COVID-19 pandemic- eight pediatric hospitals, United States, March 2020–March 2022. *MMWR, 71*(31), 1000–1001.

Kitano, T., Kitano, M., Krueger, C., Jamal, H., Rawahi, H., Lee-Krueger, R., et al. (2021). The differential impact of pediatric COVID-19 between high-income countries and low-and middle-income countries: A systematic review of fatality and ICU admission in children worldwide. *PLoS One, 16*, e0246326. https://doi.org/10.1371/journal.pone.0246326

Klover, M., Ziegfeld, S., Ryan, L., Goldstein, M., Gardner, R., Garcia, A., & Nasr, I. (2021). Increased proportion of physical abuse injuries at a level 1 pediatric trauma center during the COVID-19 pandemic. *Child Abuse & Neglect, 116*, 104756.

Lessa, A., Bitercourt, V., Crestani, F., Andrade, G., Costa, C., & Garcia, P. (2022). Impact of the COVID-19 pandemic on patient and family centered care and on the mental health of health care workers, patients, and families. *Frontiers in Pediatrics, 10*, 2–7.

McBride, D. (2021). The impact of visiting restrictions during the COVID-19 pandemic on pediatric patients. *Journal of Pediatric Nursing, 61*, 436–438.

McGough, M., Amin, K., Panchal, N., & Cox, C. (2022). *Child and teen firearm mortality in the U.S. and peer countries*. https://www.kff.org/global-health-policy/issue-brief/child-and-teen-firearm-mortality-in-the-u-s-and-peer-countries/

Otten, M., Buysse, C., Buddingh, E., Terheggen-Lagro, S., von Asmuth, E., Sonnaville, E., Ketharanathan, N., et al. (2023). Neurocognitive, psychosocial, and quality of life outcomes after multisystem inflammatory syndrome in children admitted to the PICU. *Pediatric Critical Care Medicine, 24*(4), 289–300.

Parcha, V., Booker, K., Kalra, R., Kuranz, S., Berra, L., Arora, G., et al. (2021). A retrospective cohort study of 12, 306 pediatric COVID-19 patients in the United States. *Scientific Reports, 11*(1), 10231.

Remy, K., Philip, V., Malone, J., Ruppe, M., Kaselitz, T., Lodeserto, F., et al. (2020). Caring for critically ill adults with coronavirus disease 2019 in a PICU: Recommendations by dual trained intensivists. *Pediatric Critical Care Medicine, 21*(7), 607–619.

Sanford, E., Zagory, J., Blackwell, J., Szmuk, P., Ryan, M., & Ambardekar, A. (2021). Changes in pediatric trauma during COVID-19 stay at home epoch at a tertiary pediatric hospital. *Journal of Pediatric Surgery, 56*, 918–922.

Schroeder, J., Sharron, M., Wai, K., Pillai, D., & Rastogi, D. (2023). Asthma as a comorbidity in COVID-19 pediatric ICU admissions in a large metropolitan children's hospital. *Pediatric Pulmonology, 58*, 206–212.

Shekerdemian, L., Mahmood, N., Wolfe, K., Riggs, B., Ross, C., Mckiernan, C., et al. (2020). Characteristics and outcomes of children with coronavirus disease 2019 (COVID-19) infection admitted to US and Canadian pediatric intensive care units. *JAMA Pediatrics, 174*(9), 1–6.

Slidell, M., Kandel, J., Prachand, V., Baroody, F., Gundeti, M., Reid, R., Angelos, P., et al. (2020). Pediatric modification of the medically necessary, time-sensitive scoring system for operating room procedure prioritization during the COVID-19 pandemic. *Journal of the American College of Surgeons, 231*(2), 205–215.

U.S. Food & Drug Administration. (2020, October 22). *FDA approves first treatment for COVID-19*. https://www.fda.gov/news-events/press-announcements/fda-approves-first-treatment-covid-19

Wanga, V., Gerdes, M., Shi, D., Choudhary, R., Dulski, T., Hsu, S., Idubor, O., et al. (2021). Characteristics and clinical outcomes of children and adolescents aged <18 years hospitalized with COVID-19—six hospitals, United States, July-August 2021. *MMWR, 70*(51–52), 1766–1772.

Wasserman, E., Toal, M., Nellis, M., Traube, C., Joyce, C., Finkelstein, R., et al. (2021). Rapid transition of a PICU space and staff to adult coronavirus disease 2019 ICU care. *Pediatric Critical Care Medicine, 22*(1), 55–55.

Worsely, J. (2019). *Statement on age parameters during COVID-19 pandemic.* NAPNAP. https://www.napnap.org/statement-on-age-parameters-during-covid-19-pandemic/ #:~:text=NAPNAP%20stands%20by%20its%20age,safe%20harbor%20protections%20 are%20in

Yager, P., Whalen, K., & Cummings, B. (2020). Repurposing a pediatric ICU for adults. *The New England Journal of Medicine, 382*(22), e80(1-2).

Younis, N., Zareef, R., Fakhri, G., Fadi, B., Eid, A., & Arabi, M. (2021). COVID-19: Potential therapeutics for pediatric patients. *Pharmacological Reports, 73*, 1520–1538.

Primary Care Implications: Principles for Outpatient Management

Jessica L. Peck and Mikki Meadows-Oliver

> *I've learned that people will forget what you said, people will forget what you did, but people will never forget how you made them feel.*
>
> —Maya Angelou

Introduction and Background

Pediatric primary care renders opportunity for a holistic, integrated, and collaborative approach that focuses on the whole child. Such care is family-centered and emphasizes importance of the healthcare provider (HCP) and patient/family relationship in the context of a shared decision-making model (Abrams et al., 2021; Haiek et al., 2021). Pediatric HCPs work hard to establish trusting relationships with families to meet their needs and ensure optimal child health outcomes (Leonard et al., 2021). During the COVID-19 pandemic, some of these trusted relationships were damaged due to interruptions in provision of primary care services and rising mistrust of HCPs by families who were trying to navigate rapidly changing and often conflicting health advice from entities and HCPs previously viewed as generally credible sources of information. Discussions of rising mistrust were particularly amplified in parental perception of vaccine recommendations and exploring experiences among racial and ethnic minority communities (Ash et al., 2021; Leonard et al., 2021; Smith et al., 2021; Szilaygi et al., 2021), both of which have significant impacts for primary care delivery.

J. L. Peck
Louise Herrington School of Nursing, Baylor University, Dallas, TX, USA
e-mail: jessica_peck@baylor.edu

M. Meadows-Oliver (✉)
Rory Meyers College of Nursing, NYU, New York, NY, USA
e-mail: mikki.meadows.oliver@nyu.edu

© The Author(s), under exclusive license to Springer Nature Switzerland AG 2025
J. L. Peck (ed.), *COVID-19 Impacts on Child Health*,
https://doi.org/10.1007/978-3-031-80369-7_2

The COVID-19 pandemic resulted in significant disruptions in a variety of settings across the care continuum for multiple populations (Matenge et al., 2022). Much of the attention regarding unfavorable care repercussions focused on the pandemic's impact on hospital-based and acute-care services (Huggins et al., 2023). However, the ability to provide services in primary care settings was also affected considerably during the pandemic (Basu et al., 2023). During this time, reductions in health seeking behaviors for pediatric clients were reported, including a decline in the number of well-child visits and immunizations provided in the pediatric setting. A national US survey found 41.3% of parents reported their youngest child missed a scheduled visit and one-third of parents reported missing a routine vaccination. Pediatric influenza vaccination decreased by 10% from 2020 to 2021 (Teasdale et al., 2022). Data from the US Census Bureau's Household Pulse Survey revealed that more than one-fourth of families had at least one child who missed a preventive care visit, with dramatic variations noted by state (Lebrun-Harris et al., 2021), fanning concern about outbreaks of vaccine-preventable diseases on top of the COVID-19 pandemic. Additionally, services such as routine screenings, preventive health care education, and the diagnosis and ongoing management of both acute and chronic diseases were adversely affected due to the cancelation or suspension of services in primary care settings (Basu et al., 2023; Matenge et al., 2022; Teasdale et al., 2022). Multiple factors are associated with this decrease in health care utilization, including policies designed to limit infection and caregiver concerns about seeking non-urgent care. Competing personal priorities, additional responsibilities for caregivers during the pandemic, and other psychoscoial factors seemingly influenced decisions to defer or forgo visits for well-child care, immunizations, and health screenings (Weston et al., 2021). As of 2023, some signs of recovery in preventive care and immunization were emerging but were still below pre-pandemic levels (World Health Organization [WHO], 2023).

Pediatric primary care offices play a central role in supporting access to timely, accessible, affordable care including providing preventive services, identifying and diagnosing common conditions, delivering consistent care for chronic disease, and managing behavioral health problems. In order to maintain these services and minimize effects of disruptions in care caused by COVID-19, pediatric primary care offices had to find new and often untested ways to quickly adjust to the changing circumstances and to curtail service disruptions (Matenge et al., 2022). Primary care providers (PCPs) found innovative solutions, such as increased adoption of telehealth services to adapt to meet patient and family needs and to provide needed services to their communities (Andreadis et al., 2023; Matenge et al., 2022). In finding ways to adjust to a world in which trust in medical science is at a crossroads, HCPs became more aware of disparities in health care, the effects of socioeconomic factors on access to well-child care services, and the importance of a trusting relationship in an uninterrupted, accessible care continuum between families and pediatric HCPs (Leonard et al., 2021).

Points of Care

Primary care is often the first point of access into a health system in which patients initially appear for health promotion services or the first complaints of a presenting malady. Pediatric PCPs provide holistic care to patients from diverse cultural, ethnic, and socioeconomic backgrounds. Providing holistic care allows PCPs to focus on the whole child within the context of their families and communities. These HCPs work to encourage partnerships with children and their families to deliver evidence-based, culturally responsive care that addresses unique health care needs of each patient. Because health promotion and wellness are vital components of primary care encounters, such partnerships empower patients and their families to be active participants in their care and to take responsibility for their health and wellness. A 2023 scoping review detailed continuing impacts of COVID-19 on primary care provision including demanding significant redesigns of services provided, providing continuous care for chronic illness, considering the well-being of HCPs, and raising critical questions about the very future of primary care (Khalil-Khan & Khan, 2023).

Disruption in Primary Care Service Provision

Even before COVID-19, pediatric visits to primary care were declining. In a study of commercially insured US children from 2008 to 2016, overall visits decreased by 14.4% while problem-based visits decreased 24.1% (Ray et al., 2020). In 2019, the National Health Interview Survey reported that more than one in four children had at least one visit to a retail clinic or urgent care center in the previous 12 months, suggesting parental preference for convenience and rapidity of access to care over waiting for connection to primary care (Centers for Disease Control and Prevention [CDC], 2020). When the US Department of Health and Human Services issued a declaration in 2020 allowing pharmacists to administer vaccines to children, the American Medical Association (AMA) vehemently opposed, citing concerns that families would forgo well-child visits and comprehensive preventive services offered in primary care (American Medical Association [AMA], 2020). These challenges were then further accentuated by dramatic physical barriers in the provision of primary care itself that further impeded access to pediatric primary care environments.

The COVID-19 pandemic altered the typical in-person manner in which most provider–patient interactions in the pediatric primary care setting occurred. This was largely related to infection control measures implemented in clinics including closed waiting rooms, increased time for visits to decrease crowding and facilitate lower risk of virus transmission between families, added time to don and doff extensive newly required personal protective equipment, and triaging appointments more strictly to reduce transmission (National Association of Pediatric Nurse Practitioners [NAPNAP], 2020). These significant disruptions occurred alongside parental fears of COVID-19 exposure in the clinic environment and hesitancy to come in for appointments, colloquially dubbed "corona-phobia," increasing concern for delayed diagnosis as well as increased injury and illness related to lack of prevention measures promoted during well visits (Danzinger et al., 2021; Muellers et al., 2023). In the face of pediatric patients going so-called AWOL in the early days of the pandemic, the American Academy of Pediatrics (AAP) launched a social media campaign in May of 2020 to #CallYourPediatrician, encouraging families to connect to their PCP for credible information and health guidance. The AAP president also called out the lack of financial relief assistance to pediatric primary care because of an emphasized governmental focus on Medicare (Rubin, 2020). Families who were accustomed to friendly, prompt, service in the context of community were now faced with lengthy telephone triage, delayed appointments, closed waiting rooms necessitating sitting in a parked car awaiting their turn, lengthy COVID-19 screening procedures for all appointments, and HCPs who once appeared with smiling faces now walking into an exam room in head-to-toe PPE looking unfamiliar and even frightening to children. It is difficult to express how much this sudden, catastrophic disruption and destabilization of pediatric primary care infrastructure impacted the culture and landscape of pediatric primary care delivery at the time. Emerging research has identified themes including environmental adjustments for clinics, adapting to new models of healthcare delivery, and concerns for long-term impacts (Ashley et al., 2022).

Telehealth: Innovative Disruption

This crisis of access to primary care challenged pediatric HCPs to rethink modes of primary care delivery for children to ensure continuation of care (Shibukawa et al., 2022). The swift shift to virtual care was one method initially used to minimize the pandemic's disruptive effects on patient health and on patient–provider relationships (Matenge et al., 2022). It required both patients and HCPs to quickly learn how to navigate care remotely, the complexities of which are discussed in detail in Chap. 4.

Although delays in accessing primary care were notable during the height of the pandemic, telehealth services allowed children and their families a way to continue to receive preventive care as well as care for managing chronic diseases when in-person interactions were limited (Andreadis et al., 2023; Shibukawa et al., 2022). The AAP recommended using telehealth to conduct virtual well visits, followed by an in-person visit for physical examination and vaccination, with the exclusion of newborns, for whom in-person visits were still recommended by designating specific well-child hours for clinics (AAP, 2020). It is unclear the extent to which this was an effective strategy in supporting families to access well-child care in a timely manner or how well virtual visits translated into the recommended in-person follow-ups. However, using virtual visits particularly for acute and episodic care, pediatric nurses and HCPs were able to maintain connections with existing patients in their practice and reduce risk of COVID-19 transmission (Matenge et al., 2022) while continuing to generate revenue. Video telehealth allowed HCPs to have a unique view into their patient's homes and allowed introduction to new family members during virtual visits that they otherwise might not have been able to meet. A survey of pediatric-focused Advanced Practice Registered Nurses (APRNs) found 92% of respondents reported positive benefits associated with pediatric telehealth adoption during the pandemic (Sonney & Peck, 2023).

Telehealth appointments were convenient for children and their families seeking primary care, reducing cost, and travel time (Andreadis et al., 2023). While patients enjoyed benefits of convenience, some HCPs reported their increased availability led to blurred boundaries crossing personal and professional spaces that were previously well demarcated. Although the number of primary care visits conducted via telehealth peaked in the early months of the pandemic, many pediatric primary care practices continue to offer telehealth visits to children for a variety of conditions. Although research suggests much more work is needed to leverage telehealth to effectively address health disparities (Jamison et al., 2023), these virtual visits generate possibilities for new shared experiences between pediatric patients and their PCPs that were not widely adopted before the pandemic.

Disruption of Seasonal Illness Patterns

At the beginning of the pandemic, the combination of school, work, and daycare closures along with mandatory stay-at-home orders resulted in a dramatic decrease in exposure to communicable diseases. Primary care offices normally bustling with schedules listing patient complaints of ear infections, sore throats, stomach viruses, flu, respiratory syncytial virus (RSV), and other common maladies were ghost towns. While pediatric HCPs would never wish illness upon any child or their family, quiet fears began to grow with a feeling of impending doom that these maladies would indeed return and with a vengeance. Those fears were realized as common communicable childhood diseases began to reappear with the relaxing of public health measures and lifting of isolation requirements. However, they returned in unpredictable patterns. Prior to the COVID-19 pandemic, RSV and flu both had a predictable "season" with reasonable estimations of the peak (Yang et al., 2023). Concern over "off-season" presentations grew until the so-called tripledemic of concurrent RSV, influenza, and COVID-19 (Tanne, 2022) overpowered children's hospitals, leaving many without access to timely, high-quality care (Furlow, 2023).

Preventive Care Service Disruption

Preventive services for children, routine pediatric screenings, and provision of well-child care and immunizations were all negatively affected by re-prioritization of care during the COVID-19 pandemic (Ashley et al., 2022; Matenge et al., 2022). Changes in care delivery during the pandemic created missed opportunities to discuss pertinent health issues with patients and their families (Matenge et al., 2022). The decrease in the number of well-child appointments during the pandemic provided fewer opportunities for HCPs to screen children for developmental delays and other health conditions as many screening questionnaires are self-report forms filled out in the waiting room. Pediatric PCPs also reported fewer opportunities to directly assess patients, perhaps incidentally noting issues such as development delays that parents or caregivers may not have realized (Matenge et al., 2022). In the case of developmental delays, early diagnosis and intervention are essential to prevent long-term consequences.

In addition to decreased screenings for developmental delays and mental health issues, many children and adolescents missed scheduled immunizations related to fewer in-person visits (O'Leary et al., 2022)—increasing their chances of contracting communicable diseases and fueling increasing probability of an outbreak of vaccine-preventable diseases such as measles (Kelly et al., 2023). The missed opportunities for adolescent patients were particularly concerning because teens seek health care less often than younger children and it may take them longer to catch up on any missed vaccinations (Kelly et al., 2023). Generally, pediatric PCPs expressed consensus in their willingness to recommend COVID-19 vaccination (94% of pediatricians and 84% of nurses and advanced practice nurses) (Thompson et al., 2023). Alongside immunization delays because of decreased availability of well-child visits, pediatric PCPs faced an increase in parental vaccine hesitancy, discussed in more detail in Chap. 8. One of the most beneficial health promotion interventions in primary care is supporting breastfeeding. However, both parental and provider fears emerged as little was known initially about the safety of breastfeeding in the face of suspected or confirmed maternal infection with COVID-19. The first formal recommendations advised separating the mother/baby dyad and expressing milk to be bottle-fed in favor of infection prevention, but this was later revised by the AAP to recommend direct feeding, guidance that was in contrast to other international societies at the time. Later, questions emerged about the safety of breastfeeding in the presence of mothers taking prescribed medications commonly given at the beginning of the pandemic or vitamin supplements loosely recommended for disease prevention (Cheema et al., 2023). Lack of credible information to guide decision-making along with HCP and parental anxieties about doing the right thing put pediatric PCPs in a very difficult position when making professional recommendations. Then in 2022, a severe US shortage of infant formula ensued following a voluntary recall of contaminated stock and subsequent shutdown of the factory. The national out-of-stock rate rose from 18% to 70% in 5 months as desperate parents stocked and hoarded supply much like the public had done with toilet paper in the early days of COVID-19, with high-risk, under-resourced families most severely impacted (Jung et al., 2023)). This supply chain crisis was felt more acutely in the shadow of supply chain issues created by COVID-19 and left potentially dangerous homemade concoctions circulating widely on social media. Once again, PCPs stood in the gap to communicate with their patients to guide safe, evidence-based individual feeding options, seek and distribute supplies of formula samples, and connect families to social and economic support resources to obtain formula while striving to encourage families to breastfeed.

Chronic Disease Management

Due to delays in seeking care during the height of the pandemic, chronic conditions for children with special health needs such as asthma and type 2 diabetes mellitus were exacerbated and children's overall health and functional status may have worsened. One-third of all COVID-19-related deaths in the first stage of the pandemic were in persons with diabetes, with people representing racial ethnic or minorities disproportionately impacted (Hambling et al., 2021). Additionally, new onset medical conditions had a delay in diagnosis—potentially leading to worse patient outcomes. More widely available virtual appointments increased accessibility to health services for children living with physical disabilities who often require significant transportation accommodations for clinic visits. The impacts of the pandemic on children with special health needs are discussed in greater detail in Chap. 12.

Mental Health

Mental health issues were a prominent concern and presented unique challenges in pediatric primary care during the pandemic and continuing in its aftermath (Ashley et al., 2022). Pediatric PCPs reported varying effects of the pandemic on the mental health of children and their parents who presented for care in their offices. When screening, evaluation and treatment for some mental health conditions were delayed, pediatric PCPs noticed an increase in behavioral and emotional difficulties in children and adolescents. Children with conditions such as autism spectrum disorder (Thompson et al., 2023) and attention deficit hyperactivity disorder (ADHD) may have been particularly affected by disruptions in care —in addition to factors related to the pandemic in general—such as lockdowns, school closures, and remote learning. Primary care visits for ADHD dropped 33% in the first quarter of the pandemic. While prescribing patterns for children with ongoing diagnosis and disease management remained relatively stable, first-time primary care visits and initial prescription initiation were significantly decreased when compared to pre-pandemic rates, an outcome magnified in low-income communities (Bannett et al., 2022).

Pediatric PCPs reported increased anxiety, depression, and loneliness in children and adolescents which often intersected social determinants (or drivers) of health (Lee et al., 2022). Some symptoms were attributed to increased isolation in the face of school closures. For some children and adolescents, their symptoms were related to increased time at home—especially for those living in crowded conditions where they had little space for privacy. Providers also reported that, for some children, school closures during the pandemic may have had a positive effect on mental health. Children and adolescents who were affected by social anxiety, bullying, and/ or academic challenges may have experienced relief from stressors associated with attending school when the lockdowns were in effect. However, other pediatric HCPs noted that conditions in place during the lockdowns may have reinforced avoidant behaviors in some of these children and adolescents, possibly making existing mental health conditions worse upon return to school.

In addition to mental health factors attributable to school closures, pediatric HCPs described their patients being affected by stress from their parents related to job loss and socioeconomic factors. Parents also reported mental health issues in their children including an increase in video gaming addiction, running away from home, or suicidal ideation. Many HCPs agree that the pandemic had an overall negative effect on child and adolescent mental health, and problems of access to mental health resources were exacerbated.

It is of paramount importance that more mental health care services be integrated into primary care delivery modalities. It is not practical to reasonably expect to be able to refer every child with any suspected mental health complaint for timely, affordable, accessible, specialized care, especially with the significant shortage of child and adolescent psychiatrists (Lee et al., 2022). Pediatric PCPs are often responsible for initial assessment of these complaints (Lee et al., 2022), and they must be educated and trained to provide basic mental health care for common conditions such as depression, anxiety, attention deficit disorder, self-harming, and suicidality at the point of care in primary care offices. Professional pathways and policy supports are discussed in more detail in Chap. 7.

Economic and Policy Implications for Pediatrics as a Specialty

With average pediatric primary care visit volumes dropping 70–80% at the beginning of the pandemic, economic impacts to pediatric practice sustainability were devastating (Baulkman, 2021). Lost revenue during the pandemic was particularly threatening to independent HCPs practicing outside of a health system (Basu et al., 2023) and contributed to rapid acceleration of the centralization of care through health systems, a practice that has both advantages and drawbacks. As of January 1, 2022, it was estimated that approximately 74% of physicians in the United States work for health systems or corporations (Shryock, 2022). Between 2012 and 2022, the number of physicians working in private practice fell from 60.1% to 46.7%, a decline of 13 points. Even more telling, only 22% of physicians under the age of 45 own their own practice. Four of five physicians cite unfavorable reimbursement rates as very influential in the decision to sell their practice (Kane, 2022). The American Medical Association (AMA) (Rittenhouse et al., 2021) cites advantages of private practice for both patient and physician through greater autonomy and flexibility to meet individual family needs, and more accessible relationship-based care. Independent practices and small health systems for community regional points of care are critical access points in rural communities. Rural communities are seeing health system and hospital closure at alarming rates. By 2030, the US Government Accountability Office (GAO, 2023) estimates the anticipated supply of obstetric and gynecologic care will only meet 50% of the projected need in rural areas. With today's advancements in knowledge about the impact of pre-conceptual and conceptual health, impacts on long-term child health outcomes will manifest themselves in primary care. Threats to private practice accelerating the risk for closure include significant burdens of administrative work for clinicians who feel stretched for time to practice, low and still declining reimbursements that threaten practice viability, and lack of negotiating leverage with payors. Recruiting new pediatric PCPs to private practice is also extremely costly and independent office owners find themselves competing with very attractive lucrative offers from larger health systems. Other disadvantages of private practice include lack of resources to collect and analyze data that drives evidence-based practice change, untenable costs in implementing and maintaining sophisticated electronic health record systems, feeling professionally isolated, and lack of mentorship for newer clinicians (Rittenhouse et al., 2021).

Pediatric nurse practitioners (PNPs) and other pediatric advanced practice clinicians face their own challenges in entering and maintaining practice in pediatric primary care. Of practicing physician associates (PAs) (formerly referred to as physician assistants in the professional collective), only 1.9% reported working in general pediatrics in 2020, and those numbers are not differentiated by primary, acute, or specialty care environments (National Commission on Certification of Physician Assistants [NCPAA], 2022). While PAs are trained as generalists, the NCCPA (2024) offers a Certificate of Added Qualifications (CAQ) in pediatrics, although it is unclear how many actually hold active certification. Conversely, PNPs are trained initially and exclusively for pediatric specialty throughout their graduate training and are nationally certified by the Pediatric Nursing Certification Board to practice in pediatrics (Hittle-Gigli et al., 2019). However, of the more than 385,000 nurse practitioners currently in the United States, less than 5% are certified to practice in pediatrics (American Association of Nurse Practitioners [AANP], 2024). Of the approximately 18,000 PNPs certified in pediatrics, 85% are certified in primary care while 10% are certified in acute care and 5% are certified in both (Hittle-Gigli et al., 2019) Even before the COVID-19 pandemic, the National Association of Pediatric Nurse Practitioners (NAPNAP) issued a white paper, predicting a critical shortage looming (Hittle-Gigli et al., 2019). Despite support from the American Hospital Association, the Robert Wood Johnson Foundation, the Federal Trade Commission, the Veterans Administration, and the American Association of Retired Persons among others, significant barriers for NP practice that impede patient access to care still exist in some states (Hittle-Gigli et al., 2019). Currently, more than half of US states along with the District of Columbia and other US territories allow NPs to practice to the full extent of their education and training while the remaining states require various forms of costly regulatory oversight (AANP, 2023). The National Governors Association (NGA) issued a formal paper in support of the role of NPs in meeting primary care demands as early as 2012, concluding that "NPs can perform a subset of primary care services as well as or better than physicians" and "Expanded utilization of NPs has the potential to increase access to care, particularly in historically underserved areas" (NGA, 2012, p. 11).

Pediatrics has ranked among the lowest paid medical specialties since at least 2013, making it difficult to encourage promising young medical students to be pediatricians (Baulkman, 2021). Undergraduate pediatric nursing experiences are highly influential in prompting pursuit of an advanced practice nursing care, creating opportunity for early influence to choose pediatrics as an advanced practice specialty. With health systems and health consumers increasingly recognizing the value of the specialized expertise of clinicians certified in pediatrics, it is important to leverage pragmatic and policy actions that support enhanced development of the pediatric workforce (Hittle-Gigli et al., 2019).

Barriers and Breakthroughs

While there were factors such as lockdowns and social distancing that impacted direct provision of care to pediatric patients and their families, there were several breakthroughs in the pediatric primary care setting that enhanced care. These breakthroughs included innovation and increased use of new models of care delivery to provide health care services to patients and their families (Matenge et al., 2022). In addition to enhanced relationships formed with patients in their practices, primary care clinicians reported collaborating more among themselves and leveraging their partnerships with other—especially with hospital-based specialists and community organizations for shared learning and peer support (Sirkin et al., 2023).

Pediatric primary care offices adopted new models of care delivery to ensure continuity of, as well as safe access to health care in regard to disease prevention. Widespread use of telehealth and virtual visits emerged as a breakthrough in primary care, not only as an important adjunct to providing direct care for patients and their families—but also as a way to provide support for families in need who were unable to present for care in-person for a wide variety of reasons (Matenge et al., 2022). One benefit of virtual appointments is that they reduced the need for patient and family travel (sometimes quite a distance) to the primary care office. For children and adolescents who required in-person care, many offices offered hybrid models of care, providing options for both virtual and in-person visits. Hybrid models of care were particularly helpful for children and families affected most by the disruption of health care and social services. This was particularly true for families whose parents or guardians were working long hours as front-line service providers during the pandemic to maintain critical health and safety services even during quarantine.

While the increased use of telehealth and virtual visits allowed some primary care services to continue during the lockdown, these same services were a barrier to some pediatric patients and their families. Those with low socioeconomic status, families in rural areas with limited internet service, and those with low technology literacy experienced barriers to accessing telehealth. Disparities in access to resources linked to telehealth services affected pediatric patients most at risk for adverse outcomes (Matenge et al., 2022).

While enhanced relationships with other HCPs were noted as a breakthrough, some clinicians noted concerns regarding the patient–provider connection. Providers reported challenges with engaging pediatrics patients and building relationships with new patients and families via telehealth (Matenge et al., 2022). An additional concern regarding telehealth visits was confidentiality. Clinicians noted concerns about patients' access to private spaces for health care encounters, particularly for those living in shared family homes. A lack of privacy during visits may have hampered patients' ability to be open and honest during virtual appointments. This was especially true for telehealth visits with adolescents.

A component of primary health care services not often discussed in relation to the COVID-19 pandemic is the school-based health center. While not being able to attend school was certainly a barrier for students both socially and academically, a breakthrough was that the pandemic has shed light on the importance of school-based health services access in the lives of many children. Because of the lockdown, many children lost access to social safety nets provided in the school setting. Schools are a place where children whose families suffer from food insecurity can receive two meals per day. Additionally, schools provide connections for children and adolescents to critical support services—especially those children with developmental or behavioral conditions such as autism spectrum disorder or ADHD. The absence of these services at a time when they were critically needed helped bring awareness to the crucial role that school-based health centers play in the lives of school-age children and adolescents.

Primary care clinicians and clinics did their very best in stepping forward to meet with courage, innovation, and tenacity the incredible challenges that arose. They learned to screen, test, diagnose, and manage COVID-19 in the face of scant and rapidly changing information and severe lack of access to PPE to protect their own safety (Matenge et al., 2022; Sirkin et al., 2023) before adding the complexity of vaccine recommendations and the structural and physical challenges associated with transporting, storing, and administering vaccines. They did this in the face of service disruption to every other facet of primary care and worked to helped children in their primary care services access specialty services such as cancer treatments and dialysis. However, the general feeling of the professional community was that of being blindsided. The response was reactive, and it soon became apparent that there was a terrible deficiency of a proactive strategy equipped to anticipate such disasters and respond effectively (Greenhalgh, 2023). Timely and credible guidance from trusted sources with authority to instruct primary care provision continuance of care is paramount to optimize health outcomes (Matenge et al., 2022). Other themes identified among primary care clinicians include being patient-centered, providing clinician and practice support, strategically planning for infrastructure and support, and promoting community and public health. Notably, health equity was reported across all these domains (Sirkin et al., 2023).

During the COVID-19 pandemic, many pediatric PCPs became more aware of unmet needs of pediatric patients and more knowledgeable about health disparities facing this population. Unmet needs are defined as individuals delaying care or not being able to receive medical/dental care or prescription medications due to barriers related to costs of these services. Health disparities are defined as preventable health differences experienced by socially disadvantaged populations regarding disease burden and chances to obtain their best levels of health.

Unmet Healthcare Needs

In addition to lessons learned about uses of telehealth in pediatric primary care and the importance of clinician relationships with their colleagues and with patients and their families, the pandemic helped HCPs realize the interconnection between social drivers (or social determinants) and health. Social drivers of health include factors such as language and literacy skills and access to nutritious foods and safe spaces for physical activity. For many families, social risk factors such as unemployment, housing instability, and food insecurity existed before the COVID-19 pandemic began. Economic hardships related to the pandemic disproportionally impacted populations experiencing higher levels of social risk factors (Ashley et al., 2022; David et al., 2022).

In general, unmet healthcare and social needs are associated with a variety of adverse outcomes in children and adolescents such as increased frequency of hospitalization and higher infant mortality rates. During the COVID-19 pandemic, researchers noted that patients and families with racial and ethnic minority backgrounds were more likely to report unmet health and social needs (David et al., 2022). Access to quality health care, especially mental health care, was a challenge for many patients. Families reporting a higher number of unmet needs were more likely to have delays in attending well-child visits and to use the emergency department for care rather than their PCP's office (David et al., 2022). Such health care utilization patterns led to a decrease in developmental surveillance and screenings for physical and mental health conditions. In addition to delays in receiving well-child care, many children lost access to care at school-based clinics and health centers. Previously available resources such a wellness services and resources for conditions such as learning disabilities were lost due to school closures related to the pandemic.

Health Disparities

Due to the pandemic, multiple factors directly contributing to health inequities of adults, including limited access to health care, lack of insurance coverage, and limited transportation were worsened (Azan et al., 2023). These disparities were magnified in a 2021 report, revealing more than 140,000 children had already lost a parent, custodial grandparent, or grandparent caregiver during the pandemic. Overall, one in 500 children in the United States was subjected to orphanhood or grandparent caregiver death related to COVID-19. However, 65% of those children impacted were of racial and ethnic minorities (National Institutes of Health [NIH], 2021). As of May 2022, it was estimated that 10.5 million children worldwide had experienced the death of a parent or caregiver, with the World Health Organization calling for attention to the health impacts of severely bereaved children (Bellandi, 2022). Children from minority and lower socioeconomic backgrounds, already at risk for poorer health outcomes due to health disparities and inequities, were disproportionately impacted by the COVID-19 pandemic. Pediatric patients living in low-income households, who were part of an ethnic minority group, were more likely to have pre-existing conditions associated with increased risk of illness from COVID-19. The COVID-19 pandemic raised awareness of and in some cases exacerbated pre-existing racial, ethnic, and socioeconomic health disparities in children.

The uneven impact on healthcare was noted in relation to well-child care visits and also with visits for the care of long-term health conditions. During the COVID-19 pandemic, well-child visits declined among all groups, with the most notable disparities being among Black and publicly insured children. When well-child visits are missed, that means the child is likely missing immunization opportunities and screenings for developmental conditions—such as autism spectrum disorder (Thompson et al., 2023). Researchers found that, compared to more affluent families, children from low-income families experienced more disruptions in ADHD-related care during the pandemic. Non-Hispanic Black and Hispanic patients were less likely to attend visits for ADHD, depression, and anxiety compared to White patients. These disparities in care were exacerbated by structural inequities in access to healthcare and health insurance for pediatric patients.

While many positives related to telehealth have been detailed in this chapter and in the healthcare literature, the use of telehealth visits for pediatric primary care has raised concerns about worsening disparities in children's access to care, especially those children from disadvantaged families. Researchers noted disparities in access to telehealth related to language, socioeconomic status, insurance coverage, and race and ethnicity. Studies completed in urban areas suggested that telehealth increased disparities in primary care visit attendance for historically disadvantaged populations. However, the same was not shown to hold true for pediatric patients living in rural areas. Utilization of primary health care services increased for families in rural areas when telehealth services were used. Researchers posited that eliminating the barrier of distance allowed increased access to health care services. Using telehealth in rural areas also brought challenges which may contribute to existing health care disparities. Difficulties with accessing reliable internet services were potential hindrances to starting and/or completing a telehealth visit, possibly decreasing access to care.

Previously, primary care interventions have not directly targeted populations facing health inequities. With knowledge gained during the pandemic, PCPs can work with their clinical and public health colleagues to ensure that children with unmet health care needs and/or who are socioeconomically disadvantaged continue to receive coordinated, quality care in the post-pandemic era.

Access to well-organized, excellent primary care is associated with greater odds of positive outcomes in the face of COVID-19 (Greenhalgh, 2023). The pandemic brought with it an opportunity to rethink how health care is designed and delivered. Of the many lessons learned when delivering care during the pandemic, three stand out as needing increased attention to enhance the provision of comprehensive pediatric primary care. Moving forward, partnerships between pediatric primary care clinicians and public health officials are paramount. Results of the long-term pediatric health impacts due to primary care service disruptions are still being uncovered. More comprehensive research is needed into holistic aspects of care including how to achieve a primary care redesign that makes care more equitable and responsive to the health needs of pediatric patients and their families.

Calls to Action
- Collaborate with public health entities.

Partnerships between primary care clinicians and public health entities may help to more fully address long-term health and social effects of the pandemic. Building and maintaining relationships that seek common ground and establish common goals can serve as models for more effective primary care and public health integration. Effective collaborations between public health and primary care providers have important implications for maintaining safe access to regular care during any future pandemics or wide-scale global disasters.
- Prioritize research and funding for pediatric primary care delivery.

The pandemic and its aftermath revealed several areas where more research is needed to improve care to pediatric patients. Research is needed to evaluate the effectiveness of new models of service delivery such as telehealth. The types of visits, conditions best suited for virtual visits, and ways to fully integrate telehealth visits into primary care practices need to be further studied. Other areas related to providing care via telehealth that should receive focus include perception of clinicians and patients, patient outcomes, and costs. The pediatric workforce needs policy, pragmatic and pecuniary resources to support primary care development and delivery.
- Emphasize the need for access to care for children and their families.

The COVID-19 pandemic illuminated health inequities among racial/ethnic groups, rural communities, and other socioeconomically disadvantaged populations. These populations disproportionately experienced limited access to health care, lack of insurance coverage, and limited transportation to health care facilities. Moving forward, facilitators and barriers to addressing the needs of these medically underserved populations will be an important consideration.

References

Abrams, E. M., Shaker, M., Oppenheimer, J., Davis, R. S., Bukstein, D. S., & Greenhawt, M. (2021). The challenges and opportunities for shared decision making highlighted by COVID-19. *The Journal of Allergy and Clinical Immunology. In Practice, 8*(8), 2474–2480. https://doi.org/10.1016/j.jaip.2020.07.003t

American Academy of Pediatrics [AAP]. (2020). *Guidance on providing pediatric well-care during COVID-19.* https://www.aap.org/en/pages/2019-novel-coronavirus-covid-19-infections/clinical-guidance/guidance-on-providing-pediatric-well-care-during-covid-19/#:~:text=For%20practices%20that%20have%20successfully,a%20timely%20in%2Dperson%20visit

American Association of Nurse Practitioners [AANP]. (2023). *State practice environment.* https://www.aanp.org/advocacy/state/state-practice-environment

American Association of Nurse Practitioners [AANP]. (2024). *NP fact sheet.* https://www.aanp.org/about/all-about-nps/np-fact-sheet#:~:text=There%20are%20more%20than%20385%2C000,NPs)%20licensed%20in%20the%20U.S.&text=More%20than%2039%2C000%20new%20NPs,academic%20programs%20in%202021%2D2022

American Medical Association [AMA]. (2020). *AMA opposes expanding pharmacists' ability to provide child vaccines.* [Press Release]. https://www.ama-assn.org/press-center/press-releases/ama-opposes-expanding-pharmacists-ability-provide-child-vaccines#:~:text=Aug%2021%2C%202020&text=%E2%80%9CThe%20American%20Medical%20Association%20(AMA,ages%20of%203%20and%2018

Andreadis, K., Muellers, K., Ancker, J., Horowitz, C., Kaushal, R., & Lin, J. (2023). Telemedicine impact on the patient–provider relationship in primary care during the COVID-19 pandemic. *Medical Care, 61,* S83–S88.

Ash, M. J., Berkley-Patton, J., Christensen, K., Haardorfer, R., Livingston, M. D., Miller, T., & Woods-Jaeger, B. (2021). Predictors of medical mistrust among urban youth of color during the COVID-19 pandemic. *Translational Behavioral Medicine, 11*(8), 1626–1634. https://doi.org/10.1093/tbm/ibab061

Ashley, C., Halcomb, E., James, S., Calma, K., Stephen, C., McInnes, S., Mursa, R., & Williams, A. (2022). The impact of COVID-19 on the delivery of care by Australian primary health care nurses. *Health and Social Care in the Community, 30,* e2670–e2677. https://doi.org/10.1111/hsc.13710

Azan, A., Stephens, J., Xie, X., Fiori, K., & Gover, M. (2023). COVID-19 and changes in reported social risk factors at a primary care practice in the south Bronx. *Journal of Primary Care and Community Health, 14,* 1–7. https://doi.org/10.1177/21501319221147136

Bannett, Y., Dahlen, A., Huffman, L., & Feldman, H. (2022). Primary care diagnosis and treatment of attention-deficit/ hyperactivity disorder in school-age children: Trends and disparities during the COVID-19 pandemic. *Journal of Developmental and Behavioral Pediatrics, 43,* 386–392. https://doi.org/10.1101/2021.11.03.21265902

Basu, S., Alpert, J., & Phillips, R.S. (2023). *Primary care in the COVID-19 pandemic: Improving access to high-quality primary care, accelerating transitions to alternative forms of care delivery, and addressing health disparities.* Center for Primary Care. [Harvard Medical School]. https://info.primarycare.hms.harvard.edu/primary-care-during-covid-0

Baulkman, J. (2021, May 17). *Pediatricians see drop in income during pandemic.* MDedge/Pediatrics. [Pediatric News]. https://www.mdedge.com/pediatrics/article/240217/business-medicine/pediatricians-see-drop-income-during-pandemic

Bellandi, D. (2022). Estimate: 10.5 million children lost a parent, caregiver to COVID-19. *JAMA, 328*(15), 1490. https://jamanetwork.com/journals/jama/fullarticle/2797407

Centers for Disease Control and Prevention [CDC]. (2020). *Urgent care center and retail health utilization among children: United States, 2019.* National Center for Health Statistics. https://www.cdc.gov/nchs/products/databriefs/db393.htm

Cheema, R., Partridge, E., Kair, L. R., Kuhn-Riordan, K. M., Silva, A., Bettinelli, M. E., Chantry, C. J., Underwood, M. A., Lakshminrusimha, S., & Blumberg, D. (2023). Protecting breastfeeding during the COVID-19 pandemic. *American Journal of Perinatology, 40*(03), 260–266. https://doi.org/10.10155/s-0040-1714277

Danzinger, C. R., Krause, I., Scheuerman, O., Luder, A., Yulevich, A., Dalal, I., Grisaru-Soen, G., & Bilavsky, E. (2021). Pediatrician, watch out for corona-phobia. *European Journal of Pediatrics, 180*(1), 201–206. https://doi.org/10.1007/s00431-020-03736

David, P., Fracci, S., Wojtowicz, J., McCune, E., Katyln Sullivan, K., Sigman, G., O'Keefe, J., & Qureshi, K. (2022). Ethnicity, social determinants of health, and pediatric primary care during the COVID-19 pandemic. *Journal of Primary Care and Community Health, 13*, 1–9. https://doi.org/10.1177/21501319221112248

Furlow, B. (2023). Tripledemic overwhelms paediatric units in U.S. hospitals. *Lancet Child and Adolescent Health, 7*(2), 86. https://doi.org/10.1016/S2352-4642(22)00372-8

Government Accountability Office [GAO]. (2023, May 16). *Why health care is harder to access in rural America.* https://www.gao.gov/blog/why-health-care-harder-access-rural-america

Greenhalgh, T. (2023). COVID-19 and primary care: Taking stock. *Annals of Family Medicine, 21*, 1–3. https://doi.org/10.1370/afm.2935

Haiek, L. N., LeDrew, M., Charette, C., & Bartick, M. (2021). Shared decision-making for infant feeding and care during the coronavirus disease 2019 pandemic. *Maternal & Child Nutrition, 17*, e13129. https://doi.org/10.1111/mcn.13129

Hambling, C., Patel, D. A., & Turner, B. (2021). COVID-19 and diabetes: Update for primary care in response to the ongoing coronavirus pandemic. *Journal of Diabetes Nursing, 25*, JDN172.

Hittle-Gigli, K., Beauchesne, M., Dirks, M., & Peck, J. (2019). White paper: Critical shortage of nurse practitioners predicted. *Journal of Pediatric Health Care, 33*(3), 347–355. https://doi.org/10.1016/j.pedhc.2019.02.008

Huggins, A., Husaini, M., Wang, F., Waken, R. J., Epstein, A. M., Orav, E. J., & Maddox, K. E. J. (2023). Care disruption during COVID-19: A national survey of hospital leaders. *Journal of General Internal Medicine, 38*(5), 1232–1238. https://doi.org/10.1007/s11606-022-08002-5

Jamison, S., Zheng, Y., Nguyen, L., Khan, F., Tumin, D., & Simeonsson, K. (2023). Telemedicine and disparities in visit attendance at a rural pediatric primary care clinic during the COVID-19 pandemic. *Journal of Health Care for the Poor and Underserved, 34*, 535–548. https://doi.org/10.1353/hpu.2023.0048

Jung, J., Widmar, N. O., & Ellison, B. (2023). The curious case of baby formula in the United States in 2022: Cries for urgent action months after silence in the midst of alarm bells. *Food Ethics, 8*(1), 4. https://doi.org/10.1007/s41055-022-00115-1

Kane, C.K. (2022). *Recent changes in physician practice arrangements: Shifts away from private practice and towards larger practice size continue through 2022.* Policy Research Perspectives. [American Medical Association]. https://www.ama-assn.org/system/files/2022-prp-practice-arrangement.pdf

Kelly, M., Stephens-Shields, A., Hannan, C., Rand, C., Localio, R., Shone, L., Steffes, J., Davis, K., Grundmeier, R. W., Humiston, S. G., Albertin, C., McFarland, G., Abney, D. E., Szilagyi, P. G., & Fiks, A. (2023). Missed opportunities for adolescent immunizations at well-care visits during the COVID-19 pandemic. *The Journal of Adolescent Health, 73*, 595e598. https://doi.org/10.1016/j.jadohealth.2023.05.008

Khalil-Khan, A., & Khan, M. A. B. (2023). The impact of COVID-19 on primary care: A scoping review. *Cureus, 15*(1), e33241. https://doi.org/10.7759/cureus.33241

Lebrun-Harris, L. A., Sappenfield, O. R., & Warren, M. D. (2021). Missed and delayed preventive health care visits among US children due to the COVID-19 pandemic. *Public Health Reports, 137*(2), 336. https://doi.org/10.1177/00333549211061322

Lee, C., Lutz, J., Khau, A., Lin, B., Phillip, N., Ackerman, S., Steinbuchel, P., & Mangurian, C. (2022). Pediatric primary care perspectives of mental health services delivery during the COVID-19 pandemic. *Children, 9*, 1167. https://doi.org/10.3390/children9081167

Leonard, M. B., Pursley, D. M., Robinson, L. A., Abman, S. H., & Davis, J. M. (2021). The importance of trustworthiness: Lessons from the COVID-19 pandemic. *Pediatric Research, 91*, 482–485. https://doi.org/10.1038/s41390-021-01866-z

Matenge, S., Sturgiss, E., Desborough, J., Dykgraaf, S., Dut, G., & Kidd, M. (2022). Ensuring the continuation of routine primary care during the COVID-19 pandemic: A review of the international literature. *Family Practice, 39*, 747–761. https://doi.org/10.1093/fampra/cmab115

Muellers, K., Andreadis, K., Ancker, J., Horowitz, C., Kaushal, R., & Lin, J. (2023). Provider and patient experiences of delays in primary care during the early COVID-19 pandemic. *Journal for Healthcare Quality, 45*, 169–176. https://doi.org/10.1097/JHQ.0000000000000380

National Association of Pediatric Nurse Practitioners [NAPNAP]. (2020). *NAPNAP statement on immunization outbreaks during COVID-19 outbreak*. https://www.napnap.org/napnap-statement-on-immunizations-during-covid-19-outbreak/

National Commission on Certification of PAs [NCCPA]. (2024). *Certificates of Added Qualifications (CAQs)*. https://www.nccpa.net/specialty-certificates/#pediatrics

National Governors Association [NGA]. (2012). *The role of nurse practitioners in meeting increasing demand for primary care*. [NGA Paper]. https://www.nga.org/wp-content/uploads/2019/08/1212NursePractitionersPaper.pdf

National Institutes of Health [NIH]. (2021). *More than 140,000 children lost a primary or secondary caregiver due to the COVID-19 pandemic*. [News Release]. https://www.nih.gov/news-events/news-releases/more-140000-us-children-lost-primary-or-secondary-caregiver-due-covid-19-pandemic

O'Leary, S., Cataldi, J., Lindley, M., Beaty, B., Hurley, L., Crane, L., Brtnikova, M., Gorman, C., Vogt, T., Kang, Y., & Kempe, A. (2022). US primary care providers' experiences and practices related to routine pediatric vaccination - during the COVID-19 pandemic. *Academic Pediatrics, 22*, 559–563.

Ray, K. N., Shi, Z., & Ganghuli, I. (2020). Trends in pediatric primary care visits among commercially insured US children, 2008-2016. *JAMA Pediatrics, 174*(4), 350–357. https://doi.org/10.1001/jamapediatrics.2019.5509

Rittenhouse, D., Olszuk, T., Gerteis, M., Genevro, J., Hancock, K., Li, E., Carlasare, L., Vargo, C., & Blake, K. (2021, October 21). *Supporting and promoting high-performing physician-owned private practices: Voices from the front lines*. White Paper. [American Medical Association]. https://www.ama-assn.org/system/files/mathematica-ama-white-paper.pdf

Rubin, R. (2020). COVID-19's crushing effect on medical practices: Some of which may not survive. *JAMA, 324*, 321. https://jamanetwork.com/journals/jama/fullarticle/2767633. Medical News and Perspectives

Shibukawa, B., Uema, R., Piran, C., Fonseca, B., Furtado, M., & Merino, M. (2022). Repercussions of the pandemic of COVID-19: Care of the pediatric population in primary health care. *Rev Rene, 23*, e72798. https://doi.org/10.15253/2175-6783.20222372798

Shryock, T. (2022). *Supermajority of U.S. physicians work for health systems or corporations*. Medical Economics. https://www.medicaleconomics.com/view/supermajority-of-u-s-physicians-work-for-health-systems-or-corporations

Sirkin, J., Flanagan, E., Tong, S., Coffman, M., McNellis, R., McPherson, T., & Bierman, A. (2023). Primary care's challenges and responses in the face of the COVID-19 pandemic: Insights from AHRQ's learning community. *Annals of Family Medicine, 21*, 76–82. https://doi.org/10.1370/afm.2904

Smith, A. C., Woerner, J., Perera, R., Haeny, A. M., & Cox, J. M. (2021). An investigation of associations between race, ethnicity, and past experiences of discrimination with medical mistrust and COVID-19 protective strategies. *Journal of Racial and Ethnic Disparities, 9*, 1420–1432. https://doi.org/10.1007/s40615-021-01080-x

Sonney, J., & Peck, J. (2023). The cost of caring during the COVID-19 pandemic: A clarion call to action to support the pediatric advanced practice nursing workforce. *Journal of Pediatric Health Care, 37*(6), 658–672. https://doi.org/10.1016/j.pedhc.2023.08.003

Szilaygi, P. G., Shah, M. D., Delgado, J. R., Thomas, K., Vizueta, N., Cui, Y., Vangala, S., Shetgri, R., & Kapteyn, A. (2021). Parents' intentions and perceptions about COVID-19 vaccination for their children: Results from a national survey. *Pediatrics, 148*(4), e2021052335. https://doi.org/10.1542/peds.2021-052335

Tanne, J. H. (2022). US faces tripledemic of flu, RSV, and covid. *BMJ, 379.* https://doi.org/10.1136/bmj.o2681

Teasdale, C. A., Borrell, L. N., Shen, Y., Kimball, S., Zimba, R., Kulkarni, S., Rane, M., Rinke, M. L., Fleary, S. A., & Nash, D. (2022). Missed routine pediatric care and vaccinations in US children during the first year of the COVID-19 pandemic. *Preventive Medicine, 158*, 107025. https://doi.org/10.1016/j.ypmed.2022.107025

Thompson, P., McCormick, L., Huang, Q., Gilkey, M., Dailey, S., & Brewer, N. (2023). Recommending COVID-19 vaccination for adolescents in primary care. *Family Practice, 40*, 1–8. https://doi.org/10.1093/fampra/cmac056

Weston, S. J., Condon, D. M., & Fisher, P. A. (2021). Psychosocial factors associated with preventive pediatric care during the COVID-19 pandemic. *Social Science and Medicine, 287*, 114356. https://doi.org/10.1016/j.socsmed.2021.114356

World Health Organization [WHO]. (2023, July 18). *Childhood immunization begins recovery after COVID-19 backslide.* https://www.who.int/news/item/18-07-2023-childhood-immunization-begins-recovery-after-covid-19-backslide

Yang, M., Su, Y., Chen, P., Lin, T., & Wu, J. (2023). Changing patterns of infectious disease in children during the COVID-19 pandemic. *Frontiers in Cellular and Infection Microbiology, 13*, 1200617. https://doi.org/10.3389/fcimb.2023.1200617

Telehealth: Principles of Remote Pediatric Management

Kelli Garber

The most difficult decision is the decision to act. The rest is merely tenacity. The fears are paper tigers.

—Amelia Earhart

Introduction and Background

Telehealth is considered to be the use of technology to deliver various aspects of healthcare virtually. This broad umbrella term encompasses clinical care, prevention, monitoring, health administration, and health education with the provision of medical care (Mechanic et al., 2022). Telemedicine (considered to be the fastest-growing category of telehealth) refers to using telecommunications technology to deliver medical, diagnostic, and treatment-related services across distance (Federal Communications Commission, 2023). Often, the terms *telehealth* and *telemedicine* are used interchangeably. In this chapter, the term telehealth will be used to describe the exchange of medical information across distance through electronic means. The terms remote healthcare and virtual care also refer to a broad scope of care provided across distance and may be interchanged with telehealth.

Remote healthcare emerged in the early 1900s, first in the form of telegraphs and telephone, and later integrating two-way video in the 1950s and 1960s (Gogia, 2019). Though remote care continued to evolve with advancement of the internet, widescale adoption did not occur until onset of the 2019 coronavirus disease (COVID-19) pandemic, which led to an unprecedented demand for virtual care (Brotman & Kotloff, 2021). Telehealth helps overcome barriers that prevent healthcare access, including geographic distance, limited providers in the local community, lack of transportation, poverty, and inadequate health insurance coverage (Young & Ireson, 2003). Despite these advantages, pediatric utilization was limited

K. Garber (✉)
Old Dominion University, Norfolk, VA, USA
e-mail: kgarber@odu.edu

J. L. Peck (ed.), *COVID-19 Impacts on Child Health*,
https://doi.org/10.1007/978-3-031-80369-7_3

prior to the pandemic, particularly in primary care (Barnett et al., 2018; Sisk et al., 2020; Williams et al., 2021a, 2021b). Telehealth expands access to expert pediatric care and enhances communication among healthcare providers (HCPs), leading to more efficient, higher quality, and less expensive care (Curfman et al., 2022), yet many HCPs were not early adopters.

Prior to COVID-19, the limited adoption of telehealth was often attributable to clinician's unwillingness to engage in novel modalities (Wade et al., 2014). Provider concerns included reduced quality of care, loss of the patient–provider interpersonal connection, and reduced security and privacy of patient's health information (Jumreornvong et al., 2020), along with payment and billing barriers (Sisk et al., 2020). Facilitated by the global crisis, widespread adoption of telehealth has boosted family, payor, and pediatric clinician acceptance of this important method of care delivery (Fiks et al., 2021).

The American Academy of Pediatrics recommended increasing telehealth capacity to protect both patients and HCPs from exposure to the SARS-CoV-2 virus during the COVID-19 public health emergency (PHE). Expanded Medicaid and private payor reimbursement with relaxed regulatory restrictions regarding telehealth use led to widespread adoption of virtual care (Fiks et al., 2021). According to the Centers for Disease Control and Prevention (CDC), telehealth visits increased by 154% in March 2020 (Koonin et al., 2020). Another national study including 36 million working-age individuals with private insurance showed a 766% increase in telemedicine encounters in the first 3 months of 2020 (Weiner et al., 2021). During the COVID-19 pandemic, a wide array of pediatric healthcare services shifted to virtual care, including home health, early intervention services, physical and mental health, and occupational and speech therapy (Wenderlich & Herendeen, 2021).

While the COVID-19 pandemic catapulted telehealth to the forefront of healthcare delivery, many HCPs were expected to deliver care via telehealth with little or no education or training. Few health professions programs at academic institutions included telehealth education in their curriculums prior to the pandemic (Chike-Harris et al., 2021; Rutledge et al., 2017). With telehealth expected to remain an important part of the healthcare landscape moving forward, it is essential for all pediatric HCPs to understand telehealth and related best practices to ensure safe, high-quality care is conducted virtually.

Points of Care

The Pediatric Telehealth Landscape

Though the use of telehealth in pediatrics became more mainstream during the COVID-19 pandemic, decades of work preceded this adoption of technology to establish the safety and efficacy of caring for children virtually (Wenderlich & Herendeen, 2021). Telehealth is effective at managing acute illnesses, providing positive mental health care and primary care, facilitating cardiology evaluation, and determining dermatology diagnoses, as well as enhancing rapid pediatric triage in the emergency department (Williams et al., 2021a, 2021b). Initially established to extend care to geographic areas where pediatric expertise was limited, telehealth has evolved to be used to overcome both rural and urban barriers such as loss of school time for students or work time for parents, transportation, and to ensure equitable and efficient access to care where and when it is needed (Curfman et al., 2021a; Marcin et al., 2004; McIntosh et al., 2014; McKissick et al., 2017; Williams et al., 2021b).

Telehealth Modalities

Telehealth interventions include provider-to-provider and patient-to-provider connections facilitated through synchronous, asynchronous, remote monitoring, and eHealth or mHealth technologies (Gogia, 2019) (Table 1). Additionally, some experts consider pediatric-specific telephone triage to be a component of telehealth, along with patient–provider digital communication such as text messages (Milne Wunderlich & Herendeen, 2021). Technology utilized and services provided should be dictated by patient needs, HCP discretion, and availability of connectivity. Telehealth technology should be selected as a result of the clinical care necessary to achieve desired outcomes (Valenta & Ford, 2021).

Table 1 Telehealth modalities

Telehealth modality	Description	Example
Synchronous (Brotman & Kotloff, 2021)	Live interactive encounters using both audio and video	Live patient clinical encounters
Asynchronous ("Store and Forward") (Brotman & Kotloff, 2021)	Information is captured, stored, and transmitted to a healthcare provider for later review	eVisits Evaluation of radiologic images Evaluation of dermatologic images
Remote monitoring/ telemonitoring (Brotman & Kotloff, 2021; Foster et al., 2022)	Medical and mobile technology is used to gather clinical information for transmission to a healthcare provider (oxygen saturation, spirometric measurements, blood pressure, blood glucose, weight and pulse). May be automatic or manually reported	Home monitoring • Children with special healthcare needs
Mobile health/ mHealth (Brotman & Kotloff, 2021; Park, 2016)	The use of smartphones, smartwatches, and mobile applications to support patient health	Tracking health measurements, sharing information with providers, promoting medication adherence or lifestyle management to promote health

Telehealth Practice Models

Telehealth practice models are often separated into ambulatory, hospital-to-hospital, or facility-to-facility modalities (Curfman et al., 2021b). Ambulatory telehealth, often referred to as direct-to-patient services, includes a variety of community-based originating and distant sites such as private practices, schools, childcare centers, federally qualified health centers, community centers, patient homes, and other evolving locations to meet the needs of pediatric patients (Burke et al., 2015; Curfman et al., 2021b; McIntosh et al., 2014). Hospital-based telehealth occurs between or within facilities and includes expert consultations as well as care delivery in the inpatient setting to reduce risk of exposure to infectious disease and to conserve personal protective equipment as was necessary during the COVID-19 pandemic (Bains et al., 2021; Curfman et al., 2021b).

Telehealth Applications

Teleresearch

While the COVID-19 pandemic highlighted and expanded pediatric virtual care, applications including teleresearch, tele-education, telementoring, teleconsultation, and telepractice have been utilized for years (Burke et al., 2015; Curfman et al., 2022). Teleresearch encompasses many aspects of the research process. Technology can be used to recruit study participants from the community, study an intervention, or disseminate translational research outcomes to local HCPs (Burke et al., 2015). In addition, multicenter trials have used telehealth to enhance recruitment at distant sites and to improve standardization, data dissemination, and monitoring (Kennedy et al., 2000). The pandemic disrupted clinical research worldwide while redirecting research toward COVID-19 (Weiner et al., 2021). As a result, new approaches to research design were essential, leading to implementation of a decentralized, direct-to-family study design in which recruitment, intervention, and data collection all occur remotely (Balevic et al., 2021). This form of teleresearch may improve patient recruitment, retention, and engagement in clinical trials (Khozin & Coravos, 2019).

Tele-education

Tele-education refers to education provided across distance that may be synchronous with real-time interactions between teacher and learner, one-way streaming without live interaction between teacher and student, or asynchronous interaction that delivers on-demand stored educational material (Burke et al., 2015). Virtual education, particularly for patients with chronic conditions, has been shown to be as effective, if not more effective than that delivered through traditional methods (Rush et al., 2018). Tele-education may be used to educate patients, caregivers, clinicians, or health professions students locally or globally, ensuring that barriers such as distance, transportation, and physical limitations are overcome. During the COVID-19 pandemic, tele-education was extensively utilized for medical education to ensure continuity and on-time graduation for students (Doraiswamy et al., 2020).

Telementoring

Another form of tele-education, telementoring, can be used to remotely educate HCPs on the care of children and adolescents, leading to enhanced quality of care while reducing unnecessary, invasive, and more costly care (Curfman et al., 2022). In this model, also known as Project ECHO (Extension for Community Healthcare Outcomes), knowledge rather than people is moved across distance to empower local HCPs to care for their patients in the local community (Curfman et al., 2022; Thies et al., 2021). Project ECHO incorporates didactic presentations by clinical experts, case-based learning, and guided practice to enhance the ability of HCPs to manage challenging conditions in their patients (Thies et al., 2021), limiting the need for referral to distant medical centers. At the onset of the COVID-19 pandemic, there were no guidelines for prevention, diagnosis, treatment, testing, or protection from exposure to healthcare personnel (Damian et al., 2021). Project ECHO was used extensively during the PHE to disseminate guidance about COVID-19 in a timely and scalable manner to meet the needs of primary care settings (Thies et al., 2021).

Teleconsultation

Telehealth may also be used to extend the reach of pediatric specialty care through teleconsultation. Geographic barriers and disparities in distribution of pediatric specialists across the United States have led to many inadequately resourced communities regardless of rural, suburban, or urban setting (Franca & McManus, 2017; Franca & McManus, 2018). Teleconsultation or virtually connecting patients in various settings to pediatric specialists at distant locations can expand the reach of pediatric specialty care into communities that may otherwise not have access (Curfman et al., 2022).

Teleconsultation may benefit pediatric patients in both inpatient and outpatient settings. Synchronous telehealth with use of peripheral devices such as digital stethoscopes, otoscopes, ophthalmoscopes, exam cameras, and ultrasonography can facilitate specialty consultations between specialists at distant medical centers and community or rural hospitals that may not have access to pediatric expertise (Burke et al., 2015). Approximately 20% of children experience an emergency department (ED) visit each year (National Center for Health Statistics, 2019), with the majority of EDs caring for children being nonchildren's hospitals (97%) and accounting for 82.7% of pediatric ED visits (Gausche-Hill et al., 2015). Remote consultation is especially important in time-sensitive situations such as emergency, critical care, and delivery room settings where immediate support by neonatal or pediatric experts is not available on-site (Curfman et al., 2022). Interprofessional consultation with pediatric and surgical specialists enhances care of children and youth with comparable accuracy in diagnosis, treatment, and disposition planning to an in-person consultation while reducing need for patient transfers and related cost savings (Curfman et al., 2022; Harvey et al., 2017; Heath et al., 2009; Labarbera et al., 2013). Allowing patients to remain in the local community for inpatient care may also result in less family disruption (Burke et al., 2015).

Outpatient teleconsultation can be used for less time-sensitive consultations, allowing patients to receive consultation at their local medical home, residence, or other location (Burke et al., 2015). Synchronous or asynchronous modalities may be utilized based on the type of consultation required. An emerging type of teleconsultation is that of the eConsult. An eConsult is an interprofessional consult between HCPs conducted electronically without an evaluation of the patient by the consulting HCP (Gadzinski et al., 2020). eConsults are conducted between HCPs via a shared electronic health record or secure web-based platform and do not include the patient (Vimalananda et al., 2020). The requesting HCP then communicates with the patient and continues to manage their care based on guidance provided during the consult. Like many forms of telehealth, use of teleconsultation (including eConsults) expanded following the COVID-19 pandemic, highlighting its many benefits.

Telepractice

Perhaps the largest area of telehealth expansion resulting from the COVID-19 pandemic is that of telepractice, particularly in pediatric primary care. Telepractice refers to clinical services provided directly to patients in one location by a HCP in another location (Burke et al., 2015). A variety of telehealth modalities can be implemented for telepractice including synchronous audio-video communications with or without peripheral devices (digital otoscopes, stethoscopes, and exam cameras), asynchronous or e-Visit platforms, synchronous audio-only communications, and remote patient monitoring. The technology selected depends on the care to be provided as well as the originating site and related technology assessment (Valenta & Ford, 2021). Pediatric originating sites include the patient's home, schools, daycare centers, group homes, camps, and juvenile detention facilities, among others (Burke et al., 2015; Wenderlich & Herendeen, 2021). It is important to note that no specific diagnosis, specialty, population, or care setting is fundamentally suitable or unsuitable for telehealth. Successful encounters depend on various patient factors, necessary physical exam components for medical decision-making, and the availability of resources to enhance remote examination (Curfman et al., 2021b). To determine whether a visit type is appropriate for telehealth, the clinician must determine if the standard of care can be met during a virtual visit and if not, refer to in-person care. Telehealth can be used to complete a visit entirely or may be an avenue to connect patients to care either through hybrid visits that also require in-person elements, such as a nurse visit to administer vaccines, or referral to in-person settings when additional exam elements or testing are required (Wenderlich & Herendeen, 2021). During COVID-19, the American Academy of Pediatrics endorsed a hybrid approach to well visits, dividing the components into those that could be completed remotely via telehealth and those that required a follow-up in-person visit to complete aspects requiring a physical presence (Wenderlich & Herendeen, 2021).

Pediatric ambulatory telehealth visits rose between 2015 and 2017 due to the advent of standalone virtual direct-to-consumer HCPs such as those associated with retail clinics, entrepreneurs, or insurers, but usage within pediatric primary care remained low pre-pandemic (Barnett et al., 2018; Burke et al., 2015; Curfman et al., 2021b; Fiks et al., 2022). The necessity of using telehealth during the pandemic highlighted the ability to successfully conduct pediatric telehealth visits for ambulatory care, sick visits, pre-surgical assessments, follow-up appointments, post-hospitalization or emergency department visits, chronic disease management, behavioral and mental health concerns, and speech therapy (Curfman et al., 2022; Fiks et al., 2022; Kwok et al., 2022). Evaluation demonstrates that pediatric telehealth visits are comparable to and, in some cases, more beneficial than in-person visits, particularly for conditions such as asthma, obesity, otitis media, dermatologic conditions, type 1 diabetes mellitus, cystic fibrosis-related pancreatic insufficiency, and mental health conditions including attention deficit hyperactivity disorder (ADHD) (Shah & Badawy, 2021) and autism spectrum disorders (Knopf, 2013). One early landmark study noted an 86% agreement in the diagnosis and treatment of common acute childhood illnesses between telehealth and in-person HCPs compared to a 92% agreement for duplicate in-person examinations, indicating consistency between telehealth and in-person care (McConnochie et al., 2006). Additionally, children with special healthcare needs can benefit from telehealth as it overcomes transportation barriers such as the need for special transport, and distance barriers by bringing both primary and specialty care to them while enhancing communication among the interprofessional team (Wenderlich & Herendeen, 2021). Developmentally challenged patients often experience difficulty with transitions to unfamiliar environments, such as healthcare settings which may result in anxiety, fear, and disruptive behavior. Telehealth may benefit these children by reducing the frequency of these transitions and allowing for a more effective interaction with the HCP (McConnochie et al., 2015).

Guiding Principles of Remote Pediatric Management

Telehealth Best Practices

Prior to the COVID-19 pandemic, few institutions of higher learning for healthcare professionals included telehealth education in their curriculums (Chike-Harris et al., 2021; Rutledge et al., 2017). As a result, many pediatric HCPs were thrust into conducting virtual visits with little or no training or education with the onset of

COVID-19. The rapid increase in demand for telehealth during COVID-19 limited the opportunity for this important component of telehealth program development (Williams et al., 2021a, 2021b). Essential telehealth education includes systematic and rigorous program development, integration of evidence-based practice, maintenance of standard of care, and consideration of telehealth etiquette, clinical workflows, virtual physical exam techniques, documentation, billing, and technology utilization (Curfman et al., 2021b; Rutledge et al., 2021).

Successful design and implementation of a telehealth program require detailed planning and preparation to ensure attention to each essential component, leading to long-term sustainability and achievement of positive outcomes. Often, HCPs focus on novel technology implementation rather than program development, which was often the case during the COVID-19 pandemic due to the rapid nature with which telehealth was being adopted. Following the pandemic, many practices have needed to reevaluate their programs to improve processes and procedures to enhance efficiency. Essential to a successful telehealth program are a clear focus on desired outcomes, identification of the population to be served, type of services to be provided, needs for necessary technology, and attention to pertinent legal, regulatory, and reimbursement factors impacting telehealth care at the state and national level (Rutledge et al., 2020). Various frameworks exist to facilitate development of successful programs, such as the "Four Ps of Telehealth" (Rutledge et al., 2021) and the "Telehealth Service Implementation Model (TSIM)" (Valenta & Ford, 2021). An essential component of any telehealth program is a focus on accessibility to ensure all patients have access to virtual care when needed. Technology to allow for integration of an interpreter or use of adaptive technology to facilitate communication for families with limited English proficiency and those with hearing or visual impairments should be available (Curfman et al., 2022).

Essentials of the Telehealth Encounter

When provided through the medical home, telehealth care promotes continuity of care in a cost-efficient way while fostering high-quality, high-value, coordinated care (Curfman et al., 2022). A key principle of telehealthcare is that telehealth does not change the standard of care. It is the same patient-centered, evidence-based practice that is conducted in person, just delivered across distance (Chike-Harris, 2020). Pediatric HCPs must consider the essential elements required to meet the standard of care for each telehealth encounter. If the standard of care cannot be met, the patient must be referred to in-person care, ensuring that all necessary referrals and care coordination are provided by the telehealth team (Garber et al., 2021). For example, if a specific element of a physical exam is necessary to make or confirm a diagnosis, then the diagnosis should not be made without that element. Such is the case with otitis media. If a peripheral device is not available to view the tympanic membrane and the diagnosis is suspected, the patient should be referred to in-person care for further evaluation. Much of a physical exam can be completed virtually, though the required elements will depend on the patient's history and available peripheral devices. In some cases, common household items and unique techniques can be used to facilitate the virtual exam. For example, two identical soup cans can be used to assess strength by having the patient hold one in each hand while extending the arms. Household scales, thermometers and flashlights may also facilitate components of the evaluation.

Telehealth providers benefit from patience, creativity, and flexibility. Utilizing available resources at the patient site, inviting participation of caregivers, and recognizing the importance of meeting patients where they are rather than establishing arbitrary requirements benefit the patient and provider while ensuring quality healthcare is provided virtually. Knowledge of established guidelines for telehealth related to the specific population or condition being evaluated is also essential. Additionally, ensuring up-to-date contact information is available, confirming the patient location during the virtual encounter, and establishing an emergency plan are key to maintaining safe, quality care (Garber et al., 2023a, 2023b).

Telehealth Etiquette

Contrary to popular assumptions, using everyday video technologies such as FaceTime does not adequately prepare clinicians for conducting virtual visits (Sharma et al., 2019). Specific attention must be directed at telehealth etiquette to preserve the patient–provider interaction, enhance the patient–provider experience, and ensure a successful outcome (Garber et al., 2023a, 2023b; Rutledge et al., 2020). When conducting virtual care, it is important that HCPs remember to focus on the patient rather than the technology, which at times, can be distracting. Telehealth etiquette is an essential component of a telehealth encounter. It refers to *how* care is delivered rather than *what* care is provided virtually and encompasses the critical soft skills necessary to conduct a successful virtual visit (Gustin et al., 2020). "Webside manner" refers to a clinician's way of interacting with patients to make them feel comfortable when providing care across distance (McConnochie, 2019). Telehealth etiquette and webside manner foster a trusting relationship between provider, patient, and caregiver. Establishing a patient–provider relationship based on trust fosters patient understanding and willingness to follow recommended guidance, enhances patient satisfaction, and improves outcomes (Birkhäuer et al., 2017; Kelley et al., 2014; McConnochie, 2019).

Components of telehealth etiquette include the environment, the HCP's performance, and considerations related to privacy and security (Rutledge et al., 2020). The PEP (**p**erformance, **e**nvironment, and **p**rivacy/security) framework (Fig. 1) supports HCPs in prioritizing key telehealth etiquette components which are essential to a virtual encounter (Garber et al., 2023a, 2023b). Privacy and security are the core of the PEP model and include using a secure Health Insurance Portability and Accountability Act (HIPAA) compliant platform to conduct virtual care, in addition to using vendors who agree to enter into a HIPAA business associate agreement in connection with the technology (U.S. Department of Health and Human Services, 2020). The environment includes aspects of the HCP's physical location as well as

Fig. 1 The PEP framework (Garber et al., 2023a, 2023b)

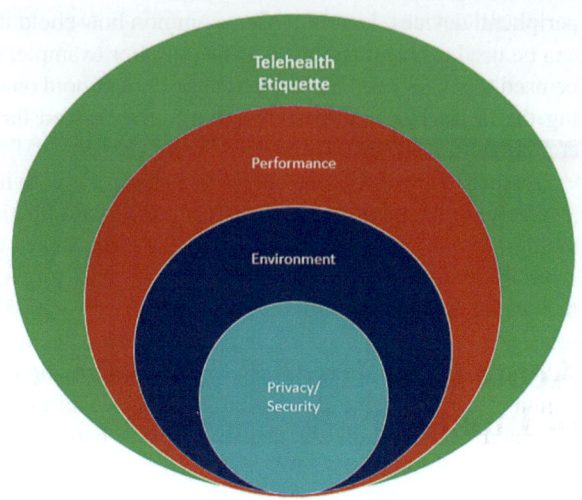

their appearance (Garber et al., 2023a, 2023b). Avoidance of visual and auditory distractions and ensuring appropriate lighting and framing are important components of the virtual visit (Sharma et al., 2019). To ensure the HCP can be seen clearly and to avoid a shadowy appearance, it is best that the light shines from behind the camera rather than behind the provider. Avoiding clutter and inappropriate items in the background, including distracting virtual backgrounds, facilitates a more focused interaction. Additionally, ensuring there are no auditory distractions such as music, email or phone alerts, television, pets, or jewelry sounds in the background is also important (Garber et al., 2023a, 2023b; Gustin et al., 2020). The HCP's personal appearance should include professional attire, visible identification, and avoidance of distracting jewelry (Garber et al., 2023a, 2023b). Technology positioning is also a key component of the HCP's environment. The computer and camera should be positioned on a stable platform with the camera at eye level with the provider's head and shoulders visible (Sharma et al., 2019) such as with a "passport view." A strong WIFI or wired internet connection is also essential to ensure there are no interruptions in the audio or video communications during the visit.

The second "P" in the PEP model refers to the provider's performance which encompasses professionalism, communication, and technology proficiency (Garber et al., 2023a, 2023b). The same professional behavior that a provider would employ in person should be followed in virtual encounters. If it wouldn't be done in an exam room, it should not be done during a virtual encounter. For example, the provider should avoid eating, drinking, and unnecessary interruptions during the visit. Being on time, establishing rapport, setting an agenda for the visit, and employing communication skills such as relationship-centered communication are essential (Garber et al., 2023a, 2023b). The inability to use touch or body language to connect with patients may be limited during telehealth encounters requiring providers to modify their communication style to emphasize the use of voice, manner, and facial expressions to convey warmth, interest, concern, and empathy (Gustin et al., 2020; McCormick, 2018).

Telehealth Quality

Telehealth visit quality encompasses the provider of the care and the technical aspects of the encounter. It is essential that HCPs caring for pediatric patients be appropriately educated in the care of children and adolescents, as well as pediatric treatment guidelines. Quality assurance guidelines apply equally to in-person and telehealth encounters necessitating adherence to recommendations for testing and treatment to be consistent (Curfman et al., 2022). Equivalence with in-person care should be the gold standard (Wenderlich & Herendeen, 2021). Ensuring the technology available is sufficient to meet evaluation and diagnostic needs of the patient while employing quality pediatric care is essential to maintaining the standard of care and to ensuring high-quality, safe telehealth encounters (Curfman et al., 2022; Wenderlich & Herendeen, 2021).

In addition to evaluating the quality of individual telehealth visits, evaluation of the telehealth program is essential to ensure high-quality, efficient, and effective care is being provided. Various frameworks exist for evaluating success of telehealth programs. The National Quality Forum (NQF) serves as a guide for evaluation and includes four key domains: (1) experience, (2) access to care, (3) effectiveness, and (4) financial impact/cost (National Quality Forum, 2017). The World Health Organization framework includes similar concepts but also considers the telehealth program's stage of maturity (World Health Organization, 2016). The American Academy of Pediatrics Section on Telehealth Care subgroup, Supporting Pediatric Research on Outcomes and Utilization of Telehealth (SPROUT), integrated concepts from these frameworks along with those from the Agency for Health Research and Quality (AHRQ) into a single framework titled "SPROUT Telehealth Evaluation and Measurement (STEM)" profile (Chuo et al., 2020). This framework includes four domains: (1) health outcomes, (2) health delivery (quality and cost), (3) experience, and (4) program implementation/ key performance indicators, which intend to communicate telehealth's value to patients, providers, health systems and payers, key stakeholders in telehealth (Chuo et al., 2020). Evaluating quality and effectiveness of patient encounters and telehealth programs will ensure that safe, quality pediatric care is being provided while promoting long-term sustainability of the telehealth program.

Barriers and Breakthroughs

Health Equity

The rapid and extensive shift to virtual care during the COVID-19 pandemic brought to light how children from underrepresented backgrounds can benefit from telehealth to overcome existing and potential inequities with telehealth. Lack of access to the internet, smartphones, or other devices and limited digital literacy may prevent patients from accessing care virtually (Crawford & Serhal, 2020; Curfman et al., 2021a, 2021b). Factors limiting access to technology include poverty, under-resourcing of health systems, homelessness, and other factors (Crawford & Serhal, 2020). Telehealth has potential to improve health inequities by reducing barriers to access to care; but without intentional effort to overcome these inequalities, they may be exacerbated. Ensuring reliable technical support for those with low digital literacy, integration of interpreters, options for families with internet-associated and device-associated barriers, and access to affordable, quality internet for all families will promote equity (Fiks et al., 2021). Since the pandemic, various programs at the federal and state level have been implemented to expand access to broadband to assist with overcoming the digital divide, though the impact of these programs on the care of traditionally underserved groups is yet to be determined (Cahan et al., 2022; Chakravorti, 2021). It is important that pediatric HCPs evaluate their patient populations and individual patients' circumstances to determine whether access to digital devices or low digital literacy may limit their ability to experience virtual care. Providing clear and simple guidance related to how to participate in telehealth encounters as well as what to expect during the visit is beneficial to the patient and provider and should be offered in a variety of modalities such as print, audio, and video.

Policy and Reimbursement

Telehealth policy is regulated by federal and state legislation and regulation, professional requirements, CMS reimbursement policies, and private payer rules (Garber et al., 2023a, 2023b). COVID-19 changed rules, regulations, and reimbursement procedures governing telehealth. Restrictions affecting reimbursement for telehealth services had traditionally limited utilization of telehealth, with many pediatric HCPs affirming these regulatory barriers to telehealth adoption and use (Sisk et al., 2020). The COVID-19 pandemic ignited need for rapid expansion of telehealth to ensure safe and ongoing healthcare for patients and providers, which necessitated alterations in these restrictions to ensure financial viability for HCPs. In March 2020, Congress implemented major changes to Medicare restrictions, including removing geographic restrictions, expanding originating sites, expanding eligible provider types, expanding reimbursable services and reimbursable telehealth modalities, and even allowing for audio-only services. This led to similar relaxations on interstate practice and privacy regulations as well. State Medicaid and private payors followed suit, leading to dramatically improved reimbursement for telehealth services (Fiks et al., 2021; Shaver, 2022). The COVID-19 federal public health emergency officially ended on May 11, 2023 and with it, many COVID-era flexibilities ceased or are evolving. Though it varies by state, many state-level modifications have already been rescinded, and yet others remain in transition. Legislation at the federal level has been introduced to extend or make permanent many of the COVID-era flexibilities (Center for Connected Health Policy, 2023) to ensure continued sustainability of telehealth initiatives. Telehealth policy continues to evolve, necessitating constant vigilance in monitoring federal and state laws and regulations to ensure HCPs remain in legal and regulatory compliance while maximizing reimbursement (Garber et al., 2023a, 2023b). Advocating for policies at the state and federal levels to support telehealth sustainability and accessibility for all patients is essential.

Lessons Learned

While telehealth has existed since the early 1900s, it was not widely used (particularly in pediatrics) until the COVID-19 pandemic necessitated its implementation. Technologies have continued to advance and will continue to do so with deployment of Artificial Intelligence (AI) in healthcare and implementation of chatbots that provide conversation-like interactions that can be used for patient triage and screening (Rokosh et al., 2021; Shah & Badawy, 2021). Widespread use affords opportunity to expand research on telehealth regarding quality, value, and best practices demonstrating telehealth care is safe, effective, and often equivalent to in-person care (Shah & Badawy, 2021) while providing comfort and stress reduction to families (McIntosh et al., 2014). Telehealth can improve access to quality pediatric healthcare for all children, but especially for those who are traditionally underserved, including people of color, rural populations, and children with special healthcare needs (Curfman et al., 2022). Extending pediatric care beyond the brick-and-mortar medical home can promote greater continuity of care, improve cost-efficiency, and reduce fragmentation of care while extending the reach of pediatric clinicians to geographic regions with limited access to these experts (Curfman et al., 2022).

The Quadruple Aim, a framework developed to enhance and optimize healthcare, includes (1) cost reduction, (2) improved population health and patient experience, and (3) improved healthcare team well-being (Arnetz et al., 2020). Telehealth supports each of these goals (Fiks et al., 2021), though prior to the widespread implementation of telehealth during the PHE few HCPs embraced virtual care (Barnett et al., 2018; Sisk et al., 2020; Williams et al., 2021a, 2021b). Integrating telehealth into the healthcare continuum can enhance pediatric care while overcoming barriers, reducing costs, and improving outcomes. It is anticipated telehealth will remain an important method of healthcare delivery moving forward. Embracing it as part of pediatric practice is essential in the near term to ensure preparedness in the event of a future PHE. To sustain this integral modality of care, it is essential that COVID-era modifications and flexibilities become permanent in addition to ensuring access to technology, broadband, and digital literacy training for all.

Calls to Action
- Increase the number of health professions students who receive education on telehealth with widespread curriculum integration.
- Improve access to telehealth care through advocacy for continued funding at the federal and state levels to expand broadband access to rural communities.
- Ensure sustainability of telehealth programs by advocating at federal and state levels for payment parity for telehealth services.
- Support continuity of care with advocacy for cross-state practice licensure exceptions for telehealth providers (waivers, compacts).

References

Arnetz, B. B., Goetz, C. M., Arnetz, J. E., Sudan, S., van Schagen, J., Piersma, K., & Reyelts, F. (2020). Enhancing healthcare efficiency to achieve the Quadruple Aim: An exploratory study. *BMC Research Notes, 13*(1), 362. https://doi.org/10.1186/s13104-020-05199-8

Bains, J., Greenwald, P. W., Mulcare, M. R., Leyden, D., Kim, J., Shemesh, A. J., Bodnar, D., Farmer, B., Steel, P., Tanouye, R., Kim, J. W., Lame, M., & Sharma, R. (2021). Utilizing telemedicine in a novel approach to COVID-19 management and patient experience in the emergency department. *Telemedicine journal and e-health: the official journal of the American Telemedicine Association, 27*(3), 254–260. https://doi.org/10.1089/tmj.2020.0162

Balevic, S. J., Singler, L., Randell, R., Chung, R. J., Lemmon, M. E., & Hornik, C. P. (2021). Bringing research directly to families in the era of COVID-19. *Pediatric Research, 89*(3), 404–406. https://doi.org/10.1038/s41390-020-01260-1

Barnett, M., Ray, K., Souza, J., & Mehrotra, A. (2018). Trends in telemedicine use in a large commercially insured population, 2005-2017. *JAMA, 320*(20), 2147–2149. https://doi.org/10.1001/jama.2018.12354

Birkhäuer, J., Gaab, J., Kossowsky, J., Hasler, S., Krummenacher, P., Werner, C., & Gerger, H. (2017). Trust in the health care professional and health outcome: A meta-analysis. *PLoS One, 12*(2), e0170988. https://doi.org/10.1371/journal.pone.0170988

Brotman, J. J., & Kotloff, R. M. (2021). Providing outpatient telehealth services in the United States: Before and during coronavirus disease 2019. *Chest, 159*(4), 1548–1558. https://doi.org/10.1016/j.chest.2020.11.020

Burke, B. L., Hall, R. W., Dehnel, P. J., Alexander, J. J., Bell, D. M., Bunik, M., Burke, B. L., & Kile, J. R. (2015). Telemedicine: Pediatric applications. *Pediatrics, 136*(1), e293–e308. https://doi.org/10.1542/peds.2015-1517

Cahan, E. M., Maturi, J., Bailey, P., Fernandes, S., Addala, A., Kibrom, S., Krissberg, J. R., Smith, S. M., Shah, S., Wang, E., Saynina, O., Wise, P. H., & Chamberlain, L. J. (2022). The impact of telehealth adoption during COVID-19 pandemic on patterns of Pediatric Subspecialty Care Utilization. *Academic Pediatrics, 22*(8), 1375–1383. https://doi.org/10.1016/j.acap.2022.03.010

Center for Connected Health Policy. (2023). *Medicare telehealth/connected health waivers post-PHE*. Retrieved June 23, 2023, from www.cchpca.org/2023/03/MEDICARE-TELEHEALTH-POLICIES-POST-PHE-AT-A-GLANCE-FINAL-MAR-2023.pdf

Chakravorti, B. (2021). How to close the digital divide in the U.S. *Harvard Business Review*. Retrieved June 23, 2023, from https://hbr.org/2021/07/how-to-close-the-digital-divide-in-the-u-s

Chike-Harris, K. E. (2020). The role of the advanced practice registered nurse in implementing telehealth practice. In P. Schweickert & C. M. Rutledge (Eds.), *Telehealth essentials for advanced practice nurses*. SLACK Books.

Chike-Harris, K. E., Durham, C., Logan, A., Smith, G., & DuBose-Morris, R. (2021). Integration of telehealth education into the Health Care Provider Curriculum: A review. *Telemedicine and E-Health, 27*(2), 137–149. https://doi.org/10.1089/tmj.2019.0261

Chuo, J., Macy, M. L., & Lorch, S. A. (2020). Strategies for evaluating telehealth. *Pediatrics, 146*(5), e20201781. https://doi.org/10.1542/peds.2020-1781

Crawford, A., & Serhal, E. (2020). Digital health equity and COVID-19: The innovation curve cannot reinforce the social gradient of health. *Journal of Medical Internet Research, 22*(6), e19361. https://doi.org/10.2196/19361

Curfman, A. L., Hackell, J. M., Herendeen, N. E., Alexander, J. J., Marcin, J. P., Moskowitz, W. B., Bodnar, C. E., Simon, H. K., & McSwain, S. D. (2021a). Telehealth: Improving access to and quality of pediatric health care. *Pediatrics, 148*(3), e2021053129. https://doi.org/10.1542/peds.2021-053129

Curfman, A., Hackell, J. M., Herendeen, N. E., Alexander, J., Marcin, J. P., Moskowitz, W. B., Bodnar, C. E., Simon, H. K., & McSwain, S. D. (2022). Telehealth: Opportunities to improve access, quality, and cost in pediatric care. *Pediatrics, 149*(3), e2021056035. https://doi.org/10.1542/peds.2021-056035

Curfman, A., McSwain, S. D., Chuo, J., Yeager-McSwain, B., Schinasi, D. A., Marcin, J., Herendeen, N., Chung, S. L., Rheuban, K., & Olson, C. A. (2021b). Pediatric telehealth in the COVID-19 pandemic era and beyond. *Pediatrics, 148*(3), e2020047795. https://doi.org/10.1542/peds.2020-047795

Damian, A., Gonzalez, M., Oo, M., & Anderson, D. (2021). A national study of community health centers readiness to address COVID-19. *Journal of American Board of Family Medicine, 34*(Supplement), S85–S94. https://doi.org/10.3122/jabfm.2021.S1.200167

Doraiswamy, S., Abraham, A., Mamtani, R., & Cheema, S. (2020). Use of telehealth during the COVID-19 pandemic: Scoping review. *Journal of Medical Internet Research, 22*(12), e24087. https://doi.org/10.2196/24087

Federal Communications Commission (FCC). (2023). *Telehealth, telemedicine and telecare: What's what?* Retrieved September 21, 2023, from https://www.fcc.gov/general/telehealth-telemedicine-and-telecare-whats-what

Fiks, A. G., Frintner, M. P., Gottschlich, E. A., & Ray, K. N. (2022). Pediatricians' experiences with telehealth in 2021. *Pediatrics, 150*(6), e2022059306. https://doi.org/10.1542/peds.2022-059306

Fiks, A. G., Jenssen, B. P., & Ray, K. N. (2021). A defining moment for Pediatric Primary Care Telehealth. *JAMA Pediatrics, 175*(1), 9. https://doi.org/10.1001/jamapediatrics.2020.1881

Foster, C., Schinasi, D., Kan, K., Macy, M., Wheeler, D., & Curfman, A. (2022). Remote monitoring of patient- and family-generated health data in pediatrics. *Pediatrics, 149*(2), e2021054137. https://doi.org/10.1542/peds.2021-054137

Franca, U., & McManus, M. (2017). Availability of definitive hospital care for children. *JAMA Pediatrics, 171*(9), e171096. https://doi.org/10.1001/jamapediatrics.2017.1096

Franca, U. L., & McManus, M. L. (2018). Trends in regionalization of hospital care for common pediatric conditions. *Pediatrics, 141*(1), e20171940. https://doi.org/10.1542/peds.2017-1940

Gadzinski, A. J., Andino, J. J., Odisho, A. Y., Watts, K. L., Gore, J. L., & Ellimoottil, C. (2020). Telemedicine and eConsults for hospitalized patients during COVID-19. *Urology, 141*, 12–14. https://doi.org/10.1016/j.urology.2020.04.061

Garber, K., Chike-Harris, K., Vetter, M. J., Kobeissi, M., Heidesch, T., Arends, R., Teall, A. M., & Rutledge, C. (2023b). Telehealth policy and the advanced practice nurse. *The Journal for Nurse Practitioners, 19*(7), 104655. https://doi.org/10.1016/j.nurpra.2023.104655

Garber, K., Gustin, T., & Rutledge, C. (2023a). Put PEP into telehealth: An etiquette framework for successful encounters. *Online Journal of Issues in Nursing, 28*(2). https://doi.org/10.3912/OJIN.Vol28No02PPT16

Garber, K., Wells, E., Hale, K. C., & King, K. (2021). Connecting kids to care: Developing a school-based telehealth program. *The Journal for Nurse Practitioners, 17*(3), 273–278. https://doi.org/10.1016/j.nurpra.2020.12.024

Gausche-Hill, M., Ely, M., Schmuhl, P., Telford, R., Remick, K., Edgerton, E., & Olson, L. (2015). A national assessment of pediatric readiness of emergency departments. *JAMA Pediatrics, 169*(6), 527–534. https://doi.org/10.1001/jamapediatrics.2015.138

Gogia, S. (2019). Fundamentals of telemedicine and telehealth. *Science Direct.* https://doi.org/10.1016/C2017-0-01090-X

Gustin, T. S., Kott, K., & Rutledge, C. (2020). Telehealth etiquette training: A guideline for preparing interprofessional teams for successful encounters. *Nurse Educator, 45*(2), 88–92. https://doi.org/10.1097/NNE.0000000000000680

Harvey, J. B., Yeager, B. E., Cramer, C., Wheeler, D., & McSwain, S. D. (2017). The impact of telemedicine on pediatric critical care triage. *Pediatric Critical Care Medicine, 18*(11), e555–e560. https://doi.org/10.1097/PCC.0000000000001330

Heath, B., Salerno, R., Hopkins, A., Hertzig, J., & Caputo, M. (2009). Pediatric critical care telemedicine in rural underserved emergency departments. *Pediatric Critical Care Medicine, 10*(5), 588–591. https://doi.org/10.1097/PCC.0b013e3181a63eac

Jumreornvong, O., Yang, E., Race, J., & Appel, J. (2020). Telemedicine and medical education in the age of COVID-19. *Academic medicine: journal of the Association of American Medical Colleges, 95*(12), 1838–1843. https://doi.org/10.1097/ACM.0000000000003711

Kelley, J. M., Kraft-Todd, G., Schapira, L., Kossowsky, J., & Riess, H. (2014). The influence of the patient-clinician relationship on healthcare outcomes: A systematic review and meta-analysis of randomized controlled trials. *PLoS One, 9*(4), e101191. https://doi.org/10.1371/journal.pone.0101191

Kennedy, C., Kirwan, J., Cook, C., Roux, P., Stulting, A., & Murdoch, I. (2000). Telemedicine techniques can be used to facilitate the conduct of multicentre trials. *Journal of Telemedicine and Telecare, 6*(6), 343–347. https://doi.org/10.1258/1357633001936030

Khozin, S., & Coravos, A. (2019). Decentralized trials in the age of real-world evidence and inclusivity in clinical investigations. *Clinical Pharmacology and Therapeutics, 106*(1), 25–27. https://doi.org/10.1002/cpt.1441

Knopf, A. (2013). School-based telehealth brings psychiatry to rural Georgia: Solution enables not only children-but working parents-to access regular treatment. *Behavioral Healthcare, 33*(1), 47–49. https://go.gale.com/ps/i.do?p=HRCA&sw=w&issn=19317093&v=2.1&it=r&id=GALE%7CA320591686&sid=googleScholar&linkaccess=fulltext.&userGroupName=anon%7E8f89fd6f&aty=open+web+entry

Koonin, L. M., Hoots, B., Tsang, C. A., Leroy, Z., Farris, K., Jolly, B., Antall, P., McCabe, B., Zellis, C., Tong, I., & Harris, A. (2020). Trends in the use of telehealth during the emergence of the COVID-19 pandemic - United States, January-March 2020. *MMWR. Morbidity and Mortality Weekly Report.* https://doi.org/10.15585/mmwr.mm6943a3. https://pubmed.ncbi.nlm.nih.gov/33119561/

Kwok, E. Y. L., Chiu, J., Rosenbaum, P., & Cunningham, B. J. (2022). The process of telepractice implementation during the COVID-19 pandemic: A narrative inquiry of preschool speech-language pathologists and assistants from one center in Canada. *BMC Health Services Research, 22*(1), 81. https://doi.org/10.1186/s12913-021-07454-5

Labarbera, J. M., Ellenby, M. S., Bouressa, P., Burrell, J., Flori, H. R., & Marcin, J. P. (2013). The impact of telemedicine intensivist support and a pediatric hospitalist program on a community hospital. *Telemed J e-health, 19*(10), 760–766. https://doi.org/10.1089/tmj.2012.0303

Marcin, J. P., Ellis, J., Mawis, R., Nagrampa, E., Nesbitt, T. S., & Dimand, R. J. (2004). Using telemedicine to provide pediatric subspecialty care to children with special health care needs in an underserved rural community. *Pediatrics, 113*(1), 1–6. https://doi.org/10.1542/peds.113.1.1

McConnochie, K. M. (2019). Webside manner: A key to high-quality primary care telemedicine for all. *Telemedicine Journal and e-Health, 25*(11), 1007–1011. https://doi.org/10.1089/tmj.2018.0274

McConnochie, K. M., Conners, G. P., Brayer, A. F., Goepp, J., Herendeen, N. E., Wood, N. E., Thomas, A., Ahn, D. S., & Roghmann, K. J. (2006). Differences in diagnosis and treatment using telemedicine versus in-person evaluation of acute illness. *Ambulatory Pediatrics, 6*(4), 187–195. https://doi.org/10.1016/j.ambp.2006.03.002

McConnochie, K. M., Ronis, S. D., Wood, N. E., & Ng, P. K. (2015). Effectiveness and safety of acute care telemedicine for children with regular and special healthcare needs. *Telemed E-Health, 21*(8), 611–621. https://doi.org/10.1089/tmj.2014.0175

McCormick, T. M. (2018, August). Three essential qualities that make a good telemedicine physician. *LinkedIn Corporation.* https://www.linkedin.com/pulse/three-essential-qualities-make-good-telemedicine-mccormick-md/

McIntosh, S., Cirillo, D., Wood, N., Dozier, A. M., Alarie, C., & McConnochie, K. M. (2014). Patient evaluation of an acute care pediatric telemedicine service in Urban Neighborhoods. *Telemed E-Health, 20*(12), 1121–1126. https://doi.org/10.1089/tmj.2014.0032

McKissick, H. D., Cady, R. G., Looman, W. S., & Finkelstein, S. M. (2017). The impact of telehealth and care coordination on the number and type of clinical visits for children with medical complexity. *Journal of Pediatric Health Care, 31*(4), 452–458. https://doi.org/10.1016/j.pedhc.2016.11.006

Mechanic, O., Persaud, Y., & Kimball, A. (2022). *Telehealth systems.* StatPearls. Retrieved May 25, 2023, from https://www.ncbi.nlm.nih.gov/books/NBK459384/

Milne Wunderlich, A., & Herendeen, N. (2021). Telehealth in pediatric primary care. *Current Problems in Adolescent and Pediatric Health Care, 51*(1), 100951. https://doi.org/10.1016/j.cppeds.2021.100951

National Center for Health Statistics. (2019). *Health, United States, Table 036.* Hyattsville, MD. Retrieved June 20, 2023, from https://www.cdc.gov/nchs/hus/data-finder.htm

National Quality Forum. (2017). *Creating a framework to support measure development for telehealth.* https://www.qualityforum.org/Publications/2017/08/Creating_a_Framework_to_Support_Measure_Development_for_Telehealth.aspx

Park, Y. T. (2016). Emerging new era of mobile health technologies. *Healthcare Informatics Research, 22*(4), 253–254. https://doi.org/10.4258/hir.2016.22.4.253

Rokosh, R. S., Lewis, W. C., Chaikof, E. L., & Kavraki, L. E. (2021). How should we prepare for the post-pandemic world of Telehealth and digital medicine? *NAM Perspectives.* https://doi.org/10.31478/202106a

Rush, K. L., Hatt, L., Janke, R., Burton, L., Ferrier, M., & Tetrault, M. (2018). The efficacy of telehealth delivered educational approaches for patients with chronic diseases: A systematic review. *Patient Education and Counseling, 101*(8), 1310–1321. https://doi.org/10.1016/j.pec.2018.02.006

Rutledge, C. M., Gustin, T. S., & Schweickert, P. (2020). Telehealth competencies: Knowledge and skills. In C. M. Rutledge & P. Schweickert (Eds.), *Telehealth essentials for advanced practice nurses.* SLACK Books.

Rutledge, C., Kott, K., Schweickert, P., Poston, R., Fowler, C., & Haney, T. (2017). Telehealth and eHealth in nurse practitioner training: Current perspectives. *Advances in Medical Education and Practice, 8,* 399–409. https://doi.org/10.2147/amep.s116071

Rutledge, C. M., O'Rourke, J., Mason, A. M., Chike-Harris, K., Behnke, L., Melhado, L., Downes, L., & Gustin, T. (2021). Telehealth competencies for nursing education and practice. *Nurse Educator, 46*(5), 300–305. https://doi.org/10.1097/NNE.0000000000000988

Shah, A. C., & Badawy, S. M. (2021). Telemedicine in pediatrics: Systematic review of randomized controlled trials. *JMIR Pediatrics and Parenting, 4*(1), e22696. https://doi.org/10.2196/22696

Sharma, R., Nachum, S., Davidson, K. W., & Nochomovitz, M. (2019). It's not just FaceTime: Core competencies for the Medical Virtualist. *International Journal of Emergency Medicine, 12*(1), 8. https://doi.org/10.1186/s12245-019-0226-y

Shaver, J. (2022). The state of telehealth before and after the COVID-19 pandemic. *Primary Care, 49,* 517–530. https://doi.org/10.1016/j.pop.2022.04.002

Sisk, B., Alexander, J., Bodnar, C., Curfman, A., Garber, K., McSwain, S., & Perrin, J. (2020). Pediatrician attitudes toward and experiences with telehealth use: Results from a national survey. *Academic Pediatrics, 20*(5), 628–635. https://doi.org/10.1016/j.acap.2020.05.004

Thies, K. M., Gonzalez, M., Porto, A., Ashley, K. L., Korman, S., & Lamb, M. (2021). Project ECHO COVID-19: Vulnerable populations and telehealth early in the pandemic. *Journal of Primary Care and Community Health, 12*, 21501327211019286. https://doi.org/10.1177/21501327211019286

U.S. Department of Health and Human Services. (2020). *Notification of enforcement discretion for telehealth | HHS.gov.* https://www.hhs.gov/hipaa/for-professionals/special-topics/emergency-preparedness/notification-enforcement-discretion-telehealth/index.html

Valenta, S., & Ford, D. (Eds.). (2021). *TSIM: The telehealth framework.* The Stationary Office (TSO).

Vimalananda, V. G., Orlander, J. D., Afable, M. K., Fincke, B. G., Solch, A. K., Rinne, S. T., Kim, E. J., Cutrona, S. L., Thomas, D. D., Strymish, J. L., & Simon, S. R. (2020). Electronic consultations (E-consults) and their outcomes: A systematic review. *Journal of the American Medical Informatics Association, 27*(3), 471–479. https://doi.org/10.1093/jamia/ocz185

Wade, V. A., Eliott, J. A., & Hiller, J. E. (2014). Clinician acceptance is the key factor for sustainable telehealth services. *Qualitative Health Research, 24*(5), 682–694. https://doi.org/10.1177/1049732314528809

Weiner, J. P., Bandeian, S., Hatef, E., Lans, D., Liu, A., & Lemke, K. W. (2021). In-person and telehealth ambulatory contacts and costs in a large US insured cohort before and during the COVID-19 pandemic. *JAMA Network Open, 4*(3), e212618. https://doi.org/10.1001/jamanetworkopen.2021.2618

Wenderlich, A., & Herendeen, N. (2021). Telehealth in pediatric primary care. *Current Problems in Pediatric and Adolescent Health Care, 51*(1), 100951. https://doi.org/10.1016/j.cppeds.2021.100951

Williams, S., Hill, K., Xie, L., Mathew, M. S., Ofori, A., Perry, T., Wesley, D., & Messiah, S. E. (2021a). Pediatric telehealth expansion in response to COVID-19. *Frontiers in Pediatrics, 9*, 642089. https://doi.org/10.3389/fped.2021.642089

Williams, S., Xie, L., Hill, K., Mathew, M. S., Perry, T., Wesley, D., & Messiah, S. E. (2021b). Potential utility of school-based telehealth in the era of COVID-19. *The Journal of School Health, 91*(7), 550–554. https://doi.org/10.1111/josh.13031

World Health Organization. (2016). *Monitoring and evaluating digital health interventions: A practical guide to conducting research and assessment.* World Health Organization.

Young, T. L., & Ireson, C. (2003). Effectiveness of school-based telehealth care in urban and rural elementary schools. Pediatrics, 112(5), 1088–1094. https://doi.org/10.1542/peds.112.5.1088.

Institutional Care Settings: Principles of Systems-Based Support

Brigit VanGraafeiland, Dawn Garzon, Cathy Woodward, Rachel Mundy Ghosh, and Jessica L. Peck

> *There can be no keener revelation of a society's soul than the way in which it treats its children.*
>
> —Nelson Mandela

Children in Foster Care

Introduction and Background

Approximately 391,000 youth were in foster care in 2022 (Child Welfare Gateway, 2022). The American Academy of Pediatrics (AAP) has determined that youth in foster care should be classified as a vulnerable population with special healthcare needs (Szilagyi et al., 2015). Additionally, studies have shown that 60% of youth who enter foster care have developmental delays; 80% have at least one medical or mental illness and chronic condition; and 40% have learning challenges (Szilagyi et al., 2015; Jee et al., 2010).

B. VanGraafeiland
Johns Hopkins School of Nursing, Baltimore, MD, USA
e-mail: bvangra1@jhu.edu

D. Garzon
Washington University Division of Child and Adolescent Psychiatry, St. Louis, MO, USA

C. Woodward
UT Health San Antonio, San Antonio, TX, USA
e-mail: woodwardc@uthscsa.edu

R. M. Ghosh
Medical and Behavioral Health Units, Franciscan Children's Hospital, Boston, MA, USA
e-mail: raghosh@franciscanchildrens.org

J. L. Peck (✉)
Louise Herrington School of Nursing, Baylor University, Dallas, TX, USA
e-mail: jessica_peck@baylor.edu

© The Author(s), under exclusive license to Springer Nature
Switzerland AG 2025
J. L. Peck (ed.), *COVID-19 Impacts on Child Health*,
https://doi.org/10.1007/978-3-031-80369-7_4

During the COVID-19 pandemic, specific populations and individuals were at greater risk for contracting and experiencing complications from COVID-19 infection and demonstrated poorer outcomes, specifically those with asthma, diabetes, and obesity (Loria et al., 2021). Of note, rates and incidence of asthma and obesity are disproportionately higher among youth in foster care (Turney & Wildeman, 2016). Furthermore, pre-pandemic child welfare and community systems were overworked and understaffed, further exacerbating health inequities during the pandemic (Wong et al., 2020).

Points of Care

COVID-19 and its variants have not only changed the world's landscape but have changed healthcare culture. As the pandemic waxed and waned over the first 3 years, youth in foster care experienced an interruption of services, lack of court engagement, and social isolation (Katz & Cohen, 2021; Whitt-Woosley et al., 2022). Whitt-Woosley et al. (2022), via a nationwide survey, identified food insecurity, mental health issues, loneliness, school issues, childcare issues, and financial problems. COVID-19 brought challenges for families in general, with schools and daycare centers closing; however, for youth in foster care, these challenges were augmented due to the lack of support, resources, and care (Shpiegel et al., 2022). Financial insecurity due to job loss, social isolation, and virtual learning highlighted disparities among foster care youth and families, increasing child maltreatment risk factors (Griffith, 2020).

For foster youth aging out of the system during COVID-19, studies found they experience more harmful outcomes as compared to pre-pandemic measures regarding housing and food stability, employment, permanency planning, and physical, mental, and behavioral health issues (Cohen & Bosk, 2020; Washburn et al., 2022; Czeisler et al., 2020). Pre-pandemic foster and transitional care youth reported low family, social, and non-familiar support levels. During the pandemic and post-pandemic, a disproportionate number of youths in care reported greater social isolation, lack of social system support, homelessness, school failure, and unmet healthcare needs (Washburn et al., 2022; LaBrenz et al., 2022).

Issues were raised during the pandemic regarding the reporting of child neglect, maltreatment, and abuse. In the presence of decreased outside social support, lack of permanency plans, implementation of stay-at-home orders, diminished childcare services, postponement of court proceedings, canceled training for biological and foster parents, shortage of primary care appointments, and no school engagement, lack of clarity emerged surrounding decreasing reports to child protection services. It was surmised that child maltreatment, abuse, and neglect reports were underreported due to a lack of encounters with mandated reporters. Conversely, there was also a supposition that reports of child maltreatment would increase due to lack of services increasing caregiver stressors and children's time in the presence of only their caregiver (Jonson-Reid et al., 2020; Musser et al., 2021). A study by Musser et al. (2021) noted that while there was a decrease in placements to foster care during the pandemic, reports of child maltreatment increased by more than 3%.

Growing concerns over lack of mental health care access during the pandemic were incredibly challenging, with 80% of youth in foster care experiencing some type of mental health illness, particularly depression and anxiety (Child Welfare Gateway, 2022). Haliwa et al. (2021) found that amid the pandemic, rates of anxiety and depression significantly increased, especially in vulnerable populations. The potential long-term effects on families include increased antisocial behavior, domestic violence, ineffective parenting, and child maltreatment (Mazza et al., 2021). Youth generally experienced increased stress, social isolation, school struggles, depression, and loneliness. Evidence supports that youth in foster care are significantly adversely impacted by the social sequelae of COVID-19 (Manzar et al., 2021; Oosterhoff & Palmer, 2020).

Barriers and Breakthroughs

One of the most significant barriers for youth in foster care during COVID-19 was a general delay in court proceedings. Legal proceedings, permanency plans, reunification goals, and delays in adoptions occurred due to closed court systems across the country (Loria et al., 2021). Additionally, questions concerning safety for youth, families, and caregivers arose due to lack of consistent contact with those professionals who generally report child maltreatment as mandated reporters (Loria et al., 2021). Further barriers were raised regarding youth who needed to enter foster care during COVID-19. Of particular concern was ensuring safe placements in light of decreased placements with caregivers in currently licensed foster homes because of the pandemic and concerns for their own overall safety and health (Loria et al., 2021).

Peterman et al. (2020) reported that pandemics are associated with increased risk factors for violence among women and children. The added vulnerability of foster care contributes to the risk of child maltreatment and emotional and physical abuse. Interruption of child welfare services and social isolation are consequences of the pandemic that generate ideal conditions for maltreatment and violence (Katz & Cohen, 2021; Bérubé et al., 2021). This service interruption significantly increases stress among families and youth who rely on visitations for reunification and a feeling of connectedness to the family unit. Child welfare workers reported that visitations stopped indefinitely for long periods during the pandemic (Crenshaw-Williams, 2023). This lack of connection mired in uncertainty affects the core element of reunification and increases the length of stay in the foster home. Evidence demonstrates that visitation with family members decreases the length of stay in foster care (Crenshaw-Williams, 2023).

The expansion of telehealth was a valuable breakthrough to engage children and their families to address the gap in care and services, particularly in rural and underserved communities. Telehealth gave healthcare providers (HCPs) a glimpse into their lives during a stressful and challenging time. Telehealth expanded care while continuing to abide by social distancing. This helped to address the lack of transportation, engagement with HCPs, and no-show rates (Loria et al., 2021). Telehealth enables collaboration and communication among HCPs, child welfare, juvenile justice, and the educational system (Loria et al., 2021). Without the option of telehealth, this collaboration would likely not occur. Virtual opportunities increased engagement between biological families and foster parents. The improved communication benefited families and youth (Loria et al., 2021).

Lessons Learned

COVID-19 taught us that it is imperative to translate best evidence into practice to support clinical practice and care from a population health perspective. Public health policies need to be developed with action plans as standard operating procedures for youth in foster care to ensure minimum disruption to services. Studies have shown that sustained access to physical and mental health care, educational opportunities, financial support, and childcare will improve the well-being of families and youth in foster care and prevent further trauma and suffering (Whitt-Woosley et al., 2022; Wilke et al., 2020). The court system must also be strategic to avoid delays and communication plans to ensure all parties continue with court recommendations and permanency plans. COVID-19 illuminated defects in the child welfare system. Advocacy for the most vulnerable youths is essential to understand the impact of COVID-19 on the physical, mental, and behavioral health and well-being of children and families immersed in the child welfare system. Systems need to assuage risk factors and identify prevention strategies to ensure the health and well-being of youth in foster care during public health crises.

Calls to Action
- Professionals who work with children in foster care must recognize that investigations, visitations, parental classes, court appearances, and problem-focused and primary care visits need to continue throughout any future pandemics and public health crises.
- There is a need for further research on vulnerable populations during global pandemics and crises to better understand the impact of events. These efforts will inform policy, address disparities, inform preparedness, and focus on prevention measures.
- Pediatric HCPs play a critical role in advocating for preventive and implementation support for children and families engaged in the child welfare system.
- Routine screening, telehealth, parenting hotlines, and online support groups are critically needed moving forward to ensure optimal care and well-being for vulnerable youth in foster care.

Inpatient Mental Health Care

Introduction and Background

Pediatric inpatient mental health care is delivered in emergency rooms to youth in acute crisis and youth who are trying to access care for chronic or untreated conditions. Inpatient care is reserved for youth who have primary medical concerns and are experiencing concurrent mental health exacerbations, youth who have acute psychiatric needs but are too medically unstable to be cared for in a psychiatric facility, and youth housed in designated psychiatric units designed to provide care for patients with acute mental health care needs primarily managed in brief stays lasting 1 week or less. Care is provided along a continuum to vulnerable children and adolescents with special attention paid to treating each individual as a member of a family unit who contributes to the patient's mental health. Prior to the COVID pandemic, the pediatric mental health system was already challenged with increasing rates of psychiatric disorders among children and adolescents, rising suicide rates and suicidal behaviors, and critical workforce and infrastructure inadequacies. Access to care was already compromised for the uninsured, those in rural settings, and for children with complex psychiatric needs (Leeb et al., 2020). The COVID-19 pandemic resulted in significant societal and healthcare changes that contributed to a joint declaration from the Children's Hospital Association of America, the American Academy of Child and Adolescent Psychiatry (AACAP), and the American Academy of Pediatrics (AAAP) of a national emergency in child and adolescent mental health in 2021 (American Academy of Pediatrics, 2021). A primary component of this statement is the explicit callout advocating to improve the availability of inpatient psychiatric beds, along with improved access to step-down programs and short-stay stabilization units (American Academy of Pediatrics, 2021).

When the COVID-19 pandemic started, pediatric inpatient resources were diverted to ensure adequate bed space was prepared to care for children ill with COVID-19. Non-essential services stopped. Overall pediatric admissions and emergency room visits decreased significantly from pre-pandemic levels (Leeb et al., 2020). Most psychiatric facilities are open units, meaning care is provided in group settings. As a result, at the height of the initial wave and until the vaccine was readily available, many group programs (including partial hospitalization programs and intensive outpatient programs) closed or shifted from in-person to virtual care delivery. Requirements were quickly enacted for children to test negative for infectious viral diseases prior to being admitted to a psychiatric unit, a requirement that remains widely enforced. At the time, this meant an even greater scarcity of available inpatient resources for youth needing inpatient psychiatric care who also tested positive for COVID-19. For example, in one particular state, there are only three facilities that accept COVID-19 positive pediatric psychiatric patients and there are no facilities in any surrounding states.

The American Psychiatric Association subsequently published guidance on admission and discharge criteria of psychiatric patients during the pandemic

(American Psychiatric Association, 2020). This document emphasizes the need for safety to guide clinical decision-making on the appropriate level of care for psychiatrically ill individuals and stresses the inherent danger of discharging patients prematurely from inpatient settings (American Psychiatric Association, 2020).

Points of Care

Pediatric patients present to emergency departments (EDs) for both routine and crisis psychiatric care, especially when they have limited access to other sources of care. Given the dearth of child and adolescent psychiatric providers and the long waitlists to access qualified pediatric psychiatric care, EDs have morphed from being sites where individuals with acute psychiatric crises like suicidal ideation or suicide attempts present for care to an overstressed safety net where families access care for non-emergent anxiety, depression, and behavioral disorders that simply disrupt school and daycare attendance. During the COVID-19 pandemic, ED utilization for psychiatric disorders increased while overall ED utilization decreased, a trend that continues until the time of the writing of this chapter (Leeb et al., 2020; Ibeziako et al., 2022).

In the fall of 2020 and 2021, child and adolescent rates of patient presentations to US EDs for depression, anxiety, severe self-injury, suicidal thoughts, and suicidal ideation increased significantly over pre-pandemic levels and in higher rates in children with no prior outpatient mental health treatment or prior psychiatric hospitalizations (Leeb et al., 2020; Ibeziako et al., 2022; Ridout et al., 2021). In 2020 alone, ED mental health visits increased 24% for 5- to-11-year-olds and 31% for 12- to 17-year-olds (Leeb et al., 2020). From 2019 to 2021, ED visits for suicide attempts increased by almost 51% in 12- to 17-year-old females (Yard et al., 2021). At the same time, the length of time youth boarded in EDs doubled, making it not uncommon for patients to wait days to more than a week for an inpatient bed (Leeb et al., 2020; Cutler et al., 2022). Younger patients, children who are most ill, children perceived as requiring the highest care level, and those assessed as the most acute tend to board longer in ED in a "reverse triage" (Morledge & Diamond, 2023). This is important to note as EDs are highly stimulating environments that are not optimal for anxious, neurodivergent, and dysregulated individuals. And, although relatively safe environments, EDs do not allow for the full array of therapies required by children requiring care in inpatient settings including psychological and other therapeutic approaches.

Consultation liaison (C/L) teams routinely manage children with psychiatric needs who are admitted to medical floors. Examples of patients managed by C/L teams include children with complex medical conditions requiring long-term hospitalization who experience anxiety, patients with eating disorders who require refeeding, adolescents who had a suicide attempt and require stabilization prior to psychiatric admission, or a patient with acute stress reaction following a traumatic injury. Due to delayed ED boarding times, there are higher volumes of patients admitted to medical floors while awaiting psychiatric placement (Leith et al., 2022). Starting in late 2020, the volume of patients seen by C/L services increased significantly over 2019 levels and illness severity for C/L patients increased by as much as four times, as measured by the need for physical restraints, as needed medications and antipsychotic medications (Leith et al., 2022). It is unclear how these rates objectively reflect increases in the severity of eating disorders, the need to place psychiatrically unstable but COVID-19+ patients on medical floors until the period of viral contagiousness passed, or increases in suicide attempts (Leith et al., 2022). The phenomenon of boarding psychiatric patients on medical floors is problematic as it is costly to the healthcare system, with that cost typically passed on to the family. Additionally, most routine medical floors are not equipped for provision of routine psychiatric care including initiating psychopharmacologic and psychologic treatments that these children require (Cutler et al., 2022).

Inpatient psychiatric care on designated psychiatric units is traditionally provided in open units that require close contact (safety monitoring) where group therapies and group meals are common as these provide opportunities for socialization and behavioral activation (Bojdani et al., 2020). On pediatric units, older children (12 years-old and older) are kept separate from younger children to provide safe, developmentally appropriate therapies and to allow for creation of a therapeutic milieu. Additionally, most psychiatric hospitals are freestanding facilities and are not associated with a medical hospital, making it difficult to care for youth with complex medical needs, meaning that medical emergencies typically require transfer to another facility for stabilization. Thus, it is common to require medical clearance for admission, including laboratory evidence of metabolic stability and evidence of the absence of infectious disease prior to psychiatric hospitalization. This was particularly challenging during a global infectious disease pandemic. A systematic review indicates that children with chronic physical conditions and neurodiversity had poorer pandemic mental health outcomes as compared to their non-affected peers, yet these patient populations are challenging to place in inpatient psychiatric settings (Bortoletto et al., 2022). Most psychiatric facilities only provide care to adolescents (youth 12 years-old and older) because of the challenges of maintaining separate units for younger and older patients. For example, in one state, there are only four facilities that provide inpatient care to children under 12 years-old. If the local facility is full, the closest facility is 2 h away and one is almost 5 h away. This places significant burden on families already in crisis and worsens with mismatch between care needs and system capacity given increasingly younger presentations of serious psychopathology and suicidality (Leeb et al., 2020).

One of the complicating factors of the pandemic, especially prior to the availability of the COVID-19 vaccine, was the need for strict infection control practices. This meant that many inpatient units ceased multidisciplinary interventions and group therapies during 2020, thus diluting program effectiveness (Bortoletto et al., 2022). Most psychiatric hospitalizations are brief (approximately a week in duration), and it is not uncommon for patients to need intensive outpatient services or partial hospitalization programs after discharge. However, many of these programs closed during the pandemic and when they reopened, support was provided only in a virtual format. This left many patients with decreased follow-up services after discharge. It is important to remember that telehealth services are not universally accessible to all. For some, broadband access is limited and it is unclear if individuals who have attention deficit hyperactivity (ADHD) and other neurodivergences respond as favorably to virtual programming (Ali et al., 2023).

Barriers and Breakthroughs

The leading barrier to inpatient psychiatric care is the increasing demand compared to inadequate system capacity. There are insufficient beds and significant workforce shortages at all levels. It is not uncommon for children to have to wait months for a new appointment with a pediatric psychiatric provider. Emergency departments are seeing record numbers of patients with psychiatric concerns, and extended ED boarding has become commonplace (Wolff et al., 2023). Loss of multidisciplinary therapies in inpatient units and closure of intensive outpatient programs interrupted care to youth post-hospitalization. However, the proliferation of telepsychiatry allowed for expansion of psychiatry services to a broader population, now no longer limited by geographical proximity. But it should be noted that telepsychiatry is not equally accessible to all and is significantly limited by state policies which often restrict nurse practitioner practice (Garber et al., 2023). In addition, research finds that telehealth for mental health services is less preferred for children when compared to their adult counterparts (Hoffnung et al., 2021).

Lessons Learned

The already strained pediatric mental health system was further challenged during the COVID-19 pandemic, resulting in widening gaps between child/family needs and resource capacity. There are insufficient psychiatric beds for children who require specialized, inpatient care and for the volume of patients currently presenting to EDs. Often, those children with the most severe disease burden, those with acutely aggressive behaviors, and those who do not have the intellectual or developmental capacity to participate in an open inpatient psychiatric milieu face extended boarding or placement on medical floors when psychiatric placement is difficulty to find. Over the last decades, the incidence of pediatric psychiatric disorders, including serious self-harm, suicidal ideation, and suicide increased, and there is no evidence that this trend is decreasing. The result is a national pediatric mental health crisis and rising suicide rates that are taking lives in a generation of our children (AAP, 2021).

Calls to Action
- Increase capacity of pediatric mental health care services at all care levels, particularly in inpatient and residential treatment care.
- Expand and increase support for the pediatric psychiatric workforce at all care levels.
- Identify novel approaches to mental health care, especially for those with complex disease and for whom inpatient placement is challenging.
- Improve access to school-based and integrated primary care mental health services to identify and treat youth prior to reaching an acute crisis.
- Expand access to telehealth and remove barriers that make telehealth challenging for many.

Refugee, Migrant and Immigrant Children

Introduction and Background

The negative impact of COVID-19 on children, initially thought to be minimal, is years later being manifested. Its bearing on already stressed refugee, immigrant and migrant children in the United States (US) is even more detrimental (Siegel, 2022). The term "immigrant" will be used to include refugee, migrant and immigrant children as descriptive of a person who was either not born in the US but is currently living in the US or children living with parent(s) who were not born in the US. The Migration Policy Institute reported that there were over 18 million immigrant children in the US in 2022 (Migration Policy Institute, 2022). This overarching term includes refugee children who were pre-screened and received medical clearance before arrival, those who arrived at US borders seeking asylum (accompanied by family or traveling unaccompanied), and children and their families currently living in the country who are undocumented. There are estimated to be 11 million unauthorized immigrants in the US with 1 in 5 being under 18 years of age (Baker, 2021). The largest group of immigrant children in the US are children of unauthorized immigrants who have fled their home country due to poverty, violence, and/or to seek a better life (Abu-Shamsieh & Maw, 2022).

The Organization for Economic Cooperation and Development reported that immigrant populations are more likely to contract COVID-19, manifest severe illness requiring hospitalization, and experience mortality than non-immigrant persons in neighboring communities (Organization for Economic Co-operation and Development, 2020). Immigrant children tend to live in lower socioeconomic communities, poor housing, and overcrowded conditions and are more likely to experience inequity with respect to healthcare access, which made the effects of the COVID-19 pandemic in immigrant populations especially severe (Đoàn et al., 2021).

As with all children during the pandemic, the pivot from in-person care to tele-health was less than successful in keeping children up-to-date with routine immunizations and was worse for immigrant children (Greenburg et al., 2021). Immigrant families who did not have resources or adequate understanding of the healthcare system in the US were more likely to have children who missed vaccine doses, well-child visits, and information on how to prevent and treat COVID-19 illness. Some immigrant children whose families were undocumented were afraid they would be arrested and deported if they went to vaccine centers (Greenburg et al., 2021).

Mental health of already traumatized immigrant children was compounded during the pandemic. Immigrant children were already at risk for mental health issues due to adverse childhood experiences (ACEs) associated with leaving their country of birth and their often harrowing transit to the US. Changes associated with the pandemic such as school closings, illness, death of caregivers, and caregiver job loss created worsening anxiety during an already anxious period in their lives (Claypool, 2021). The explosive combination of worries about immigration, inequity in healthcare, and family loss due to the pandemic created burdens on families who were the least likely to have resources to adapt.

During the pandemic, institutions which might have provided some services for immigrant children, such as schools and/or faith-based and social organizations were either physically closed or limited to virtual options. Immigrant children without access to digital infrastructure of home computers, reliable internet connection, and digital literacy were not able to participate equitably with their non-immigrant peers (Lin et al., 2023). In addition, for younger school age children, caregivers were expected to serve as computer helpers for their children although their caregivers often had little or no digital skill and less than adequate language skills to assist (Đoàn et al., 2021). The necessary pandemic illness mitigation strategies led to missed learning opportunities for this extremely vulnerable group of children.

Points of Care

Immigrant children who are identified as refugees arrive in the US having had a pre-arrival medical exam and as of 2021 must have received at least the primary series of COVID-19 vaccine (if available) in their home country. The Centers for Disease Control and Prevention (CDC) established a guideline for decision-making about when to accept a vaccine given in a foreign country and when revaccination is warranted (Centers for Disease Control and Prevention, 2023). If the child has received COVID-19 vaccines that are either not FDA-authorized or among those not listed for emergency use authorization (EUA) by the World Health Organization (WHO), they should start an age-appropriate primary vaccine series on arrival to the US.

Immigrant children arriving as asylum seekers or unaccompanied minors may or may not have had any COVID-19 vaccine. Unaccompanied children in the custody of the Office of Refugee Settlement are given the COVID-19 vaccine within days of their arrival if they do not have any documentation of vaccination (Office of Refugee

Resettlement, 2021). Additionally, all asylum seekers or persons in custody of the Border and Customs Protection agency are now offered the COVID-19 vaccine upon arrival in the US (Department of Homeland Security, 2022). In the interest of public health, any child presenting to a clinic using federally provided vaccines can and should be given the COVID-19 vaccine without charge regardless of their ability to pay or insurance status.

Barriers and Breakthroughs

Lack of health insurance coverage continues to be a barrier to immigrant children. The Migration Policy Institute reported in 2022 that over 1 million immigrant children were either ineligible for health insurance due to their undocumented status or were eligible but not currently covered. Immigrant families may not have understood that COVID-19 vaccines were available to everyone living in the US regardless of immigration and insurance status. States were encouraged and provided federal funds to expand coverage for immigrant children who became ill with COVID-19 during the pandemic and 34 states did expand access to health care for these children (Lacarte, 2022). Despite this expanded available coverage for some immigrant families, afraid accepting this help will make them ineligible for permanent status, did not apply, leaving their children without adequate healthcare.

Throughout the pandemic, various communities recognized the unique problems immigrant children and their families were suffering and sought to diminish the barriers encountered. With grant funding from the federal government, local community resources were mobilized to seek out immigrant families with information on COVID-19 in their own languages (Greenburg et al., 2021). Vaccine clinics were offered in lower socioeconomic communities, free transportation was provided to clinics on city buses, and COVID-19 testing kits were made available to community resource groups (City of Philadelphia Department of Public Health, 2023). One city government group created free hot-spots for internet available in parking lots of schools and libraries (City of San Antonio Initiative, 2020).

The barriers to education and healthcare during the pandemic presented challenges for the entire country but marginalized immigrant children experienced additional social burdens (Hill et al., 2021). As city and state governments address barriers to learning and healthcare experienced by immigrant families, it is critical to recognize immigrant populations deserve special attention and focus.

Lessons Learned

Care of immigrant children was neglected prior to the pandemic and their particular vulnerabilities in social and healthcare networks were magnified during COVID-19 (Hill et al., 2021). To be ready for the inevitable next pandemic, communities need to take meaningful action now to mitigate the spread of contagious illness and improve dissemination of information to immigrant communities to decrease disease transmission and improve health outcomes (Clark et al., 2021). Lack of equity in digital resources, glaringly evident during the pandemic, encouraged school systems to work with community partners to provide not only computers but also access to reliable internet service for all school age children (Lin et al., 2023). Improvement in internet access will improve access to both telehealth and translator services, creating greater access to healthcare and education for immigrant children.

Call to Action
- Another pandemic is inevitable. Communities must include immigrant families and/or their representatives in community-wide mitigation and crisis planning as well as planning for equitable vaccination campaigns.

Incarcerated Youth in Juvenile Justice Systems-Based Care

Introduction and Background

On any average day, around 44,000 youth under the age of 18 years are detained or incarcerated in the US (Sawyer, 2019). As with the adult justice system population, the majority of detained youth are from lower income families and racial or ethnic minority groups. Detained and incarcerated youth have higher medical and mental health morbidity than the general adolescent population. Combined with the containment model of the justice system, these youth are more susceptible to infectious outbreaks, such as COVID-19. People who are involved with the justice system broadly have about five times the prevalence of COVID-19 infection and three times the related mortality rate compared to the general population (Montoya-Barthelemy et al., 2020; Saloner et al., 2020).

By October 2020, attempts to reduce crowding in congregate care settings for infection control resulted in about a 25% overall decline in youth incarceration (Blumberg et al., 2021). While youth generally do not experience the same degree of physical illness severity risk with COVID-19, mental health impacts are only beginning to be studied and understood. However, youth involved in juvenile justice have a much higher prevalence of pre-existing conditions or co-morbidities such as asthma, high cholesterol, and atopy (Staples-Horne et al., 2021). Even more concerning is the high incidence of mental health diagnoses including anxiety, depression, attachment disorders, post-traumatic stress disorder, mood disorder, ADHD, conduct disorder, bipolar disorder, and substance use disorder (Underwood & Washington, 2016). During the height of the COVID-19 pandemic, upon entry to a detention facility, youth would be placed immediately into quarantine. This often meant they had to isolate within their cell for up to 10 days, depending on the current recommendations by the CDC and the local epidemiology patterns of COVID-19 outbreaks. If a youth tested positive for COVID-19, initially they were isolated for 14 days. The isolation time eventually was shortened to 5 days, but this reduction in isolation days happened slowly over the past 3 years.

Points of Care

Compounding this experience in the shadowy complexities of a global pandemic accelerated development of a mental health crisis. The effects of this continue to be seen in detained and incarcerated youth with emerging concerns for an increase in recidivism, greater risk for substance misuse when in the community, and more aggressive behaviors within facilities (National Commission on Correctional Health Care—NCCHC, 2022).

The standard of care for youth detained within the juvenile justice system includes receiving necessary medical, mental health, and dental care, whether it is acutely needed or not (NCCHC, 2022). During the COVID-19 pandemic when many specialties adopted telehealth care modalities, youth within juvenile justice facilities were able to experience virtual visits if there were HCPs and staff willing and able to support this process. Previously, youth who needed specialty care generally required transport to an outside facility while wearing handcuffs and shackles in the custody of juvenile detention staff. Staff shortages and active COVID-19 infection presented barriers to traditional in-person appointments requiring transportation. Replacing this stressful and often traumatic experience with telehealth access was an unintended benefit of the pandemic repercussions. Incarcerated youth have a higher prevalence of dental abscess, dental extraction, and caries. Dental care for justice involved youth is imperative as they often have not received preventive or tertiary care (Staples-Horne et al., 2021). This meant that some of these youth, who do have a higher prevalence of dental abscess, dental extractions, and caries, were possibly not receiving needed care for upwards of 2 years.

Vaccinations are part of necessary medical care, according to the NCCHC, the American Academy of Pediatrics, the National Association of Pediatric Nurse Practitioners, and the CDC. In a congregate care setting, being vaccinated is an important part of disease prevention and health promotion. Vaccinations, specifically the COVID-19 vaccine, have not been mandated within the juvenile justice setting for residents due to the varying state laws around child and adolescent consent (Shpiegel et al., 2022).

Barriers and Breakthroughs

Although quarantine and isolation are often used interchangeably, there are differences in the terms. Quarantine involves isolating from others to assess for symptoms after a personal exposure to limit other's exposure to possible illness. Isolation separates and restricts persons who are already ill or have tested positive for an illness. Being quarantined to a home or a bedroom, even with access to one's typical comforts, technology, and home-cooked meals, can be stressful. However, quarantine or isolation within an 8 × 10 ft. cell or smaller, with just a bed, a toilet, and a sink and without any personal comforts or contacts nearby is a very stressful and traumatic experience for youth. Often, there is almost no contact with other people except for brief interactions through a locked door. Punitive solitary confinement for juveniles was banned on the federal level in 2016 and therefore is not allowed today per the National Commission on Correctional Healthcare (NCCHC) guidelines; however, medical quarantine or isolation, though not punitive, remains a form of solitary confinement in how it impacts mental health by causing depression, anxiety, or psychosis (Rousseau & Miconi, 2020). In addition to imposed isolation or solitary confinement during COVID-19, family visits were also suspended indefinitely for a time. This combination of social isolation plus lack of family contact exacerbated already prevalent pre-existing mental health conditions within this vulnerable cohort (Simkins et al., 2014). Many facilities allowed youth to have video visits with their families; however, the combination of limited technology accessibility combined with significant staffing shortages during the pandemic made these video visits challenging and irregular.

Incarcerated youth still generally require parental or guardian consent for vaccination. In some states, youth can consent to receiving vaccinations without a guardian's consent (Sharko et al., 2022). When youth are within the carceral system, care must be applied to make certain that they and their guardians feel safe within the health system offered. They must not ever feel like they have been bribed or forced into a vaccination, testing, or a procedure.

Many youth are behind in their education upon entering the juvenile justice system. This has been true for many years, though the pandemic amplified learning difficulties. When youth are detained, they are required to be provided with public school education. During the COVID-19 pandemic, many youth were given uniform paper packets for self-study, despite many youth having Individualized Education Plans (IEPs) and need for other, more specialized and individualized instruction (Barnert, 2020). Some teachers used e-learning platforms, but inability to effectively capture youth attention through a static screen led to many disruptions and frustrations.

Lessons Learned

Throughout the COVID-19 pandemic, youth within the juvenile justice system were more vulnerable to both physical ailments and deteriorating mental health. Contributing factors include crowded facilities, locked confinement, increased social and physical isolation, racial injustices, inequities in social determinants of health, and higher rates of underlying trauma and mental health conditions (Zalla et al., 2022). Staffing shortages and remote learning also contribute to significant hardships for this cohort. In the future, more care and deliberation must be taken to avoid detrimental holistic health impacts.

Calls to Action
- Reduce the number of youth sent to court-ordered out-of-home placements.
- Increase the number of community-based programs.
- Employ family-focused, multidisciplinary therapy models of care.
- Increase access to cognitive behavioral therapy in detention centers.
- Expand access to telehealth services to minimize the need for traumatic transport.

References

Abu-Shamsieh, A., & Maw, S. (2022). Pediatric care for immigrant, refugee, and internationally adopted children. *Pediatric Clinics of North America, 69*(1), 153–170.

Ali, M. M., West, K. D., Bagalman, E., & Sherry, T. B. (2023). Telepsychiatry use before and during the COVID-19 pandemic among children enrolled in Medicaid. *Psychiatric Services, 74*(6), 644–647.

American Academy of Pediatrics. (2021). *AAP-AACAP-CHA declaration of a national emergency in child and adolescent mental health.* https://www.aap.org/en/advocacy/child-and-adolescent-healthy-mental-development/aap-aacap-cha-declaration-of-a-national-emergency-in-child-and-adolescent-mental-health/

American Psychiatric Association. (2020). *Guidance on admittance, discharge of psychiatric patients during COVID-19.* https://www.psychiatry.org/File%20Library/Psychiatrists/APA-Guidance-Admittance-Discharge-of-Patients-COVID-19.pdf

Baker, B. (2021). *Estimate of the unauthorized immigrant population residing in US.* Population Estimates Department of Homeland Security. https://www.dhs.gov/sites/default/files/publications/immigration-statistics/Pop_Estimate/UnauthImmigrant/unauthorized_immigrant_population_estimates_2015_-_2018.pdf

Barnert, E. S. (2020). COVID-19 and youth impacted by juvenile and adult criminal justice systems. *Pediatrics, 146*(2), e20201299. https://doi.org/10.1542/peds.2020-1299

Bérubé, A., Clément, M.-È., Lafantaisie, V., LeBlanc, A., Baron, M., Picher, G., Turgeon, J., Ruiz-Casares, M., & Lacharité, C. (2021). How societal responses to COVID-19 could contribute to child neglect. *Child Abuse & Neglect, 116*, 104761.

Blumberg, S., Lu, P., Hoover, C. M., Lloyd-Smith, J. O., Kwan, A. T., Sears, D., Bertozzi, S. M., & Worden, L. (2021). Mitigating outbreaks in congregate settings by decreasing the size of the susceptible population. *medRxiv [Preprint].* https://doi.org/10.1101/2021.07.05.2126004 3. Update in: PLoS Comput Biol. 2022; 18(7):e1010308. https://doi.org/10.1371/journal.pcbi.1010308.

Bojdani, E., Rajagopalan, A., Chen, A., Gearin, P., Olcott, W., Shankar, V., Cloutier, A., Solomon, H., Naqvi, N. Z., Batty, N., Festin, F. E. D., Tahera, D., Chang, G., & DeLisi, L. E. (2020). COVID-19 pandemic: impact on psychiatric care in the United States. *Psychiatry Res., 289*, 113069. https://doi.org/10.1016/j.psychres.2020.113069

Bortoletto, R., Gennaro, G., Antolini, G., et al. (2022). Sociodemographic and clinical changes in pediatric in-patient admissions for mental health emergencies during the COVID-19 pandemic: March 2020 to June 2021. *Psychiatry Research Communications, 2*(1), 100023. https://doi.org/10.1016/j.psycom.2022.1000023

Centers for Disease Control and Prevention. (2023, May 12). *Interim clinical considerations for use of COVID-19 vaccines: appendices, references, and previous updates appendix A. people who received COVID-19 vaccine outside the United States*. Retrieved from https://www.cdc.gov/vaccines/covid-19/clinical-considerations/interim-considerations-us-appendix.html#appendix-a

Child Welfare Gateway. (2022). *Foster care statistics 2022*. Washington, DC: U.S. Department of Health and Human Services. Administration for Children and Families, Children's Bureau. https://www.childwelfare.gov/

City of Philadelphia Department of Public Health. (2023). *Providing services, support, and guidance to reduce the spread of COVID-19 in Philadelphia*. https://www.phila.gov/programs/coronavirus-disease-2019-covid-19/

City of San Antonio Initiative. (2020). *Connected beyond the classroom*. Retrieved from: https://covid19.sanantonio.gov/What-Were-Doing/Connected-Beyond-the-Classroom

Clark, E. H., Fredricks, K., Woc-Colburn, L., Bottazzi, M. E., & Weatherhead, J. (2021). Preparing for SARS-CoV-2 vaccines in US immigrant communities: strategies for allocation, distribution, and communication. *American Journal of Public Health, 111*(4), 577–581.

Claypool, N. M. (2021). The influence of adverse childhood experiences (ACEs) including the Covid-19 pandemic, and toxic stress on development and health outcomes of Latinx children in the USA: a review of the literature. *International Journal on Child Maltreatment, 4*(S1), 257–278.

Cohen, R. I. S., & Bosk, E. A. (2020). Vulnerable youth and the COVID-19 pandemic. *Pediatrics, 146*(1), e20201306.

Crenshaw-Williams, N. (2023). The impact on foster care children and working with their families during and after COVID-19. *Youth, 3*(3), 800–808.

Cutler, G. J., Bergmann, K. R., Doupnik, S. K., Hoffmann, J. A., et al. (2022). Pediatric mental health emergency department visits and access to inpatient care: a crisis worsened by the COVID-19 pandemic. *Academic Pediatrics, 22*(6), 889–891. https://doi.org/10.1016/j.acap.2022.03.015

Czeisler, M. É., Lane, R. I., Petrosky, E., Wiley, J. F., Christensen, A., Njai, R., Weaver, M. D., Robbins, R., Facer-Childs, E. R., Barger, L. K., Czeisler, C. A., Howard, M. E., & Rajaratnam, S. M. W. (2020). Mental health, substance use, and suicidal ideation during the COVID-19 pandemic - United States, June 24-30, 2020. *MMWR Morb Mortal Wkly Rep., 69*(32), 1049–1057. https://doi.org/10.15585/mmwr.mm6932a1

Department of Homeland Security. (2022). *FACT SHEET: DHS preparations for a potential increase in migration*. https://www.dhs.gov/news/2022/03/30/fact-sheet-dhs-preparations-potential-increase-migration

Đoàn, L., Chong, S., Misra, S., Kwon, S., & Yi, K. (2021). Immigrant communities and COVID-19 strengthening the public health response. *American Journal of Public Health, 111*(S3), S224–S231.

Garber, K., Chike-Harris, K., Vetter, M. J., Kobeissi, M., Heidesch, T., Arends, R., Teall, A. M., & Rutledge, C. (2023). Telehealth policy and the advanced practice nurse. *The Journal for Nurse Practitioners, 19*(7), 104655. https://doi.org/10.1016/j.nurpra.2023.104655

Greenburg, M., Grow, K., Heredia, S., Monin, K., & Workie, E. (2021). *Strengthening services for unaccompanied children in U.S. communities*. Migration Policy Institute. Retrieved from: https://www.migrationpolicy.org/research/services-unaccompanied-children-us-communities

Griffith, A. K. (2020). Parental burnout and child maltreatment during the COVID-19 pandemic. *Journal of Family Violence, 37*(5), 725–731.

Haliwa, I., Wilson, J., Lee, J., & Shook, N. J. (2021). Predictors of change in mental health during the COVID-19 pandemic. *Journal of Affective Disorders, 291*, 331–337.

Hill, J., Rodriguez, D., & McDaniel, P. (2021). Immigration status as a health care barrier in the USA during COVID-19. *Journal of Migration and Health, 4*, 100036. Retrieved from https://www.ncbi.nlm.nih.gov/pmc/articles/PMC7979269/m

Hoffnung, G., Feigenbaum, E., Schechter, E., Guttman, D., Zemon, V., & Schechter, I. (2021). Children and telehealth in mental healthcare: what we have learned from COVID-19 and 40,000+ sessions. *Psychiatric Research and Clinical Practice, 3*(3), 106–114. https://doi. org/10.1176/appi.prcp.20200035

Ibeziako, P., Kaufman, K., Scheer, K. N., & Sideridis, G. (2022). Pediatric mental health presentations and boarding: first year of the COVID-19 pandemic. *Hospital Pediatrics, 12*(9), 751–760. https://doi.org/10.1542/hpeds.2022-006555

Jee, S. H., Szilagyi, M., Ovenshire, C., Norton, A., Conn, A. M., Blumkin, A., & Szilagyi, P. G. (2010). Improved detection of developmental delays among young children in foster care. *Pediatrics, 125*(2), 282–289.

Jonson-Reid, M., Drake, B., Cobetto, C., & Ocampo, M. (2020). *Child abuse prevention month in the context of COVID-19.* Center for Innovation in Child Maltreatment Policy, Research and Training. https://cicm.wustl.edu/child-abuse-prevention-month-in-the-context-of-covid-19/

Katz, C., & Cohen, N. (2021). Invisible children and non-essential workers: child protection during COVID-19 in Israel according to policy documents and media coverage. *Child Abuse & Neglect, 116*, 104770.

LaBrenz, C., Yu, M., Washburn, M., Palmer, A., Jenkins, L., & Kennedy. (2022). Experienced of perceived support post discharge among foster care alumni: difference among LGBTQ+ youth and youth of color. *Journal of Public Child Welfare, 17*(3), 569–594.

Lacarte, V. (2022). *Immigrant children's medicaid and CHIP access and participation: a data profile.* Migration Policy Institute. Retrieved from https://www.migrationpolicy.org/sites/default/files/publications/mpi_chip-immigrants-brief_final.pdf

Leeb, R. T., Bitsko, R. H., Radhakrishnan, L., Martinez, P., Njai, R., & Holland, K. M. (2020). Mental health–related emergency department visits among children aged< 18 years during the COVID-19 pandemic—United States, January 1–October 17, 2020. *Morbidity and Mortality Weekly Report, 69*(45), 1675.

Leith, T., Brieger, K., Malas, N., et al. (2022). Increased prevalence and severity of psychiatric illness in hospitalized youth during COVID-19. *Clinical Child Psychology and Psychiatry, 27*(3), 804–812. https://doi.org/10.1177/13591045221076889

Lin, N. T., Molgaard, M., Wishard Guerra, A., & Cohen, S. (2023). Young children and families' home literacy and technology practices before and during COVID-19. *Journal of Early Childhood Research, 21*, 341. https://doi.org/10.1177/1476718X231164132

Loria, H., McLeigh, J., Wolfe, K., Conner, E., Smith, V., Greeley, C., & Keefe, R. (2021). Caring for children in foster and kinship care during a pandemic: lessons learned and recommendations. *Journal of Public Child Welfare, 12*(1), 1–24.

Manzar, M. D., Albougami, A., Usman, N., & Mamun, M. A. (2021). Suicide among adolescents and youths during the COVID-19 pandemic lockdowns: a press media reports-based exploratory study. *Journal of Child and Adolescent Psychiatric Nursing, 34*(2), 139–146.

Mazza, M., Marano, G., Lai, C., Janiri, L., & Sani, G. (2021). Danger in danger: interpersonal violence during COVID-19 quarantine. *Psychiatry Research, 289*, 113046.

Migration Policy Institute. (2022). *Children in US immigrant families, tabulation of US census bureau's 2021 American Community Survey.* Retrieved from https://www.migrationpolicy.org/programs/data-hub/charts/children-immigrant-families

Montoya-Barthelemy, A. G., Lee, C. D., Cundiff, D. R., & Smith, E. B. (2020). COVID-19 and the correctional environment: The American prison as a focal point for public health. *American Journal of Preventive Medicine., 58*(6), 888. https://doi.org/10.1016/j.amepre.2020.04.001

Morledge, M. D., & Diamond, J. (2023). Child and adolescent mental health boarding without transfer. *Journal of the American Academy of Child and Adolescent Psychiatry, 62*, 1073. https://doi.org/10.1016/j.jaac.2023.03.023

Musser, E., Riopelle, C., & Latham, R. (2021). Child maltreatment in the time of COVID-19: changes in the Florida foster care system surrounding the COVID-19 safer-at-home order. *Child Abuse & Neglect, 116*, 104945.

NCCHC. (2022). *Standards for health services in juvenile detention and confinement facilities*. NCCHC.

Office of Refugee Resettlement. (2021). *Field guidance #17—COVID-19 vaccination of Unaccompanied Children (UC) in ORR care*. https://www.acf.hhs.gov/sites/default/files/documents/orr/Field_Guidance_17_COVID-19_Vaccination_6-10-21.pdf

Oosterhoff, B., & Palmer, C. A. (2020). Attitudes and psychological factors associated with news monitoring, social distancing, disinfecting, and hoarding behaviors among U.S. adolescents during the COVID-19 pandemic. *Archives of Pediatrics & Adolescent Medicine, 174*(12), 1184–1190.

Organization for Economic Co-operation and Development. (2020, Oct 19). *What is the impact of the Covid-19 pandemic on immigrants and their children?* Retrieved from https://www.oecd.org/coronavirus/policy-responses/what-is-the-impact-of-the-covid-19-pandemic-on-immigrants-and-their-children-e7cbb7de/

Peterman, A., Potts, A., O'Donnell, M., et al. (2020). *Pandemics and violence against women and children*. Centre for Global Development. https://www.cgdev.org/publication/pandemics-and-violence-against-women-and-children

Ridout, K. K., Alavi, M., Ridout, S. J., Koshy, M. T., Awsare, S., Harris, B., Vinson, D. R., Weisner, C. M., Sterling, S., & Iturralde, E. (2021). Emergency department encounters among youth with suicidal thoughts or behaviors during the COVID-19 pandemic. *JAMA Psychiatry, 78*(12), 1319–1328.

Rousseau, C., & Miconi, D. (2020). Protecting youth mental health during the COVID-19 pandemic: A challenging engagement and learning process. *Journal of the American Academy of Child & Adolescent Psychiatry, 59*(11), 1203–1207.

Saloner, B., Parish, K., Ward, J. A., DiLaura, G., & Dolovich, S. (2020). COVID-19 cases and deaths in federal and state prisons. *Journal of the American Medical Association., 324*, 602–603. https://doi.org/10.1001/jama.2020.12528

Sawyer, W. (2019). *Youth Confinement: The Whole Pie 2019*. Prison Policy Initiative.

Sharko, M., Jameson, R., Ancker, J. S., Krams, L., Webber, E. C., & Trent Rosenbloom, S. (2022). State-by-state variability in adolescent privacy laws. *Pediatrics, 149*(6), e2021053458. https://doi.org/10.1542/peds.2021-053458

Shpiegel, S., Aparicio, E., Ventola, M., Doig, A., Jasczynski, M., Martinez-Garcia, G., Smith, R., Sanchez, A., & Robinson, J. (2022). Experiences of young parents with foster care backgrounds during the COVID-19 pandemic. *Child Abuse & Neglect, 131*(2), 105527.

Siegel, J. (2022). The covid-19 pandemic: health impact on unaccompanied migrant children. *Social Work, 67*, 218. https://doi.org/10.1093/sw/swac014

Simkins, S., Beyer, M., & Geis, L. (2014). The harmful use of isolation in juvenile facilities: The need for post disposition representation. *Washington University Journal of Law and Policy, 38*(24).

Staples-Horne, M., Faiver, K. L., & Wimberly, Y. (2021). Juvenile corrections and public health collaborations: Opportunities for improved health outcomes. In R. B. Greifinger (Ed.), *Public health behind bars*. Springer. https://doi.org/10.1007/978-1-0716-1807-3_22

Szilagyi, M., Rosen, D., Rubin, D., & Zlotnik, S. (2015). Health care issues for children and adolescents in foster care and kinship care. *Pediatrics, 136*(4), 1142–1166.

Turney, K., & Wildeman, C. (2016). Mental and physical health of children in foster care. *Pediatrics, 138*(5), 1–10.

Underwood, L. A., & Washington, A. (2016). Mental illness and juvenile offenders. *International Journal of Environmental Research and Public Health, 13*(2), 228. https://doi.org/10.3390/ijerph13020228

Washburn, M., Yu, M., LaBrenz, C., & Palmer, A. (2022). The impacts of COVID-19 on LGBTQ+ foster youth alumni. *Child Abuse & Neglect, 133*, 9.

Whitt-Woosley, D., Sprang, G., & Eslinger, J. (2022). Foster care during the COVID-19 pandemic: a qualitative analysis of caregiver and professional experiences. *Child Abuse & Neglect, 124*(12), 105444.

Wilke, N. G., Howard, A. H., & Pop, D. (2020). Data-informed recommendations for service providers working with vulnerable children and families during the COVID-19 pandemic. *Child Abuse & Neglect, 110*(Pt 2), 104642.

Wolff, J. C., Maron, M., Chou, T., Hood, E., Sodano, S., Cheek, S., Thompson, E., Donise, K., Katz, E., & Mannix, M. (2023). Experiences of child and adolescent psychiatric patients boarding in the emergency department from staff perspectives: patient journey mapping. *Administration and Policy in Mental Health, 50*(3), 417–426. https://doi.org/10.1007/s10488-022-01249-4

Wong, C. A., Gifford, E. J., & Gifford, E. J. (2020). Mitigating the impacts of the COVID-19 pandemic response on at-risk children. *Pediatrics, 146*(1), e20200973.

Yard, E., Radhakrishnan, L., Ballesteros, M. F., et al. (2021). Emergency department visits for suspected suicide attempts among persons ages 12-25 years before and during the COVID-19 pandemic- United States, January 2019–May 2021. *MMWR, 70*, 888–894.

Zalla, L. C., Mulholland, G. E., Filiatreau, L. M., & Edwards, J. K. (2022). Racial/ethnic and age differences in the direct and indirect effects of the COVID-19 pandemic on US mortality. *American Journal of Public Health, 112*, 154–164. https://doi.org/10.2105/AJPH.2021.306541

Non-Pharmacologic Interventions: Developmental Considerations for Pandemic Preparedness

Michelle Yu-Brillhart, Anna Goddard, and Patricia Stinchfield

In the midst of every crisis, lies great opportunity.

—Albert Einstein

Perspectives on Child Development

Introduction and Background

Child development and behavior frame the field of pediatrics in healthcare (Richmond, 1967). The processes of child development are complex—occurring in a sequential, linear, and predictable pattern immediately after conception and continuing into adulthood (High et al., 2018). Decades of scientific evidence have sifted the processes to two broad concepts: nature versus nurture (AAP Section on Developmental and Behavioral Pediatrics et al., 2018). Nature is intrinsic (i.e., a child's genetic makeup), and nurture is extrinsic (i.e., a child's experiences in the physical world) (Richmond, 1967; High et al., 2018; AAP Section on Developmental and Behavioral Pediatrics et al., 2018; Committee on Integrating the Science of Early Childhood Development, 2000; Plomin et al., 1994; Burt, 2009; Ackerman, 2018).

M. Yu-Brillhart (✉)
Clinical Instructor/Nurse Practitioner, Department of Pediatrics,
Baylor College of Medicine, Houston, TX, USA
e-mail: mtyu1@texaschildrens.org

A. Goddard
Goddard Quality Healthcare Consulting, LLC, Old Saybrook, CT, USA
e-mail: anna@goddardconsulting.org

P. Stinchfield
Independent Consultant, Excelsior, MN, USA

J. L. Peck (ed.), *COVID-19 Impacts on Child Health*,
https://doi.org/10.1007/978-3-031-80369-7_5

In January 2020, the novel virus, SARS-CoV-2 (COVID-19), became a pandemic, and countries around the globe hurriedly implemented containment actions that uprooted normalcy. This chapter explores the many lessons learned from data collected between 2019 and 2022. Given that developmental pediatrics provides the foundational science of the pediatric discipline (Bartek et al., 2021), pediatric healthcare providers (HCPs) should stay apprised of the most recent research to provide holistic care and effective anticipatory guidance for adverse event preparedness response.

Nature versus Nurture

Nature (i.e., genetics) endows physical and psychological characteristics, and nurture is the physical environment and situations experienced (Richmond, 1967; High et al., 2018; AAP Section on Developmental and Behavioral Pediatrics et al., 2018; Committee on Integrating the Science of Early Childhood Development, 2000; Plomin et al., 1994; Burt, 2009; Ackerman, 2018). This section will examine how nature and nurture influence child development.

Nature: Intrinsic Factors

During conception, a zygote is formed when an oocyte is fertilized by a sperm. The zygote undergoes rapid cell division, each new cell has 23 chromosomes (i.e., bundles of deoxyribonucleic acid fibers (DNA)) governing the of organization of cells into functioning organs, and passing psychological and physiological traits to an offspring via gene expression (Marlow, 1999). Gene expression makes our anatomy and physiology alike and unique from one person to another (Marlow, 1999). At times, an aberrant gene expression may produce one or multiple genetic disorder(s) (Amorosi et al., 2008). For example, a homozygous mutation in the FOXN1 gene is associated with anencephaly and immunodeficiency (Amorosi et al., 2008). Anencephaly is a devasting neural tubal defect that causes immunodeficiency and a baby to be born without parts of the brain, spine, or skull (Amorosi et al., 2008). Many fetuses identified with FOXN1 homozygous mutation end in fetal demise, stillborn, or multiple congenital anomalies and neurodevelopmental disorders that are nonmodifiable (Amorosi et al., 2008). Another example is Attention-Deficit/Hyperactivity Disorder (ADHD), which causes symptoms of inattention, hyperactivity, impulsivity, and poor executive functioning skills, impairing relationships with peers, life skills, occupational and academic performance in numerous settings (Committee on Integrating the Science of Early Childhood Development, 2000; Plomin et al., 1994; Burt, 2009). ADHD has a heritability of 74%—meaning a child who has a parent diagnosed with ADHD has a 74% probability of receiving a diagnosis of ADHD (Committee on Integrating the Science of Early Childhood Development, 2000; Plomin et al., 1994; Burt, 2009).

Nurture: Extrinsic Factors

Brain research from animal models provides invaluable data on the impact of the environment on brain structure and neuroplasticity (Volkmar & Greenough, 1972; Koizumi et al., 2018). Research conducted by Volkmar and Greenough (1972) utilized homogenous laboratory-bred rats of the same age and size, with equal number of males and females are used to ensure homogeneity (Volkmar & Greenough, 1972). Each rat received individual pre- and post-tests to minimize confounding variables (Volkmar & Greenough, 1972). After the pretest, the rats were randomly assigned to one of three environments for one month: enrichment group (EG), social group (SG), and isolation group (IG) (Volkmar & Greenough, 1972). Twelve rats in the EG lived in a large wooden box with various toys and had daily free play outside the box (Volkmar & Greenough, 1972). SG rats were housed in pairs in identical metal cages without toys or free play (Volkmare & Greenough, 1972). IG rats lived alone in identical metal cages without toys or free play (Volkmar & Greenough, 1972). All three groups received the same amount of water, food, and light-out schedule [a]Volkmar & Greenough, 1972). Pre-and post-test scores from EG and SG rats were not statistically significant. Rats from the IG showed variations in their problem-solving skills, slower completion time, and increased clumsiness during the post-test. IG post-test results deviated from their baseline (i.e., pretest) and statistical significance compared to EG and SC (Volkmar & Greenough, 1972). Postmortem exams found larger brains with complex dendritic branching and synapses in the EC compared to both SC or IC, suggesting that brain plasticity can be impacted by either positive or negative experiential factors (Volkmar & Greenough, 1972). Unlike animal protocols, human brains are not so readily available for experimentation. Over the decades, data from neuroimaging obtained from children with adverse childhood experiences (ACEs) (e.g., neglect, abuse, malnutrition, toxic stress, and poverty) also exhibits dendritic shrinkage, small brain size, and smooth brain appearence (i.e., lissencephaly) compared to their unaffected peers. (Committee on Integrating the Science of Early Childhood Development, 2000; Gilmore et al., 2018; Nemeroff, 2016).

The accumulation of ACEs begins in utero (High et al., 2018). A pregnant woman has a 20% increased risk of experiencing adverse event(s) compared to a nonpregnant women (High et al., 2018; Committee on Integrating the Science of Early Childhood Development, 2000; Burt, 2009; Ackerman, 2018). The following adverse events are commonly reported by pregnant women: experiencing homelessness, loss of income, interruption of education, intimate-partner violence, vitamin deficiency, lack of access to prenatal care, and risky behaviors (Committee on Integrating the Science of Early Childhood Development, 2000; Plomin et al., 1994; Burt, 2009; Ackerman, 2018; Marlow, 1999; Jaan & Rajnik, 2023; Genetic Alliance; District of Columbia Department of Health, 2010). Risky behaviors include substance abuse (e.g., exposure to teratogens), unprotected sexual intercourse with new partners, and nicotine and alcohol consumption exposure (Committee on Integrating the Science of Early Childhood Development, 2000; Plomin et al., 1994; Burt, 2009; Ackerman, 2018; Marlow, 1999; Jaan & Rajnik, 2023; Genetic Alliance; District of Columbia Department of Health, 2010). Unprotected sexual intercourse and inoculation of a pathogen via paraphilia (e.g., contaminated needles) with or without prenatal care increase the chance of acquiring TORCH Complex (i.e., toxoplasmosis, others [syphilis, hepatitis B, human immunodeficiency virus (HIV), parvovirus, varicella virus], rubella, cytomegalovirus (CMV), and herpes simplex (HSV)) (Committee on Integrating the Science of Early Childhood Development, 2000; Plomin et al., 1994; Burt, 2009; Ackerman, 2018; Marlow, 1999; Jaan & Rajnik, 2023; Genetic Alliance; District of Columbia Department of Health, 2010).

Epigenetics

While ACEs negatively impact brain anatomy and physiology, emerging epigenetic data suggest that a nurturing (i.e., enriched) environment can mitigate further neurodevelopmental damages (High et al., 2018; AAP Section on Developmental and Behavioral Pediatrics et al., 2018; Committee on Integrating the Science of Early Childhood Development, 2000; Plomin et al., 1994; Burt, 2009; Ackerman, 2018; Marlow, 1999; Volkmar & Greenough, 1972; Koizumi et al., 2018; Gilmore et al., 2018; Nemeroff, 2016). Epigenetic data from monozygotic twins (MT) who were raised apart (i.e., different environments, social and religious practices, SES, diets, and lifestyles) have different DNA methylation sequences, causing each twin to exhibit or inhibit hereditary traits (Sahu & Prasuna, 2016). Genetic and environmental research has identified numerous synthetic chemicals increases congenital deformities in humans, animals, and cancers (High et al., 2018). For example, per- and polyfluoroalkyl substances (PFAS) was commonly found in cookware coated with Teflon, various tapes, body care, and kitchen ware. Repeat exposure led to a build up of PFAS in human and animal cells that induced cell death and neoplasms (High et al., 2018; Committee on Integrating the Science of Early Childhood Development, 2000; Plomin et al., 1994; Gilmore et al., 2018; Nemeroff, 2016).

While genetics governs cellular function and organ development necessary for a healthy brain and body, our environment incites synaptic pruning and methylation, affecting brain plasticity and development. Pearls for addressing developmental and behavioral concerns include start by obtaining a thorough prenatal and birth history, medical history, and family medical and psychosocial history, followed by an extensive developmental history, including the child's age, when developmental milestones are mastered. Carefully review the comprehensive history to construct a developmental profile(s) (e.g., delays, deviations, plateaus, and regressions) and refer for a comprehensive neurodevelopmental assessment as indicated with early intervention (i.e., EI and ECI), local education agency (i.e., a public school within your district), physical therapy, speech therapy, occupational therapy, pediatric psychologist, developmental behavior pediatrician, neurodevelopmental disorder specialist, and/or pediatric psychiatrist. For instance, Learning Disability (LD) is commonly diagnosed in school-age children who had multiple years of failures in one or more academic subjects (e.g., reading, writing, and math) compared to their peers (Turkeimer et al., 2003; Soto-Icaza et al., 2015). Children with LD do not have intellectual disability (ID), yet they consistently score at least two standard deviations below their peers in academics (High et al., 2018; AAP Section on Developmental and Behavioral Pediatrics et al., 2018; Turkeimer et al., 2003; Soto-Icaza et al., 2015). A child with LD is 75% more likely to report a familial history of LD (Turkeimer et al., 2003; Soto-Icaza et al., 2015). MT studies found that MT with a familial history of LD performed lower in academic achievement than MT without such history (High et al., 2018; AAP Section on Developmental and Behavioral Pediatrics et al., 2018; Turkeimer et al., 2003; Soto-Icaza et al., 2015). However, genetics alone does not determine the outcome of a child with a familial history of LD (High et al., 2018; AAP Section on Developmental and Behavioral Pediatrics et al., 2018; Turkeimer et al., 2003; Soto-Icaza et al., 2015). The child's environment is fundamentally developing pre-academic and academic skills throughout childhood (High et al., 2018; AAP Section on Developmental and Behavioral Pediatrics et al., 2018; Turkeimer et al., 2003; Soto-Icaza et al., 2015). For example, children with multiple ACEs, untreated mental (i.e., ADHD, anxiety, and schizophrenia) or medical disorders (i.e., hyperopia and absence seizures), language barriers, and/or survivors of traumatic brain injuries also have the same probability of developing LD as children with a familial history (High et al., 2018; AAP Section on Developmental and Behavioral Pediatrics et al., 2018; Turkeimer et al., 2003; Soto-Icaza et al., 2015). Moreover, children of low SES raised in a nurturing environment performed similarly to peers of high SES (High et al., 2018; AAP Section on Developmental and Behavioral Pediatrics et al., 2018; Turkeimer et al., 2003; Soto-Icaza et al., 2015). Primary care providers should assess for LD risk factors via family history during newborn exams and routine well-child check-up (WCC) exams, essential for early intervention and parental guidance that may positively alter the academic trajectory. The "wait and see" approach is strongly discouraged by the American Academy of Pediatrics (AAP) in the presence of identified concerns, aberrations, or anomalies (High et al., 2018; AAP Section on Developmental and Behavioral Pediatrics et al., 2018; Schering & Writer, 2022; CDC, 2023).

Key Points of Care
- Nature and nurture affect child development and outcome equally.
- Accumulation of ACEs starts en utero; maternal and fetal ACEs affect synaptic pruning and DNA methylation.
- A nurturing environment may be more beneficial than heritability or SES.

Points of Care

COVID-19 Containment Efforts

In the fall of 2019, healthcare leaders from Asia and Europe began sharing their harrowing experiences of caring for people infected with COVID-19 and its impact on their society and infrastructure. Their testimonies stunned HCPs and leaders around the globe as reports of the number of cases multiplied day after day. Disturbingly, many patients were asymptomatic for days to weeks before the sudden onset of severe fatigue, increased work of breathing, dyspnea, and loss of smell and taste. Diagnostics would reveal advanced destruction of the lung parenchyma, cardiopulmonary dysfunction, and coagulopathies. Despite emergent interventions, homeostasis failed to return in many people. Hospitals in Asia and Europe began diverting patients until neighboring hospitals followed suit. Medical supplies, medicine, equipment, personal protective equipment (PPE), diagnostics and laboratory equipment, hospital beds, and human resources became scarce and exhausted. Within months, Asian and European governments and healthcare leaders acknowledged an impending collapse of their medical infrastructure (CDC, 2023; CDC COVID-19 Response Team, 2020; Centers for Disease Control and Prevention, 2021).

To slow transmission, Asian and European governments mandated social distancing measures, self-quarantining, closure of nonessential businesses (restaurants, plazas, shops, places of worship, schools, etc.), and cessation of both public and private gatherings until further notice. Essential businesses and personnel (e.g., hospitals, healthcare workers, mail services, government, food distributors, environmental services, first responders, and law enforcement) operated under curfews and restrictions to provide services under the constant threat of contracting the virus (CDC, 2023; CDC COVID-19 Response Team, 2020; Centers for Disease Control and Prevention, 2021).

In February 2020, the Centers for Disease Control and Prevention (CDC) warned the American public that a stay-at-home order was imminent to prevent the spread of COVID-19 (CDC, 2023; CDC COVID-19 Response Team, 2020; Centers for Disease Control and Prevention, 2021). By mid-March 2020, all US territories, Washington D.C, and all 50 states reported at least one positive case of COVID-19 in person(s) without travel history, particularly in densely populated cities (CDC, 2023; CDC COVID-19 Response Team, 2020; Centers for Disease Control and Prevention, 2021). Small and large hospital systems began diverting patients to neighboring states while medical supplies and human resources stretched to near breaking-points (CDC, 2023; CDC COVID-19 Response Team, 2020; Centers for Disease Control and Prevention, 2021). Droves of healthcare systems pleaded for federal aid, medical supplies, medicine, ventilators, and human resources (CDC, 2023; CDC COVID-19 Response Team, 2020; Centers for Disease Control and Prevention, 2021). Due to a lack of available beds, some hospitals raised temporary treatment structures (i.e., tents erected in vacant parking lots, utilizing medical offices, clinics, stadiums, and malls as temporary inpatient beds), halted elective surgeries, and reassigned HCP's roles and expanded credentials (e.g., pediatric outpatient or specialty care clinicians were reassigned to inpatient services while other pediatric specialists were tasked with caring for adults) to care for the avalanche of COVID-19 patients(CDC, 2023; CDC COVID-19 Response Team, 2020; Centers for Disease Control and Prevention, 2021). Many primary and specialty care clinics lacked resources to deliver care safely, prompting clinic closures and disrupting crucial medical services. Many HCPs shifted to telemedicine in attempt to provide care, likewise, many patients adapted to a virtual delivery of healthcare (CDC, 2023; CDC COVID-19 Response Team, 2020; Centers for Disease Control and Prevention, 2021).

Impact on Family and Livelihood

At the pinnacle of the stay-at-home orders, schools, colleges, and daycares were suspended, groups of six or more people were widely prohibited in a public or private setting, a person traveling in public must maintain a 6 ft. distance from another person, travelers from COVID-19 burden zones were restricted entry to the US, and mandatory face coverings (i.e., facemasks) were worn by person(s) 2 years or older in public (CDC, 2023; CDC COVID-19 Response Team, 2020; Centers for Disease Control and Prevention, 2021). These containment actions stemmed from extensive infection control data from past epidemics and pandemics procedures historically used to mitigate disease transmission (Centers for Disease Control and Prevention, 2021). However, for many families, these containment actions caused a sudden loss of childcare, income, health insurance, social networks, normalcy, religious practices, healthcare services, and education. Over time, many HCPs, educators, and social service providers predicted an uptick in child maltreatment, family discord, and domestic violence, given the aforementioned stressors.

The National Bureau of Economic Research (2022) found that working person(s) had reduced working hours along with pay reduction in response to business closures affected by stay-at-home orders (Patel et al., 2020; Garcia & Cowan, 2022; Bowleg, 2020; The Nation's Report Card, n.d.; Ryan, 2018). Notably, women were more likely to take time off to care for children in part or throughout the stay-at-home order (Patel et al., 2020; Garcia & Cowan, 2022; Bowleg, 2020; The Nation's Report Card, n.d.; Ryan, 2018). Married and single women with and without dependent(s) experienced higher rates of furlough, reduced hours, reduced pay, and unemployment than married and single men (Patel et al., 2020; Garcia & Cowan, 2022; Bowleg, 2020; The Nation's Report Card, n.d.; Ryan, 2018). Additionally, caregivers or young adults without a college degree and a work-from-home option were more likely to experience furlough, unemployment, and financial hardship (Patel et al., 2020; Garcia & Cowan, 2022; Bowleg, 2020; The Nation's Report Card, n.d.; Ryan, 2018).

Child maltreatment (e.g., physical abuse, sexual abuse, emotional abuse, and neglect) is a pervasive problem (U.S. Department of Health & Human Services,

2020; Bullinger et al., 2021; Abramson, 2020; Sege & Stephens, 2022; Mann, 2021; Zviedrite et al., 2021; EdWeek, 2020). However, in 2020, the number of child protective services (CPS) requests for investigations reduced by 331,000 cases compared to 2019—the most significant decline in a decade (U.S. Department of Health & Human Services, 2020; Bullinger et al., 2021; Abramson, 2020; Sege & Stephens, 2022; Mann, 2021; Zviedrite et al., 2021; EdWeek, 2020). Epidemiologists compared CPS data collected during and after natural disasters to understanding the sudden drop in CPS referrals, despite preexisting stressors compounded by new stressors (i.e., unemployment or strained finances, disconnection from social support systems, displacement, and limited social resources). CPS data from natural disasters consistently demonstrated an increased reporting of domestic violence and child maltreatment (U.S. Department of Health & Human Services, 2020; Bullinger et al., 2021; Abramson, 2020; Sege & Stephens, 2022; Mann, 2021; Zviedrite et al., 2021; EdWeek, 2020). Two plausible theories for the decline in CPS requests are (1) underreporting and (2) a positive change in home dynamics, which are more fully explored in chapter "Children with Special Care Needs: Principles of Management for Complex Patients".

The first theory is that due to social isolation, loss of social network, monitoring of children by school and HCPs, and lack of wraparound services, children who suffered maltreatment may not have been identified; thus, the decline reflected underreporting (Ryan, 2018; U.S. Department of Health & Human Services, 2020; Bullinger et al., 2021; Abramson, 2020; Sege & Stephens, 2022; Mann, 2021; Zviedrite et al., 2021). The second theory is having an increased parental presence at home due to furlough or work-from-home opportunities. This new parental presence may have enhanced the parent–child relationship, allowing parent involvement in schoolwork, e-learning, and fostering bonding and attachment (Ryan, 2018; U.S. Department of Health & Human Services, 2020; Bullinger et al., 2021; Abramson, 2020; Sege & Stephens, 2022; Mann, 2021; Zviedrite et al., 2021). Additionally, household provider(s) who became unemployed or had a salary reduction became eligible for government stimulus programs and social programs (e.g., Medicaid, CHIP, food stamps) as part of the COVID-19 Relief Programs executed by Federal and State legislations may have alleviated daily stress and access to healthcare and mental health services accessible via virtual platforms (Ryan, 2018; U.S. Department of Health & Human Services, 2020; Bullinger et al., 2021; Abramson, 2020; Sege & Stephens, 2022; Mann, 2021; Zviedrite et al., 2021).

However, small-scale data sets from nine pediatric trauma centers reported that victims of child maltreatment ages 5 years and older tripled compared to the previous pre-pandemic data (U.S. Department of Health & Human Services, 2020; Bullinger et al., 2021; Abramson, 2020; Sege & Stephens, 2022; Mann, 2021; Zviedrite et al., 2021; EdWeek, 2020). The family-centered approach is indispensable in rapport building and patient–parent engagement. Primary care and other HCPs should regularly engage caregivers by asking open-ended questions such as, "How are things going at home?" in addition to caregiver screens (e.g., Edinburgh Postnatal Depression Screening [EPDS]). If the screener result is concerning or the caregiver endorses difficulties with parenting and bonding, it is critical to perform a safety assessment and provide resources for mental health services. As mentioned before, established and emerging data are necessary to understand the social impact of COVID-19 truly. The implications on families related to school closures are extensively covered in the chapter "Abuse and Neglect: Risk Management, Early Identification, and Evaluation".

Barriers and Breakthroughs

The information on developmental milestones in this section was adapted from Bright Futures and the Capute Scales: Cognitive Adaptive Test/Clinical Linguistic and Auditory Milestones Scale (CAT/CLAMS).

Developmental milestones are the building blocks for cognition, communication, personality, socialization, learning, and mobility (Richmond, 1967; High et al., 2018; Accordo & Captue, 2005). Attainment of developmental milestones occurs in an orderly, sequential, and predictable manner, typically acquiring "easier" milestones before "harder" milestones (Accordo & Captue, 2005). Hence, the "easier" milestone is the bedrock for the ensuing "harder" milestone. For example, a 1-month-old infant can lift his chin off a surface in a prone position and visually fixate on an object momentarily (Accordo & Captue, 2005). By 2 months of age, the infant can visually track an object horizontally and vertically and lift his chest and shoulders off a surface in a prone position (Accordo & Captue, 2005).

Social and emotional development can be quantified as early as 2 months of age by inquiring about an infant's ability to be soothed, make eye contact, interpret tone of voice, and return a social smile (Accordo & Captue, 2005; Duby, 2018). The development and mastery of social and emotional development milestones hinge on a delicate balance between temperament and attachment between a child and parent, later child and peer interactions (Accordo & Captue, 2005; Duby, 2018). Temperament is the innate element driving individualism, and preferences affect sociability (Thomas & Chess, 1977; Hong & Park, 2012). During infancy, attachment can be achieved by creating a sense of safety, security, and trust/predictability by addressing the individual needs and preferences of a child (Thomas & Chess, 1977; Hong & Park, 2012). The crux of attachment and temperament can be examined in the following exemplar scenario. A baby girl cries, and her father quickly attempts to soothe her by picking her up and then processes through a list of interventions tailored to his daughter's preference. Her father warms her bottle of formula to room temperature, followed by a diaper change before swaddling her with a lightweight cotton blanket. The father's timely response to her cries and knowledge of her preference quickly alleviates her distress.

Thomas and Chess (Thomas & Chess, 1977) categorized temperament into three types: easy/flexible, complex/feisty/inflexible, and slow-to-warm-up/fearful type (Thomas & Chess, 1977). For example, the father forgot to warm the bottle, and when he presented it, she cried and pushed it away (i.e., inflexible); she continued to cry despite her father returning with a room-temperature bottle. As she ages, her rigidness begins to disrupt family meals; her father cannot dine at the same table because she fears his food is too hot. Social and behavioral development is complex and multidimensional; the above scenario demonstrates a narrow view of social and behavioral red flags that may be pathological (Duby, 2018; Thomas & Chess, 1977; Hong & Park, 2012).

Social and emotional development builds on synergistic interactions with family and peers. The ability to perceive and interpret social cues (e.g., eye contact, facial expressions, body gestures, and intonation) and reciprocate began with mimicry during infancy and toddlerhood (Curby et al., 2012; Drimalla et al., 2019; Franco et al., 2014; Van den Berg et al., 2021; Boutzoukas et al., 2022). Multiple components of the COVID-19 containment effort prohibited a child's ability to observe and practice social skills with people outside of their family, causing parents, educators, and HCPs to question its benefit to child development, especially the effect obstructing facial features via masking (Calderon, 2020; Stoekle & Herve, 2020; CDC, 2022).

The masking mandate required anyone 2 years and older to wear a facial covering or surgical mask securely around the nose, mouth, and chin in public. By doing so, a person can reduce the expulsion while limiting inhalation of droplets and particles during conversations, coughing, and sneezing (Van den Berg et al., 2021; Boutzoukas et al., 2022). Some masking data affirmed that properly fitted and adherent masking along with other preventive health measures reduced some transmission of COVID-19 and common viral illnesses (e.g., influenza and respiratory syncytial virus), resulting in an acute drop in pediatric acute care visits and hospitalization (Van den Berg et al., 2021; Boutzoukas et al., 2022). However, emerging data from adults and children (3–8 years of age) also found that facial coverings hindered interpretation of a stranger's emotions (e.g., disgust, anger, sadness, and happiness) despite maintaining eye contact (Curby et al., 2012; Drimalla et al., 2019; Franco et al., 2014). Preschoolers demonstrated the most difficulty interpreting and perceiving emotions in strangers with facial covers compared to infants, adolescents, and teenagers (Curby et al., 2012; Drimalla et al., 2019; Franco et al., 2014; Van den Berg et al., 2021; Bourke et al., 2023; Chronaki et al., 2015; Li et al., 2023). Interestingly, using facial coverings did not interfere with sociability or social-emotional development between parent(s) or sibling(s) living within the same household (Curby et al., 2012; Drimalla et al., 2019; Franco et al., 2014; Van den Berg et al., 2021; Bourke et al., 2023; Chronaki et al., 2015; Li et al., 2023).

Lessons Learned

Developmental-behavioral disorders are among the most common medical disorders in pediatrics, affecting about 1 in 6 children in the US (Schering & Writer, 2022; Houtrow et al., 2020). As previously mentioned, the COVID-19 containment effort essentially interrupted health services, causing delays in annual well-child check-ups that ensure health and development (Schering & Writer, 2022; Houtrow et al., 2020). At each WCC, parent(s) complete developmental screeners such as Parents' Evaluation of Development Status (PEDS) or Ages and Stages Questionnaire (ASQs). Developmental-behavioral screeners are administered at specific ages. For example, the Modified Checklist for Autism in Toddlers and Revised with Follow-Up (MCHAT -MCHAT R/F) are administered at 18 and 24 months, respectively (Schering & Writer, 2022; Houtrow et al., 2020; Macias & Lipkin, 2018). Each screener has questions targeted at four developmental domains: motor (i.e., gross and visual-fine), cognitive, social-emotional, and language enhancing early detection of atypical developmental (Schering & Writer, 2022; Houtrow et al., 2020; Macias & Lipkin, 2018).

Atypical development may present as delayed (i.e., not mastered by expected age), dissociated (i.e., differences between one and more developmental domains (e.g., speech/language vs. gross motor), and deviation (i.e., acquiring milestones in non-sequential order) (High et al., 2018; Schering & Writer, 2022; Houtrow et al., 2020; Macias & Lipkin, 2018). Evidence of delay, dissociation, and deviation may indicate neurodevelopmental and neurobehavioral disorders warranting an immediate referral for neurodevelopmental assessment and diagnostics to establish an etiology and early intervention (Schering & Writer, 2022; Macias & Lipkin, 2018). The American Academics of Pediatrics (AAP) and CDC strongly advise against the "wait-and-see" method (Schering & Writer, 2022; Macias & Lipkin, 2018). Early diagnosis with targeted therapy can prevent irreversible loss of functional skills necessary for activities of daily living and social-emotional development for individuality and independence (Schering & Writer, 2022; Houtrow et al., 2020; Macias & Lipkin, 2018). Pediatric HCPs should be alert and attentive to possible alterations across the aforementioned planes of development in the wake of COVID-19, recognizing the impact this global crisis may have for years to come.

Calls to Action
- Pediatric experts' routine developmental and mental health surveillance is essential and requires additional check-ins during social isolation.
- If there are developmental delays and regression concerns, refer for neurodevelopmental evaluation and therapy.
- Conduct safety, trauma, neglect, abuse, and exploitation assessment during all medical visits.

Trauma-Informed Care

Introduction and Background

COVID-19 created worldwide, simultaneous, massive suffering across the globe. Public health implications related to COVID-19 preventative efforts, transmission, and management created long-term, pediatric developmental trauma exposure for youth. COVID-19 left the healthcare system and individuals receiving care with chronic stress, documented trauma, complicated grief, secondary stress syndrome; and critical challenges to pediatric HCPs long term. Further, COVID-19 caused health, social, and economic repercussions including exposure to Adverse Childhood Experiences (ACEs).

Adverse Childhood Experiences

ACEs are traumatic events that occur in childhood before 18 years of age. Originally identified ACEs include experiencing violence, abuse, or neglect; witnessing violence in the home; and having a family member attempt or die by suicide as first coined by Felitti and Anda at Kaiser Permanente (Felitti et al., 1998). This study is now recognized as one of the largest investigations of childhood abuse, neglect, and household dysfunction and is further known for connecting later life health and well-being in adulthood to traumas from childhood (Burke et al., 2011; Harris, 2018).

ACEs increase cortisol and adrenaline in the body, causing long-term damage to physical and mental health and correlate with greater risk of long-term addiction, autoimmune disease, chronic illness such as COPD, asthma, allergies, and behavioral/emotional consequences such as domestic violence, self-harm, suicide, teenage pregnancy, anxiety, depression, and post-traumatic stress disorder (PTSD) (Anda et al., 2006; Bryan, 2019; Goddard, 2020; Goldin & Salani, 2020). Decades of research from the original ACEs study recognize school and community violence, forced displacements, war, terrorism, political violence as well as natural disasters including COVID-19 as ACEs causing long-term dysfunction to the body's well-being (Burke et al., 2011; Anda et al., 2006; Bryan, 2019; Alexandra et al., 2005; Zarse et al., 2019). The ACE pyramid is often used conceptually to understand and model the long-term physical and mental health outcomes from experiencing early adverse childhood experiences (Fig. 1).

Trauma has devastating effects on children from delay in acquiring milestones, mild to severe aggression with siblings and other children, and parental detachment (Goldin & Salani, 2020; Alexandra et al., 2005; Perry, 2002). School-aged youth often experience difficulty in skill acquisition, short-term memory losses, fighting, disruptions in the classroom, difficulty with academic school work including reading and writing and remembering details, and loss of memories and fine details (Lee, 2020). The epigenetic changes that occur with traumatic and cumulative toxic stress have long-lasting adverse effects on children (Zarse et al., 2019; Shonkoff & Garner, 2012). Hypothalamic-pituitary-adrenal and epigenetic changes from ACEs are consistent with poorer adult health outcomes including heart disease, stroke, diabetes, and depression (Anda et al., 2006; Goldin & Salani, 2020).

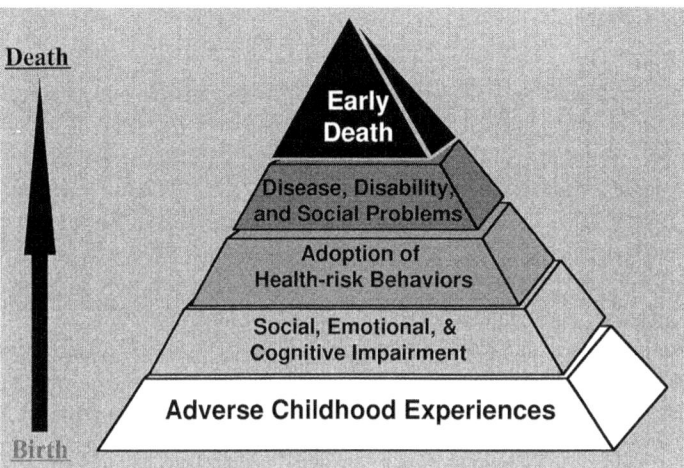

Fig. 1 The ACE pyramid. With permission from (Felitti et al., 1998)

COVID-19 Impacts on Childhood Trauma

COVID-19 amplified the risk of ACES through increased household stress, disrupted support systems, mental health individual and system challenges, and educational disruptions to learning (Bartek et al., 2021; Bryan, 2019; Lee, 2020; Bryant et al., 2020). Devasting economic consequences of job insecurity, financial instability, school and child care closures, and business closures all created significant social and economic hardships which resulted in mental distress and implication for what is currently known about the impact of ACEs (Lee, 2020; Bryant et al., 2020). Cumulative ACEs further affect the short- and long-term child and adolescent development progression and show additional neurobiological effects ranging from brain abnormalities to stress hormone dysregulation (Anda et al., 2006; Bryan, 2019; Shonkoff & Garner, 2012; Perry, 2009).

COVID-19 further disrupted normal protective factors for individuals who have experienced ACEs such as social support and consistent caregiving (Bartek et al., 2021; Bryant et al., 2020). Children and adolescents were deprived of vital support networks in the school systems due to lockdowns, school closures, and social interaction limitations (Lee, 2020). Further, the educational disruptions of remote learning, academic setbacks, and interrupted school routines thwarted children's educational progress and created significant social isolation (Bartek et al., 2021). Addressing the impact of COVID-19 and providing trauma-informed care will be crucial in mitigating the long-term consequences on children's well-being.

Points of Care

Trauma-informed care is a recognized practice requiring constant attention, awareness, sensitivity, and cultural change at an organizational level (Goddard et al., 2022). First defined by the Substance Abuse and Mental Health Services Administration (SAMHSA) (Substance Abuse and Mental Health Services Administration, 2014) and mainstreamed through Dr. Nadine Burke Harris's work with ACEs (2018), trauma-informed care presumes universal precaution for a presumed history of trauma for all individuals seeking care through a comprehensive, multi-disciplinary approach to care.

Trauma-informed care is most often explained using the SAMHSA (Substance Abuse and Mental Health Services Administration, 2014; Substance Abuse and Mental Health Services Administration, 2018) "4-Rs" framework of "Realize, Recognize, Respond, and Resist Re-traumatization." See Fig. 2.

1. Realize represents conceptual understanding of the impact of trauma beyond just the visible consequences of physical and sexual abuse and the neurological, physiological, biological, and psychological effects across one's lifetime that may result (see Fig. 1).

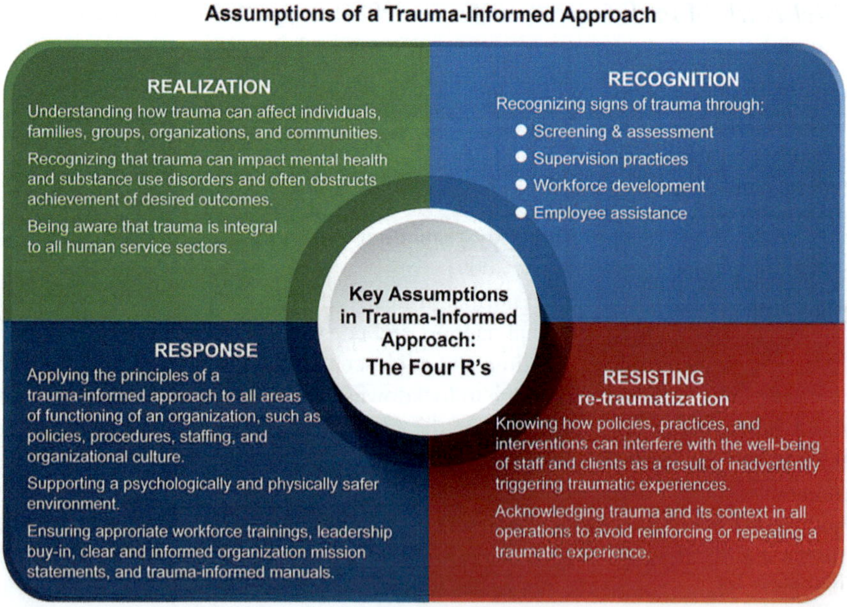

Assumptions of a Trauma-Informed Approach

REALIZATION
Understanding how trauma can affect individuals, families, groups, organizations, and communities.
Recognizing that trauma can impact mental health and substance use disorders and often obstructs achievement of desired outcomes.
Being aware that trauma is integral to all human service sectors.

RECOGNITION
Recognizing signs of trauma through:
- Screening & assessment
- Supervision practices
- Workforce development
- Employee assistance

Key Assumptions in Trauma-Informed Approach: The Four R's

RESPONSE
Applying the principles of a trauma-informed approach to all areas of functioning of an organization, such as policies, procedures, staffing, and organizational culture.
Supporting a psychologically and physically safer environment.
Ensuring approriate workforce trainings, leadership buy-in, clear and informed organization mission statements, and trauma-informed manuals.

RESISTING re-traumatization
Knowing how policies, practices, and interventions can interfere with the well-being of staff and clients as a result of inadvertently triggering traumatic experiences.
Acknowledging trauma and its context in all operations to avoid reinforcing or repeating a traumatic experience.

Fig. 2 The four Rs of trauma-informed care. **Public domain notice:** All material appearing in this publication is in the public domain and may be reproduced or copied without permission from SAMHSA. Citation of the source is appreciated

2. Recognize the signs, symptoms, and different presentations of trauma in both clients and oneself providing care to assess for potential differentials related to trauma and complex co-morbidities that may present (e.g., disordered eating, sleep concerns, and developmental delays).

3. Responding involves screening and asking questions related to trauma and mental health concerns (e.g., depression, anxiety, PTSD, and other presenting symptoms of mental health) and referring and coordinating care within the established community system. This includes referrals to and coordination with the education system, housing and social support, as well as community supports (Goddard et al., 2022; Substance Abuse and Mental Health Services Administration, 2014; Substance Abuse and Mental Health Services Administration, 2018). Trauma-based management for families may include further screening for social determinants of health, anticipatory guidance, and setting up practices with protocols for universal screening in primary care (Goddard et al., 2022; Substance Abuse and Mental Health Services Administration, 2014; Substance Abuse and Mental Health Services Administration, 2018).

4. Resisting re-traumatization refers to the clinical approach in both client care and at the HCP and organizational level. This involves supporting care practices for HCPs delivering care and giving support to the community and clients experiencing care (Substance Abuse and Mental Health Services Administration, 2014; Substance Abuse and Mental Health Services Administration, 2018). Understanding the role protective factors have in buffering the effects of chronic trauma is paramount in resisting re-traumatization. These protective factors include nurturing caregiving, maintaining sleep regimens and sleep hygiene, and promoting nutrition and physical activity in families and individuals. Practicing self-awareness and mindfulness, taking medication if and as prescribed, and seeking mental health services are also key interventions to effectively respond to the impacts of trauma and ACEs as part of trauma-informed care (Harris, 2018; Goddard et al., 2022; Substance Abuse and Mental Health Services Administration, 2018).

Trauma-informed care is crucial in the post-COVID-19 era. Taking a trauma-informed approach requires addressing pandemic-related trauma, recognizing the collective trauma of communities as a whole, supporting HCPs providing said care, promoting resilience building and coping strategies, providing community supports and connection, and addressing continuing inequities in the healthcare system (Goddard et al., 2022).

Addressing pandemic-related trauma starts with recognizing the significant impact COVID-19 left on individuals' mental health and well-being. As a caring approach, recognizing the impact of trauma creates a safe and supportive environment for all individuals affected, including HCPs and caregivers delivering care for others (Goddard, 2020; Substance Abuse and Mental Health Services Administration, 2018). Creating a non-judgmental and empathetic atmosphere for children and adolescents to express emotions and experiences is critical to identify individuals impacted by COVID-19 related ACEs (Bryant et al., 2020). Earlier identification allows for appropriate interventions through screening for trauma and signs and symptoms of pediatric mental health distress. Psychoeducation to individuals, families, and communities including the potential short- and long-term effects of COVID-19 and how ACEs impact well-being normalizes trauma experiences, reduces self-blame, and enhances understanding (Bartek et al., 2021; Burke et al., 2011; Bryant et al., 2020).

Healthcare workers are experiencing immense burnout and trauma from working frontline during the pandemic. Trauma-informed care includes supporting and providing tailored resources for healthcare professionals to address their own trauma experienced, so that they can continue to provide care for the community (Peck & Sonney, 2021). Health systems should seek to build empowerment for those seeking care, as well as the caregivers providing care, to nurture trusting, collaborative, and supportive relationships. Trauma-informed care is centered around empowering individuals to actively participate in their own care and decision-making processes to restore a sense of control and create further empowerment and collaboration (Goddard, 2020; Substance Abuse and Mental Health Services Administration, 2018). Children and their caregivers, along with HCPs providing care, need to be equipped with effective coping and stress management strategies. Building emotional regulation skills help supports one's ability to navigate and cope with the effects of COVID-19 (Bartek et al., 2021; Bryant et al., 2020). Responding with trauma-informed care coordination and collaboration across healthcare, education, social services, and community organizations ensures a holistic approach and comprehensive support.

Barriers and Breakthroughs

One of the biggest barriers to universal implementation of trauma-informed care is continued misunderstanding and limited knowledge about trauma and its impact on individuals and communities. This barrier alone significantly hinders adoption of trauma-informed practices in organizational and community culture. Healthcare organizations do not prioritize time, resources, and support for trauma-informed care, further constraining forward momentum to a trauma-informed care paradigm shift. Healthcare providers face significant time constraints that do not allow for engagement in trauma-informed approach (Peck & Sonney, 2021). Often the organizational structure lacks policies, protocols, and training programs among other systemic barriers to trauma-informed care.

Before the barriers of stigma and fear from individuals seeking care to disclose trauma, structural system-based barriers must first be addressed. COVID-19 left the US healthcare system with further fragmentation in care as well as gaps in access to care for specialized services (Bartek et al., 2021; Bryant et al., 2020; Peck & Sonney, 2021). The pediatric clinician workforce experienced significant HCP burnout and compromised mental health from pandemic-related trauma on themselves during COVID-19 (Bartek et al., 2021; Peck & Sonney, 2021). The pandemic altered previously established norms of pediatric care delivery in the US with pediatric practices experiencing significant disruption in care provision including aberrations in patient presentation, clinical practices, immunization adherence, and revenue streams. Providers were also furloughed or laid off (Peck & Sonney, 2021). Not only do HCPs need adequate training on trauma-informed care to identify and respond to individuals who need further intervention, many need healing and trauma-informed support for themselves.

While the pandemic has presented numerous challenges for children, it has also provided an opportunity for resilience, adaptability, and growth. Breakthroughs include increased awareness and understanding of trauma-informed care with greater emphasis on healthcare settings embracing a more integrative approach. Responses to COVID-19 increased mental health support funding streams and access points for therapy, including funding for School-Based Health Centers where students can access physical and mental health care directly in their schools (Bryant et al., 2020; Goddard et al., 2022). Policy makers are creating access points to these critical platforms needed prior to the pandemic that are now harboring attention in addressing trauma, anxiety, and mental health challenges from the pandemic through trauma-informed care (Bryant et al., 2020).

Trauma-informed screening and assessments improve the identification of individual symptoms and needs. Increased recognition of trauma as a public health issue has led to development of guidelines supporting trauma-informed care and recognition of policies to promote more standardized practices, training requirements for HCPs, and funding sources for trauma-related and mental health services. Further, COVID-19 created a catalytic propulsion into embracing telehealth. Telehealth reduces many barriers for care including access to mental health services and is discussed further in chapter "Telehealth: Principles of Remote Pediatric Management".

While telehealth allowed for increased access for some communities, it also highlighted health disparities and inequities nationwide (Xian et al., 2021). Many marginalized communities were unable to access care through the virtual environment and were already disproportionately impacted by the pandemic. Addressing health inequity requires more equitable access to both care and resources post-COVID-19 (Xian et al., 2021). Recognizing the barriers and breakthroughs to trauma-informed care helps guide a strategic plan for the future for more effective interventions to improve outcomes for trauma survivors.

Lessons Learned

COVID-19 highlighted the importance of trauma-informed care as well as the prevalence of trauma worldwide. The pandemic caused traumatic loss to individuals and communities and prompted recognition of the impact on short- and long-term health outcomes of trauma and the prevalence of trauma, further necessitating the importance of a universal approach to trauma-informed care.

School Impacts

In youth, prolonged stress exposure and school absences with decreased classroom instruction time are associated with developmental and cognitive delays (Bartek et al., 2021; Goldin & Salani, 2020; Alexandra et al., 2005). Educators and pediatric experts report adverse linguistic, academic, and social functioning in preschooler and early school-aged cohorts following the COVID-19 pandemic. School systems are now charged with developing social and emotional learning programs which include implementing evidence-based social and emotional skills building programs in schools. Children need coping mechanisms and re-establishment of positive relationships (Lee, 2020). Further, strengthening support networks in communities such as establishment of mentorship programs, parent support, groups, and community centers can build a sense of belonging and connection.

Raising awareness and providing educational resources for parents, caregivers, and health professionals about the impact of ACEs and embracing trauma-informed care help identify and address ACEs early on (Bryant et al., 2020). Collaborative efforts include access to basic needs such as food, clothing, shelter, and healthcare to ensure access to health services, nutritious foods, and stable housing, which reduce the stress and vulnerabilities that exacerbate ACEs (Goddard, 2020; Bryant et al., 2020; Goddard et al., 2022).

Personal Impacts for Clinicians

Attention to resources for morale and well-being of the healthcare workforce are starting to be acknowledged, including programmatic efforts to cultivate holistic wellness (Peck & Sonney, 2021). The need for connection and social support were amplified, especially as COVID-19 restrictions tore apart support networks and systems. Promoting social support systems as part of the holistic trauma-informed care approach is now highlighted as a need to address long-term quality of life functioning (Bartek et al., 2021).

Trauma-informed care and "resisting re-traumatization" expand the importance of self-care for clients and practitioners. Scientific advances in epigenetics, neurobiology, and emotional regulation of the body continue to support the importance of healthy attachments and connection as a core component to healing (Anda et al., 2006; Zarse et al., 2019; Perry, 2002; Shonkoff & Garner, 2012; Perry, 2009). Mindfulness around compassion fatigue and burnout as well as vicarious traumatization is noteworthy for working in stressful environments, of which healthcare is no exception. Compassion fatigue refers to emotional exhaustion and "care depletion" from continuing to care for others. Meanwhile, burnout often refers to the helper moving beyond compassion fatigue and completed resources to be supportive to others. Vicarious traumatization is a secondary traumatic stress in which the HCP develops trauma responses from the constant exposure to traumatic experiences by helping others. Engagement in purposeful, healthy routines, and connections can ensure supportive practices and working conditions for employees.

Healthcare administrators at a systematic level should collaboratively monitor their staff for compassion fatigue and provide support for employee engagement and self-care practices. Encouragement of using paid-time-off to resist as well as de-stigmatizing the need for HCPs to seek their own mental health treatment and counseling and decrease both burnout and treat vicarious traumatization for providers. Practicing HCPs should not only be practicing trauma-informed care with individuals receiving services, but also with themselves. In 2022, the National Association of Pediatric Nurse Practitioners [NAPNAP] issued a statement on resilience in the pediatric workforce and issued calls to action on three levels: (1) individual clinician; (2) employers and health leaders; and (3) professional organizations and communities. Strategies for professional resilience cannot rest within the sole plain of power of the individual clinician. Rather, employers, leaders, and systems must take accountability in contributing (unintentionally or not) to trauma experiences of its direct care providers and other clinical workforce. It is essential that policies be leveraged to catalyze culture change to nurture health systems that recognize the human frailty of its members and seek to provide an environment in which trauma impacts are minimized, mitigated, and addressed honestly with skill and compassion while promoting a sense of belonging (Hittle-Gigli et al., 2022).

Calls to Action
- As the world and all human beings have collectively experienced the trauma of a life-threatening and fatalistic pandemic, it necessitates healthcare systems embracing a paradigm shift to adopt principles of trauma-informed care. When ACES and developmental traumas are not addressed, subsequent developmental issues cause long-term suffering across the lifespan including digestion, appetite, sleep, and immune system dysregulation. All HCPs should be trained in trauma-informed care to avoid re-traumatizing both the patient and the providers who respond to trauma.
- Addressing health inequities related to trauma, particularly regarding access to mental health care and disparities, needs to be prioritized by organizations, leaders, and policy makers.
- Screening and addressing ACEs and pediatric mental health in primary care are one of the first critical steps for public health response. Primary care providers need training, appropriate reimbursement, and resources for interventions (such as additional training to provide point-of-care mental health services, and available mental health providers and psychiatry specialists for referrals) to meet system-level capacity needs.
- Multi-disciplinary and interprofessional healthcare curricula must include awareness and background for ACEs including the assessment, diagnosis, and management of mental health diagnoses, and incorporate trauma-informed care into core competencies for providers.

Through trauma-informed care as an intervention to initiate culture change, we can reduce ACEs and subsequently decrease the risk of long-term behavioral and physical health outcomes.

Disaster-Preparedness Planning

Children deserve unique physiological, psychological, immunologic, developmental, social, and ethical considerations in times of disasters, yet are underrepresented in disaster planning, including pandemic planning (Gilchrist & Simpson, 2019; Chiu et al., 2022). Because families and children have special needs during crises such as the COVID-19 pandemic, they must be heard and actively engaged in pandemic planning, partnering with pediatric and public health experts.

Introduction and Background

Pandemic preparedness is a dynamic activity that occurs in four phases: (1) mitigation, (2) preparedness, (3) response, and (4) recovery. (see diagram A, citation 2) This is the model of emergency management the Federal Emergency Management Agency (FEMA) has followed since 1979 for universal public disasters of all types (Herstein et al., 2021).

Points of Care

Mitigation begins before the event (Herstein et al., 2021) with the attempt to prepare for and reduce adverse impacts of the emergency. In infectious disease outbreaks for which planning efforts consider children through a developmental lens, mitigation could include handwashing sessions in schools, teaching children how to "sneeze in their sleeve," teaching basic germ theory, and why staying home from school and work when a child is sick is so important. Preparing children in the mitigation phase could also consider providing nutritionally sound meals at school, maintaining a healthy weight and keeping up-to-date on all vaccines including annual influenza vaccine so children are most effectively immunologically protected for their age range as recommended by the most current immunization schedule published by the Centers for Disease Control and Prevention (CDC).

Pandemic preparedness requires direction of leaders, input from the community, physical and intellectual resources, physical spaces for community response, and practice by all parties involved. Emergency management partnerships are essential to weather an infectious disease storm. Because children physically intersect many societal sectors such as home, school, childcare settings, places of worship, sporting team events, and entry level public facing jobs broadly including retail, fast-food, and assisted living facilities, etc., effective cross-sector, interprofessional collaboration is essential to create a comprehensive preparedness plan for children. This degree of mobility and cross-sector exposure is especially critical to consider when children can be the nidus of infection and have higher risk of viral transmission because of lack of awareness for or attention to basic hygiene protection factors. As with COVID-19, children still may be contagious while appearing less symptomatic than their adult counterparts, subconsciously lowering perception of risk of infection.

Preparedness consists of a wide array of comprehensive questions posed by contributors from potentially affected communities, entities, and sectors.

Examples of these questions include:

- What is the most effective way to communicate with children to prepare them for vaccination in a mass inoculation setting? How would a child cope with receiving a vaccine in a public setting?
- What must be considered to support psychological and physical safety?
- Will schools be stocked with proper fitting masks for each age-group and hand sanitizer, etc., or will families be responsible to provide their own supplies?
- How can ventilation be improved?
- What communication will occur if a student is home ill with a novel infection?
- How would social distancing work inside the school without detriment to psychological or emotional health?
- What downsides are there to distance learning spanning domains such as emotional, social, nutritional, psychological, and educational?

The preparedness phase ideally considers such things in a preventive manner before an emergency occurs. Setting realistic expectations and repeating them often for children in a developmentally congruent manner are critical in this phase. In infectious disease outbreaks, knowledge of the novel virus emerges slowly, and interventions change based on new information, which can frustrate parents and reduce trust in public health experts. Communities must be forewarned of ambiguity and changing recommendations as new knowledge about the emerging infection is gained and should be transparently reassured with all available facts.

The final two stages of emergency management (response and recovery) occur during and after the outbreak, respectively (Herstein et al., 2021). In response, the pandemic is increasing or at its peak and responses are focused on saving as many lives as possible by preventing direct infection or indirect effects of the outbreak such as prolonged wait times in hospital emergency departments. Emergency preparedness plans are being put into action for children and families and the entire community in this phase. There may be a time when infection is so widespread that minimizing interactions with others in social settings is wise. This may include isolation (separates sick people with a contagious disease from those who are not sick) or quarantine (separates people who have been exposed to a contagious disease from all others to prevent potential spread to other vulnerable people) (www.cdc.gov/quarantine/index.html). This is often the most difficult phase for adults and children as their social support systems may be altered or limited. Children also thrive on routine, consistency, and schedules, which are often altered during this time. Advising families on developmentally appropriate interventions such as having a regular sleep and wake time with a simple bedtime routine can be calming in the face of calamity. Families and healthcare professionals alike experience stress but must still make every attempt to calmly explain, in developmentally appropriate language, the rationale for the changes in a child's everyday life.

Once the pandemic subsides, the recovery phase is also a significant time for families. The focus is how do we return to normal? What is normal? Do we want to go back to normal or should we start completely anew? What went well during the time of social distancing? What do we hope never happens again? Is it safe to interact with our community again, or fly for vacation somewhere, or visit our grandparents? This phase monitors local, regional, national, and international epidemiologic data and makes local-level risk/benefit decisions because much of pandemic response is based on regional nuances such as vaccination and hospitalization rates, weather patterns, and wastewater organism level trends (https://www.cdc.gov/mmwr/volumes/70/wr/mm7036a2.htm). Decision-making based on data at the local and community level is best for children and families. The recovery phase can be weeks, months, or even years long after a traumatic event such as a global pandemic. Families should be offered support and understanding for as long as they require. There will be another pandemic, and HCPs would be wise to debrief on lessons learned.

Considerations for Holistic Health

To best meet the needs of children and families, leaders planning the pandemic response must include children and families themselves in addition to pediatric experts who know developmental nuances and can apply that knowledge skillfully through the lens of their expertise. Resources should include supplies and equipment suitable for children such as personal protective equipment that fit properly for various age-groups, and testing kits approved for pediatric use. Space planning for such things as mass vaccination or testing sites must be child-friendly, including separating those waiting from those being vaccinated or tested so visual lines of sight are disrupted and pre-procedure anxiety is reduced. Bringing pandemic response services to familiar surroundings such as vaccination in their own car, a comfortable non-clinical setting, or at their school is also child-friendly, especially when supported by personnel already familiar to children including parents, teachers, and other school staff. Pandemic preparedness requires early and frequent communications with children and families in invited capacities like a hospital youth advisory committee or family advisory council at a school to discuss what to expect, family needs and processes while incorporating child voice.

Case Study

Early in 2020, directors of infection control from children's hospitals across the country met by video conference to discuss best practices to prevent spread of the novel virus within pediatric hospitals and clinics. One of the most beneficial outcomes of these meetings was hosting parents of children with special needs in local hospitals for "listening sessions" as was done at Children's Minnesota. These were critical early dialogues that opened communications, set expectations of frequently changing interventions as knowledge of the virus evolved and clearly documented parental minimum standards of how and when they and their family would be able to visit a child hospitalized with COVID-19. Parents on advisory councils strongly emphasized their expectation to remain with their hospitalized child with COVID-19, prompting hospitals to adapt their policies. Rather than opposing their concerns, hospitals invited these parents to join the COVID-19 visitor guidance committee, integrating them into the hospital incident command system (HICS) meetings. It seems adult hospitals and long-term care facilities did not broadly have such policies, which caused separation of loved ones at the time of great illness and even death. The needs of children were put first with risk/benefit analyses being recalculated regularly during the pandemic. Parents agreed to limit siblings if a parent was allowed to stay with their hospitalized child, with all parties wearing masks for the duration of the visit and not visiting other patient rooms or public areas. With proper fitting masks, this reduced parent exposure risk for staff and allowed psychological comfort to the child during hospitalization. Parents and teens frequently reminded hospital leaders during pandemic response planning: "Nothing about me without me."

Barriers and Breakthroughs

In their succinct and helpful article, *Children in Disasters*, Chiu and colleagues (Chiu et al., 2022) highlight the need for a national discussion on children and disasters. In the COVID-19 pandemic, we did not start with realistic expectations for how long the pandemic may last and its impact to daily life, nor could we have anticipated the struggles children, families, the nation, and even the world would have over mask mandates, vaccines, work-from-home orders, and distance learning. We could not have anticipated how politically charged this health emergency would become, with the resultant consequences framing literal boundaries of life and death. The world would do well to resist this conflicted, polarized, and politicized path in future infectious emergencies. However, one bright breakthrough was the use of telemedicine, which has been accepted by patients and clinicians alike as a convenient mode of seeking health care during an outbreak and is discussed in multiple contexts throughout this textbook. The bottom line is that non-pharmaceutical interventions specifically for children must be considered from a holistic social, psychological, intellectual, developmental, and physical standpoint.

Lessons Learned

The COVID-19 pandemic taught us to consider the tremendous psychological impacts of public health interventions on children, not just the infection prevention outcomes. The adverse mental health implications of the non-pharmacologic interventions imposed by the COVID-19 pandemic will be felt and studied for many years to come. While public health officials focus on prevention of virus transmission, pediatric clinician voices need to be raised with children and their families and other key stakeholders to take a broader look at holistic health impacts.

Early misinformation about SARS-CoV2 disease in children persisted throughout the COVID-19 pandemic in multiple arenas delivered in multiple forums. Early messaging emphasizes that it is expected for information in pandemics to evolve. Patience is required when considering the advice of public health, infectious disease, and pediatric experts for advice. Children are not little adults and deserve considerations of application of new knowledge with a different lens and process than adults. In COVID-19, it was adults, especially older individuals and the immune suppressed who showed severe symptoms first. Children were largely spared from severe physical impacts but a wider lens considers more complexities related to pediatrics. Newborns, toddlers, preschoolers, school-aged children, and adolescents have different vulnerabilities as immune systems in each of these stages are developmentally different and therefore could respond to a novel organism uniquely. In the future, all infectious outbreaks need pediatric infectious disease specialists at the helm as part of an interdisciplinary response team. Studies in children and pregnant women should not wait in the midst of a life-threatening crisis. These populations should be invited to participate as early as possible with appropriate informed consent in clinical trials on testing, vaccines, anti-viral medications, antibodies, etc.

The American Academy of Pediatrics provides a list, as noted in Chiu's article (Chiu et al., 2022), of how we can improve the care of children in disasters of all types.

In part, it lists:

- "National, state, tribal, local, and regional disaster planning must address the unique physical, mental, behavioral, developmental, communication, therapeutic, and social needs of all children.
- Pediatricians [and other pediatric experts] should participate in disaster planning, response, and recovery efforts as subject matter experts, agents of public health surveillance, healthcare providers, and representatives of practices or institutions.
- Inpatient, outpatient, and emergency services facilities should develop operational preparedness and resiliency planning, both individually and collaboratively, to continue providing care for children during and after disasters.
- Pediatricians [and other pediatric experts] should work collaboratively with local hospitals, public health agencies, emergency management teams, volunteer emergency responders, educators and school personnel, childcare programs, foster care agencies and the juvenile justice system, medical societies, and behavioral health providers, as well as nongovernmental organizations and other agencies that serve children, to effectively meet children's needs in the context of disaster.
- Equipment, medications, and supplies for children should be available to meet children's needs during a disaster in parity with similar adult needs. Where parity does not exist, research, development, and procurement must be undertaken in a timely manner.

- Federal, state, academic, and private institutions should conduct more research on identifying gaps in knowledge of treatment of children in disasters and identifying best practices in addressing these deficiencies. Federal grants and funding support for such research need to increase accordingly. The federal government is encouraged to continue developing the infrastructure to facilitate ethical and timely research and data collection in a disaster environment...".

Calls to Action

Infectious outbreaks are dynamic, especially in the context of a worldwide pandemic. Information changes regularly and quickly, early assumptions must be tested and reassessed to determine the best non-pharmaceutical interventions for children and families, with patience to allow scientific research to reinforce best practices over time through studies with high scientific rigor.

- Children and families deserve early involvement in planning and implementing outbreak specific guidelines in schools, clinics, and communities because of their unique developmental considerations—*"Nothing about me without me."*
- Emergency management has four phases of response. Any entity which serves children, such as schools, childcare centers, clinics, and children's hospitals should be familiar with the FEMA response phases, and have written plans which are reviewed and practiced regularly and collaboratively with pediatric partner experts and community stakeholders (https://training.fema.gov/emiweb/downloads/is111_unit%204.pdf).
- School closures, hospital visiting guidelines, and cancelation of youth activities, etc. require holistic considerations of both individual and public health risks and must be inclusive of physical and mental health impacts, using evidence-based decision-making.

References

AAP Section on Developmental and Behavioral Pediatrics, Voigt, R. G., Macias, M. M., Myers, S. M., & Tapia, C. D. (2018). Child development: the basic science of pediatrics. In *AAP developmental and behavioral pediatrics* (pp. 1–4). American Academy of Pediatrics.

Abramson, A. (2020, April 8). *How COVID-19 may increase domestic violence and child abuse.* https://www.apa.org/topics/covid-19/domestic-violence-child-abuse.

Accordo, P. J., & Captue, A. J. (2005). *The capute scales: Cognitive adaptive test/clinical linguistic and auditory milestones scale (CAT/CLAMS).* Paul H. Brookes Publishing Co.

Ackerman, S. (2018). The development and shaping of the brain. In *Discovering the brain* (pp. 86–103). National Academies Press.

Alexandra, C., Joseph, S., Julian, F., Cheryl, L., Margaret, B., Marylene, C., Ruth, D., Rebecca, H., Richard, K., Joan, L., Karen, M., Erna, O., & van der Kook, B. (2005). Complex trauma in children and adolescents. *Psychiatric Annals, 5,* 390. https://doi.org/10.1002/jclp.21990

Amorosi, S., et al. (2008). FOXN1 homozygous mutation associated with anencephaly and severe neural tube defect in human Athymic nude/SCID fetus. *Clinical Genetics, 73*(4), 380–384. https://doi.org/10.1111/j.1399-0004.2008.00977.x

Anda, R., Felitti, V., Bremner, J., et al. (2006). The enduring effects of abuse and related adverse experiences in childhood. A convergence of evidence from neurobiology and epidemiology. *European Archives of Psychiatry and Clinical Neuroscience, 256*(3), 175–186. https://doi.org/10.10007/s0046-005-0624-4

Bartek, N., Peck, J., Garzon, D., & Van Cleve, S. (2021). Addressing the clinical impact of COVID-19 on pediatric mental health. *Journal of Pediatric Health Care, 35*(4), 377–386. https://doi.org/10.1016/j.pedhc.2021.03.006

Bourke, L., Lingwood, J., Gallagher-Mitchell, T., & López-Pérez, B. (2023). The effect of face mask wearing on language processing and emotion recognition in young children. *Journal of Experimental Child Psychology, 226*, 105580. https://doi.org/10.1016/j.jecp.2022.105580

Boutzoukas, A. E., Zimmerman, K. O., Benjamin, D. K., Chick, K. J., Curtiss, J., & Høeg, T. B. (2022). Quarantine elimination for K-12 students with mask-on-mask exposure to SARS-CoV-2. Pediatrics (Evanston). *Pediatrics, 149*(12). https://doi.org/10.1542/peds.2021-054268L

Bowleg, L. (2020). We're not all in this together: on COVID-19, intersectionality, and structural inequality. *American Journal of Public Health (1971), 110*(7), 917. https://doi.org/10.2105/AJPH.2020.305766

Bryan, R. (2019). Getting to why: adverse childhood experiences impact on adult health. *The Journal for Nurse Practitioners, 15*(2), 153–158.

Bryant, D., Oo, M., & Damian, A. (2020). The risk of adverse childhood experiences during the COVID-19 pandemic. *Psychological Trauma, 12*(S1), S 193.

Bullinger, L. R., Raissian, K. M., Feely, M., & Schneider, W. J. (2021). The neglected ones: time at home during COVID-19 and child maltreatment. *Children and Youth Services Review, 131*, 106287. https://doi.org/10.1016/j.childyouth.2021.106287. Epub 2021 Nov 9.

Burke, N., Hellman, J., Scott, S., Weems, C., & Carrion, V. (2011). The impact of adverse childhood experiences on an urban pediatric population. *Child Abuse & Neglect, 35*(6), 408–413. https://doi.org/10.1016/j.chiabu.2011.02.006

Burt, S. A. (2009). Rethinking environmental contributions to child and adolescent psychopathology: a meta-analysis of shared environmental influences. *Psychological Bulletin, 135*, 608–637.

Calderon, V.J. (2020). *US parents say COVID-19 harming child's mental health.*

CDC. (2022). *Data and statistics on children's mental health.* Retrieved from https://www.cdc.gov/childrensmentalhealth/data.html

CDC. (2023). *CDC museum COVID-19 timeline.* Retrieved from https://www.cdc.gov/museum/timeline/covid19.html

CDC COVID-19 Response Team. (2020). Geographic Differences in COVID-19 Cases, Deaths, and Incidence - United States, February 12-April 7, 2020. *MMWR. Morbidity and Mortality Weekly Report, 69*(15), 465–471. https://doi.org/10.15585/mmwr.mm6915e4

Centers for Disease Control and Prevention. (2021). *Use masks to slow the spread of covid-19.* Centers for Disease Control and Prevention. https://www.cdc.gov/coronavirus/2019-ncov/prevent-getting-sick/masks.html.

Chiu, M., Goodman, L., Palacios, C. H., & Dingelein, M. (2022). Children in disasters. *Seminars in Pediatric Surgery, 31*(5), 151219. https://doi.org/10.1016/j.sempedsurg.2022.151219. Epub 2022 Oct 26.

Chronaki, G., Hadwin, J. A., Garner, M., Maurage, P., & Sonuga-Barke, E. (2015). The development of emotion recognition from facial expressions and non-linguistic vocalizations during childhood. *The British Journal of Developmental Psychology, 33*(2), 218–236. https://doi.org/10.1111/bjdp.12075

Committee on Integrating the Science of Early Childhood Development. (2000). *From neurons to neighborhoods: the science of early childhood development.* National Academies Press.

Curby, K. M., Johnson, K. J., & Tyson, A. (2012). Face to face with emotion: holistic face processing is modulated by emotional state. *Cognition & Emotion, 26*(1), 93–102.

Drimalla, H., Landwehr, N., Hess, U., & Dziobek, I. (2019). From face to face: the contribution of facial mimicry to cognitive and emotional empathy. *Cognition & Emotion, 33*, 1672.

Duby, J. (2018). Social and emotional development. In R. Voigt, M. Marcias, S. Myers, & C. Tapia (Eds.), *Developmental and behavioral pediatrics* (pp. 223–250). American Academy of Pediatrics.

EdWeek Research Center Survey. (2020 [updated Oct 27, 2020]). *Survey tracker: Monitoring how K-12 educators are responding to coronavirus.* Available from: https://www.edweek.org/teaching-learning/survey-tracker-monitoring-how-k-12-educators-are-responding-to-coronavirus/2020/04

Felitti, V., Anda, R. F., Nordenberg, D., Williamson, D. F., Spitz, A., Edwards, V., Koss, M., & Marks, J. (1998). Relationship of childhood abuse and household dysfunction to many of the leading causes of death in adults: the adverse childhood experiences (ACE) study. *American Journal of Preventive Medicine, 14*(4), 245–258.

Franco, F., Itakura, S., Pomorska, K., Abramowski, A., Nikaido, K., & Dimitriou, D. (2014). Can children with autism read emotions from the eyes? The eyes test revisited. *Research in Developmental Disabilities, 35*(5), 1015–1026.

Garcia, K. S. D., & Cowan, B. W. (Revised 2022, October). *The impact of U.S. school closures on labor market outcomes during the COVID-19 pandemic.* NBER; 2022, January. https://www.nber.org/papers/w29641

Genetic Alliance; District of Columbia Department of Health. (2010, Feb 17). *Understanding genetics: A District of Columbia guide for patients and health professionals.* Washington, DC: Genetic Alliance. Appendix D, Teratogens/Prenatal Substance Abuse. Available from: https://www.ncbi.nlm.nih.gov/books/NBK132140/

Gilchrist, N., & Simpson, J. N. (2019). Pediatric disaster preparedness: identifying challenges and opportunities for emergency department planning. *Current Opinion in Pediatrics, 31*(3), 306–311. https://doi.org/10.1097/MOP.0000000000000750

Gilmore, J. H., et al. (2018). Imaging structural and functional brain development in early childhood. *Nature Reviews. Neuroscience, 19*(3), 123–137. https://doi.org/10.1038/nrn.2018.1

Goddard, A. (2020). Adverse childhood experiences and trauma-informed care. *Journal of Pediatric Health Care, 35*, 145–155. https://doi.org/10.1016/j.pedhc.2020.09.001

Goddard, A., Jones, R., & Etcher, L. (2022). Trauma informed care in nursing: a concept analysis. *Nursing Outlook, 00*(00), 1–11. https://doi.org/10.1016/j.outlook.2021.12.010

Goldin, D., & Salani, D. (2020). Parental alienation syndrome: what health care providers need to know. *The Journal for Nurse Practitioners, 16*(5), 344–348. https://doi.org/10.1016/j.nurpra.2020.02.006

Harris, N. (2018). *The deepest well: health the long-term effects of childhood adversity.* Houghton Mifflin Harcourt.

Herstein, J. J., Schwedhelm, M. M., Vasa, A., Biddinger, P. D., & Hewlett, A. L. (2021). Emergency preparedness: what is the future? *Antimicrobial Stewardship & Healthcare Epidemiology, 1*(1), e29. Published 2021 Oct 13. https://doi.org/10.1017/ash.2021.190

High, P., Kelly, C., Robles, A., Thompson, B., & Dreyer, B. (2018). Environmental influences on child development and behavior. In R. Voigt, M. Macias, S. Myers, & C. Tapia (Eds.), *AAP developmental and behavioral pediatrics* (pp. 21–42). American Academy of Pediatrics.

Hittle-Gigli, K., Sonney, J., Lee, A. M., McNamara, M., Hunter, J., & Peck, J. L. (2022). NAPNAP position statement on resilience and the postpandemic pediatric nurse practitioner workforce. *Journal of Pediatric Health Care*, (36), 205–209. https://doi.org/10.1016/j.pedhc.2021.11.002

Hong, Y. R., & Park, J. S. (2012). Impact of attachment, temperament and parenting on human development. *Korean Journal of Pediatrics, 55*(12), 449–454. https://doi.org/10.3345/kjp.2012.55.12.449

Houtrow, A., Harris, D., Molinero, A., Levin-Decanini, T., & Robichaud, C. (2020). Children with disabilities in the United States and the COVID-19 pandemic. *Journal of Pediatric Rehabilitation Medicine, 13*(3), 415–424. https://doi.org/10.3233/PRM-200769

https://www.cdc.gov/mmwr/volumes/70/wr/mm7036a2.htm. Accessed 13 Aug 2023.

https://training.fema.gov/emiweb/downloads/is111_unit%204.pdf.   FEMA,   Emergency
  Management in the United States. Accessed 21 July 2023.
Jaan, A., & Rajnik, M. (2023). TORCH complex. [Updated 2023 Jul 17]. In *StatPearls [Internet]*.
  StatPearls Publishing. Available from: https://www.ncbi.nlm.nih.gov/books/NBK560528/
Koizumi, R., Kiyokawa, Y., Mikami, K., Ishii, A., Tanaka, K. D., Tanikawa, T., & Takeuchi,
  Y. (2018). Structural differences in the brain between wild and laboratory rats (Rattus nor-
  vegicus): potential contribution to wariness. *The Journal of Veterinary Medical Science, 80*(7),
  1054–1060. https://doi.org/10.1292/jvms.18-0052
Lee, J. (2020). Mental health effects of school closures during COVID-19. *The Lancet Child &
  Adolescent Health, 4*, 421.
Li, B., Blijd-Hoogewys, E., Stockmann, L., & Rieffe, C. (2023). The early development of emo-
  tion recognition in autistic children: decoding basic emotions from facial expressions and
  from emotion-provoking situations. *Development and Psychopathology, 36*, 1–12. https://doi.
  org/10.1017/S0954579423000913
Macias, M. M., & Lipkin, P. H. (2018). Developmental and Behavioral surveillance and screening
  within the medical home. In *Developmental and behavioral pediatrics* (pp. 135–163). essay,
  American Academy of Pediatrics.
Mann D. Social media is a public health crisis - U.S. news & world report. Study: Child Abuse
  Rose During COVID Pandemic; 2021, October 8. https://www.usnews.com/news/health-news/
  articles/2021-07-20/social-media-is-a-public-health-crisis.
Marlow, J. L. (1999). Keith L. Moore T.V.N. Persaud the developing human: clinically ori-
  ented embryology 6th Edition 1998 W.B. Saunders Philadelphia. *Journal of the American
  Association of Gynecologic Laparoscopists, 6*(1), 125–125. https://doi.org/10.1016/
  S1074-3804(99)80054-1
National Bureau of Economic Research. (2022). The impact of stay-at-home orders on working
  hours and pay during the COVID-19 pandemic. Retrieved from https://www.nber.org
Nemeroff, C. B. (2016). Paradise lost: the neurobiological and clinical consequences of child
  abuse and neglect. *Neuron, 89*(5), 892–909. https://doi.org/10.1016/j.neuron.2016.01.019t
Patel, J. A., Nielsen, F. B. H., Badiani, A. A., Assi, S., Unadkat, V. A., Patel, B., & Wardle, H. (2020).
  Poverty, inequality and COVID-19: the forgotten vulnerable. Public health (London). *Public
  Health, 183*, 110–111. https://doi.org/10.1016/j.puhe.2020.05.006
Peck, J., & Sonney, J. (2021). Exhausted and burned out: COVID19 emerging impacts threaten the
  health of the pediatric advanced practice nursing workforce. *Journal of Pediatric Health Care,
  35*(4), 414–424. https://doi.org/10.1016/j.pedhc.2021.04.012
Perry, B. (2002). Childhood experiences and the expression of genetic potential: what childhood
  neglect tells us about nature and nurture. *Brain and Mind, 3*, 79–100.
Perry, B. (2009). Examining child maltreatment through a neurodevelopmental lens: clinical application of the neurosequential model of therapeutics. *Journal of Loss and Trauma, 14*, 240–255.
  https://doi.org/10.1080/153250209030043350
Plomin, R., Owen, M. J., & McGuffin, P. (1994). The genetic basis of complex human behaviors.
  Science, 264(5166), 1733–1739.
Richmond, J. B. (1967). Child development: a basic science for pediatrics. *Pediatrics, 39*(5),
  649–658.
Ryan, C. (2018). *Computer and internet use in the United States: 2016*. Census.gov. https://www.
  census.gov/content/dam/Census/library/publications/2018/acs/ACS-39.pdf
Sahu, M., & Prasuna, J. G. (2016). Twin studies: a unique epidemiological tool. *Indian Journal of
  Community Medicine, 41*(3), 177–182. https://doi.org/10.4103/0970-0218.183593
Schering, S, Writer, S. (2022). *CDC, AAP update developmental milestones for surveillance
  program*. Retrieved from https://publications.aap.org/aapnews/news/19554/CDC-AAP-
  update-developmental-milestones-for
Sege, R., & Stephens, A. (2022). Child physical abuse did not increase during the pandemic. *JAMA
  Pediatrics, 176*(4), 338–340. https://doi.org/10.1001/jamapediatrics.2021.5476

Shonkoff, J., & Garner, A. (2012). The lifelong effects of early childhood adversity and toxic stress. *Pediatrics, 129*(1), e232–e246. https://doi.org/10.1542/peds.2011-2663

Soto-Icaza, P., et al. (2015). Development of social skills in children: neural and Behavioral evidence for the elaboration of cognitive models. *Frontiers in Neuroscience, 9*, 333–333. https://doi.org/10.3389/fnins.2015.0033

Stoekle, H., & Herve, C. (2020). COVID-19: act first, think later. *The American Journal of Bioethics, 20*(7), W1. https://doi.org/10.1080/15265161.2020.1761199

Substance Abuse and Mental Health Services Administration. (2014). *SAMHSA's concept of trauma and guidance for trauma-informed approach*. SAMHSA's Trauma and Justice Strategic Initiative. HHS publication no. (SMA), pp. 14–4884. https://store.samhsa.gov/sites/deafutl/files/d7/priv/sma14-4884.pdf

Substance Abuse and Mental Health Services Administration. (2018). *Trauma informed approach and trauma specific interventions*. Accessed from https://www.samhsa.gov/nctic/trauma-interventions

The Nation's Report Card. (n.d.). *The nation's report card*. https://www.nationsreportcard.gov/.

Thomas, A., & Chess, S. (1977). *Temperament and development* (pp. 1–270). Brunner/Mazel.

Turkeimer, E., Haley, A., Waldron, M., D'Onofrio, B., & Gottesman, I. I. (2003). Socioeconomic status modifies the heritability of IQ in young children. *Psychological Science, 14*(6), 623–628.

U.S. Department of Health & Human Services, Administration for Children and Families, Administration on Children, Youth and Families, Children's Bureau. (2020). *Child maltreatment 2018*. https://www.acf.hhs.gov/cb/resource/child-maltreatment-2018

Van den Berg, P., Schechter-Perkins, E., Jack, R. S., Epshtein, I., Nelson, R., Oster, E., & Branch-Elliman, W. (2021). Effectiveness of 3 versus 6 ft of physical distancing for controlling spread of coronavirus disease 2019 among primary and secondary students and staff: a retrospective, statewide cohort study. Clinical infectious diseases. *Clinical Infectious Diseases, 73*(10), 1871–1878. https://doi.org/10.1093/cid/ciab230

Volkmar, F. R., & Greenough, W. T. (1972). Rearing complexity affects branching of dendrites in the visual cortex of the rat. *Science (American Association for the Advancement of Science), 176*(4042), 1445–1447. https://doi.org/10.1126/science.176.4042.1445

www.cdc.gov/quarantine/index.html. Accessed 05 Aug 2023.

Xian, Z., Saxena, A., Javen, Z., et al. (2021). COVID-19 related state wide racial and ethnic disparities across the USA: an observational study based on publicly available date from the COVID tracking project. *BMJ Open, 11*(6), e048006.

Zarse, E., Negg, M., Yoder, R., Chambers, J., Chambers, R., & Schumacher, U. (2019). The adverse childhood experiences questionnaire: two decades of research on childhood trauma as a primary cause of adult mental illness, addiction, and medical disease. *Cogent Medicine, 6*(1), 1–9. https://doi.org/10.1080/2331205X.2019.1581447

Zviedrite, N., Hodis, J. D., Jahan, F., Gao, H., & Uzicanin, A. (2021). COVID-19-associated school closures and related efforts to sustain education and subsidized meal programs, United States, February 18-June 30, 2020. *PLoS One, 16*(9), e0248925. https://doi.org/10.1371/journal.pone.0248925

Nutrition, Exercise, and Sleep: Impacts on Health Promotion and Illness Prevention

Alison Bray, Amee Moreno, Donna Schultz, and Jessica L. Peck

In any moment of decision, the best thing you can do is the right thing.
The worst thing you can do is nothing.

—Theodore Roosevelt

Introduction and Background

While the national dialogue on COVID-19 is primarily preoccupied with vaccines, availability of prescriptive therapies, and the politics of restrictive measures, dialogue concerning a critical element of health promotion is being severely neglected. Fundamental health promotion behaviors encompassing sleep, nutrition, and exercise have well-established evidence as predictors of general measures of overall mental and physical health (Wickham et al., 2020). The better the general health of children, the less likely they are to have comorbidities or risk factors that contribute to susceptibility to viral transmission and complications ensuing from resultant infections. The COVID-19 pandemic has likely altered self-management behaviors such as sleep, nutrition, and exercise that promote health outcomes (Plevinsky et al., 2020). Overarching policies and recommendations concerning transmission mitigation efforts focused on elements of vaccine administration, mandated social distancing, and school and recreational activity closures, and played a crucial role in return to normalcy, including school. Throughout this time, pediatric providers, caregivers, parents, and teachers worked tirelessly to adapt and promote children's health. However, dialogue on the importance of simple but time-tested measures of health promotion including effective sleep hygiene, well-balanced, nutritious diets, and healthy body movement and exercise were often overlooked. Without access to

A. Bray (✉) · A. Moreno · D. Schultz · J. L. Peck
Louise Herrington School of Nursing, Baylor University, Waco, TX, USA
e-mail: alison_bray@baylor.edu; amee_moreno@baylor.edu;
donna_schultz@baylor.edu; jessica_peck@baylor.edu

J. L. Peck (ed.), *COVID-19 Impacts on Child Health*,
https://doi.org/10.1007/978-3-031-80369-7_6

109

school playgrounds and with unlimited access to screen time, many children were more sedentary. Fear of viral transmission prevented families from going to the grocery store. Supply chain issues contributed to grocery shortages and soaring food prices. Anxiety, poor nutrition, excess screen time, and a myriad of other factors contributed to sleep disruption (Burkhart et al., 2021; Khalil & Elsayed, 2020; Martinez-de-Quel et al., 2021). The post-pandemic impact on nutrition, exercise, and sleep remains apparent and poses challenges to optimizing health outcomes.

Nutrition

Points of Care

At the writing of this chapter, 4 years into the COVID-19 global pandemic, clinical and epidemiological evidence suggests that children are less likely to suffer from severe COVID-19 infections and mortality but have experienced other significant health implications. There are critical points of care to consider for pediatric health-care providers (HCPs) in practice regarding global pandemics and their impact on children's nutrition. These points include addressing food insecurity, considering immediate mobilization of alternative food resources, promoting breastfeeding, addressing possible formula shortages, and continuous screening for malnutrition at every visit to ensure children receive adequate nutrient intake (Chaves et al., 2022).

Addressing Food Insecurity

Food insecurity can be defined as inadequate access to adequate food in terms of quality and quantity (Becker et al., 2017; Paslakis et al., 2021). The United States Department of Agriculture (USDA) estimated in 2015, before the COVID-19 global pandemic, approximately 15.8 million households were food insecure (Coleman-Jensen et al., 2022). The early stages of the pandemic led to a 20.4% spike in food insecurity in US households leveling off to 8.9% by March 2021 (Kim-Mozeleski et al., 2023). When the pandemic reached global proportions in early 2020, some 194 countries, including the United States, closed school doors to reduce the spread of COVID-19, leaving many children without access to affordable, nutritious meals (Hetrick et al., 2020). It is estimated that 35 million children in the United States, primarily low- to middle-income, rely on school meals and various nutritional programs to provide food and subsequent protection from food insecurity (Mayurasakorn et al., 2020; Tan, 2021). With school no longer offered in-person, children could not receive the bulk of their physical activity and social interaction with peers at school as in the past nor rely on the schools for nutritious meals (Wechsler et al., 2000) or structured exercise. While stay-at-home orders were also critical for reducing the spread of COVID-19, children's well-being and mental health have suffered detrimentally. Children could no longer play in the neighborhood parks with friends, leading to feelings of isolation and depression (Tan, 2021). During the pandemic, food insecurity among households with children under 18 years at least doubled, if not tripled, from pre-pandemic levels. Food insecurity levels are increased by 130% from 2018 to 2020, including one in five households with children (Bauer, 2020). Even short bouts of food insecurity can have lasting effects on children. Children who are food insecure in the summer months are more likely to lose reading skills, gain excessive weight, and suffer from behavioral problems (Karpman et al., 2023).

The American Academy of Pediatrics (AAP) urges all pediatric HCPs to screen children for food insecurity at every outpatient and emergency department visit and at least once during inpatient stays (Hetrick et al., 2020). Use of the simple two-question validated screening tool, Hunger Vital Sign, during healthcare visits will aid in the identification of children at risk for food insecurity using a sensitive approach (Gitterman et al., 2015). Studies have shown that during the COVID-19 pandemic, children, adolescents, and young adults gained excessive weight with respect to their estimated weight gain for age due to inadequate nutrition, stress, and lack of exercise (Hetrick et al., 2020; Thacker et al., 2022).

Breastfeeding Promotion and Formula Shortages

The AAP continues to recommend and support promotion of breastfeeding exclusively for the first 6 months of life and continued breastfeeding with addition of complementary foods until at least the age of 12 months. Breastfeeding may last longer than 2 years if desired by mother and child (Meek & Noble, 2022). Discussions of breastfeeding practices and formula shortage possibilities must be addressed in the hospital or birthing center before discharge. Pediatric HCPs should not wait for these discussions in the primary care setting. While breastfeeding and human milk are considered optimal for infant feeding decisions, not all parents want to breastfeed or are unable for various reasons. Human milk provides immune-boosting properties, hormones, antibodies, and growth factors that cannot be produced in commercially prepared formulas (Meek & Noble, 2022). Despite human milk being the optimal infant nutrition choice, breastfeeding is not the default choice in the United States (Bartle & Harvey, 2017). Breastfeeding success is primarily influenced by positive support at home and in the community. Women may feel pressure to choose formula feeding over breastfeeding due to inadequate support from HCPs, peers, employers, as well as lack of health policies (Bartle & Harvey, 2017). A study by Imboden et al. (2023), conducted during the COVID-19 pandemic, found breastfeeding rates increased by approximately 10% during the formula shortage in the study's sample of 600 newborn mothers. According to Imboden et al. (2023), ongoing research is needed to determine the lasting effects the pandemic has had on breastfeeding outcomes and feeding decisions among parents. Pediatric HCPs must be proactive in breastfeeding and infant feeding discussions.

While formulas offer a sustainable alternative to breastfeeding, it is not without its complications. Infant formula shortages and recalls are no new problem in the United States. At the onset of the pandemic, some hoarded infant formula, like many household staples, making formula scarce and in high demand (Asiodu,

2022). In addition to the already short formula supply from its increased demand, Abbott Nutrition instituted a voluntary recall and ceased production at a plant in Michigan because of a US Food and Drug Administration (FDA) investigation into a foodborne illness, thus negatively impacting the nation's formula supply (Abrams & Duggan, 2022; U. S. Food and Drug Administration, 2022). Out of desperation and from lack of commercial formulas, some families resorted to recipes for home-made formulas, purchased imported formulas, and introduced cow's milk earlier than AAP recommendations of introduction at 1 year of age (Abrams & Duggan, 2022; Imboden et al., 2023). Formula recalls and supply shortages may lead new and expecting parents to a lack of trust in the quality and sustainability of infant formulas, negatively affecting feeding choices. Healthcare providers should respect parents in making feeding choices while serving as a source of evidence-based information to help parents make informed feeding decisions.

Screening for Malnutrition

The pandemic caused an increased need for HCPs to screen for malnutrition and ensure children are receiving adequate nutrients. Malnutrition is defined by social, economic, and environmental factors (Thacker et al., 2022). One sustainable development goal (SDG) of the World Health Organization (WHO) is to decrease/eliminate child malnutrition and mortality by 2030 (World Health Organization [WHO], 2023). The COVID-19 pandemic makes meeting this target even more challenging than before. The pandemic contributed to an increase in child malnutrition resulting from decreased access to routine health services and cuts to parental wages (Thacker et al., 2022). Low-income families spend about 70% of their wages on food and have limited access to financial resources (Kakaei et al., 2022). A recent study showed mothers of newborns restricted their own eating habits related to loss of wages and interruptions in the farm-to-fork food supply chain, which negatively impacts their children's nutritional status (Paslakis et al., 2021). Restrictive child-feeding patterns are linked to pediatric obesity risk, which is further complicated by stresses of the pandemic (Armstrong et al., 2020). Healthcare providers, families, and the community must address food security and healthy eating patterns and behaviors to ensure positive well-being of children and adolescents.

Exercise

Points of Care

The American Academy of Pediatrics recommends at least 60 min of moderate to vigorous (MTV) daily physical activity for children at least 5 years of age and adolescents (National Center for Education in Maternal and Child Health (U.S.), & Story, M, 2002). Before the COVID-19 pandemic, insufficient physical activity in youth was a recognized concern, with only 24% of children and adolescents participating in 60 min of daily physical activity (Centers for Disease Control and Prevention, 2022). Decreased levels of physical activity are associated with negative impacts on overall health systems and individual quality of life (World Health Organization [WHO], 2022). Childhood physical activity is associated with improved academic performance and mental health, bone health, and reduced adiposity (World Health Organization [WHO], 2022).

The COVID-19 pandemic profoundly impacted physical activity in the pediatric population, compounding the established problem and resulting in residual effects that continue to impact children's health. Both children who contracted COVID-19 and those who did not contract the virus experienced negative effects of the pandemic related to transmission mitigation strategies (Dayton et al., 2021). At the writing of this chapter, physical activity in children has not returned to pre-pandemic levels. Pediatric HCPs should be aware of implications of reduced physical activity from the COVID-19 pandemic and examine opportunities to improve pediatric health.

Pandemic Impact on Exercise

Youth physical activity levels were insufficient to meet recommended levels before the arrival of the COVID-19 pandemic in 2019 (Do et al., 2022). As restrictions and lockdowns were implemented, children were mandated to stay home to mitigate risk of virus transmission, further reducing physical activity. It is estimated that school closures impacted approximately 1.5 billion children worldwide (Neville et al., 2022). A systematic review and meta-analysis found that children experienced a 17-min daily decrease in MTV activity from baseline before the COVID-19 pandemic compared to during the pandemic (Neville et al., 2022). Activities such as school attendance, recreational sports and clubs, and summer camps were restricted throughout the pandemic, decreasing sun exposure associated with increased vitamin D and serotonin levels (Dayton et al., 2021; Wang et al., 2023).

The COVID-19 pandemic highlighted existing social disparities. Beckelman et al. found that among their diverse study sample of children, financial concerns and food insecurity were associated with decreased physical activity and shorter sleep duration (Bekelman et al., 2023). Their study revealed that non-Hispanic Black children were 61% less likely to engage in high levels of physical activity compared to children who were non-Hispanic white, exacerbating health disparities (Bekelman et al., 2023).

As the COVID-19 pandemic swept the globe, businesses and schools rapidly transitioned to an online format. Many children began online schooling, contributing to an increase in leisure screen time and social media usage, with a corresponding increase in sedentary behaviors (Sheldrick et al., 2023). The home environment accommodated electronic means of work, school, and entertainment. Media equipment in the home increased by 10% and by 29% in children's bedrooms, likely contributing to increased alone time and decreased physical activity (Sheldrick et al., 2023). Home activity equipment such as table tennis and trampolines created opportunities to decrease sedentary behavior, in addition to popularization of active video games (Sheldrick et al., 2023). Previous research has documented negative effects of sedentary behaviors on children's physical and mental health (Viner et al., 2020). COVID-19 and its resulting confinement negatively impact insulin resistance levels and increase total and abdominal fat in sedentary children, leading to excess weight gain and an increase in morbidity and mortality (Medrano et al., 2021).

One factor that impacted youth exercise levels was decreased availability of recreational centers. While the virus continued to spread, schools, recreational centers, and extra-curricular facilities closed to slow the spread of the virus, closure of playgrounds and other outdoor recreational spaces that promote physical activity and socializing in children minimized opportunities for exercise (Neville et al., 2022). The extent to which families relied on these activities for physical activity became apparent as children lost access to these activities. The reliance on school for physical activity in children was magnified with school closures, further amplifying the existing exercise deficit (Do et al., 2022).

Many caregivers and parents transitioned to remote work due to social distancing precautions. Although they were physically present in the home, the burden of ensuring their child's education and maintaining employment created a significant barrier to physical activity promotion (Riazi et al., 2021; Arbour-Nicitopoulos et al., 2022). However, one study revealed that children from families with at least one parent who changed their work schedule to care for children at home had 82 fewer minutes per day of screen time and engaged in more family activities (Bekelman et al., 2023). Adherence to social distancing measures and parental fear of viral transmission to their children contributed to declining youth activity levels during the pandemic (Riazi et al., 2021). Parents were challenged to create opportunities for physical activity for their children. One effective strategy for increasing exercise levels in youth is parental engagement in physical activities with their children (Xiang et al., 2022).

Long-Term Impact on Exercise

The effects of the pandemic-related pediatric exercise decline in youth can be found throughout childhood health. Dayton et al. reported that a decrease in the exercise capacity of their sample of healthy children is measured by a decrease in the maximum amount of oxygen that a person can utilize during intense physical activity in healthy children before and after the COVID-19 pandemic (Dayton et al., 2021). Access to services needed to promote physical activity in children and youth with disabilities, such as physical and occupational therapy, was limited throughout the pandemic, impacting their physical ability (Arbour-Nicitopoulos et al., 2022).

Regular physical activity contributes to healthy sleep cycles in children. Pandemic lifestyle changes altered daily routines and regular physical activity and exercise. Children's sleep patterns were negatively impacted, compounding the impact on physical and mental health. Burkart et al. found an almost 2-h shift in sleep timing during the COVID-19 pandemic attributed to lessened daily structure (Burkhart et al., 2021). Sleep timing, including sleep onset, is associated with obesity (Burkhart et al., 2021).

The negative impact on physical wellness, compounded by increased screen time, directly impacted mental health of children and adolescents (Xiang et al., 2022). Children's mental health was negatively impacted, including increased suicide among youth (Schnitzer et al., 2023). The mental health of children and adolescents was a significant area of concern pre-pandemic; however, the pandemic exacerbated the persistent feelings of hopelessness in youth, spotlighting the pre-existing inadequate access to mental health care (Centers for Disease Control and Prevention, 2022).

Adaptation to the Impact on Exercise

Caregivers, parents, teachers, and pediatric HCPs adapted to new ways of everyday life mandated by the COVID-19 pandemic and utilized opportunities to promote physical wellness in children and adolescents. Teachers transformed traditional in-person physical education activities into online classes, promoting exercise and socialization among classmates. Despite these innovative approaches to physical education, youth spent less time in physical education classes, contributing to overall decline in pediatric exercise during the pandemic (Pavlovic et al., 2021). Recreational activities created an online platform for youth to create communities with others who share their interests and engage in physical activity (Calcaterra et al., 2021).

As COVID-19 vaccination levels increased, infection levels decreased, resulting in relaxation of mandated restrictions. The world transitioned toward a post-pandemic era, and various strategies were implemented to improve physical activity levels of children and adolescents, including online practices such as exercise communities and telemedicine. Tele-exercise emerged as a popular platform to promote physical activity and mitigate the risk of viral transmission. Tele-exercise remains an innovative approach to combatting barriers to physical exercise and improving childhood obesity (Calcaterra et al., 2021).

Sleep

COVID-19 affected every continent on the globe (Zahid & Perna, 2021). While necessary, strategies to mitigate the spread of the virus had profound effects on the pediatric population worldwide. Many terms were used to describe the strategy to mitigate the spread, including "shelter-in-place," "stay-at-home," and "lockdown," depending on the area of the world. Some countries were stricter with mandates than others, but globally, the health of children is significantly impacted by this biological pandemic.

The literature is rich with evidence that correlates good sleep hygiene with overall physiologic health. Quality sleep is associated with improved immunity, healthier body mass index (BMI), lower incidence of chronic illness, and decreased anxiety (Besedovsky et al., 2019; Stone et al., 2021). Quality sleep also directly influences emotional regulation and functioning (Altena et al., 2020). Chronic sleep disruptions and disturbances can influence a persistent, low-grade inflammatory response in the body, decreasing overall immunity and facilitating inflammatory disease processes such as increased blood pressure and insulin resistance (Besedovsky et al., 2019). Sleep timing is also linked to adverse health outcomes such as obesity, lower aerobic fitness, and increased triglyceride levels (Burkhart et al., 2021). Decreased sleep quality, especially in infants and toddlers, can also increase the risk of mental health issues and maladaptive behaviors (Markovic et al., 2021). An overall decrease in sleep hygiene also places children at increased risk for severe COVID-19 infection (Zhang et al., 2020).

Daily Schedules

Quality sleep is directly affected by circadian rhythm, which is affected by daylight, mealtimes, and physical exercise. High-quality light exposure causes increased melatonin release at night, which has a positive effect on quality sleep. Decreased physical activity (such as what people experienced when confined to their homes in March, April, and May of 2020) negatively affects sleep quality, and prolonged poor sleep quality correlates with increased incidence of post-traumatic stress disorder (PTSD) (Altena et al., 2020).

During the initial months of confinement, routines were changed, physical activity and social interaction were restricted, and diets and meal timing changed. Strict sheltering in place for both children and adults radically altered daily schedules. Parents who previously worked out of the home found themselves working from home, many times with longer hours and in more stressful conditions (Altena et al., 2020). They needed to adjust to their new work schedules to accommodate a new homeschooling schedule for their children, often moving into the primary educator role. All these changes to regular routines profoundly impacted overall family function and increased overall anxiety, all of which impacted overall quality of sleep (Stone et al., 2021; Wearick-Silva et al., 2022).

Pediatric Sleep

Wearick-Silva et al. (2022) used validated tools to assess children's sleep in three age categories. Children aged 0–3 years had increased nighttime awakenings (an average of three or more), increased nighttime wakefulness, and received less than the recommended overall sleep duration based on the Brief Infant Sleep Questionnaire (BISQ). Children in the 4- to 12-year-old age-group had issues with sleep initiation, sleep-wake transition, and problems with overall sleep maintenance. Adolescents aged 13-to-17 years had an overall decrease in sleep quality (measured by the Pittsburgh Sleep Quality Index [PSQI]).

Infant and Toddler Sleep Patterns

The American Academy of Sleep Medicine (AASM) and the WHO recommend that infants have 12–16 h of sleep and toddlers have 11–14 h of sleep (including naps) daily (American Academy of Sleep Medicine, 2016; World Health Organization [WHO], 2019). Parental anxiety during the initial lockdown phase directly impacted the sleep quality of infants and toddlers; the more anxiety parents had, the decrease in overall sleep quality of the child (Markovic et al., 2021). Cassanello et al. (2022) found that bedtimes during the lockdown phase of the pandemic for the infant and toddler age-groups were significantly later ($P < 0.001$), and that total sleep time was less (but not statistically significant; $P = 0.078$). Shorter sleep duration and poor sleep quality are associated with decreased emotional regulation and cognitive development (World Health Organization [WHO], 2019).

There were some protective factors found to facilitate sleep quality. If there was more than one child in the household (especially if the other children were in child-care), these infants had better overall sleep quality (Markovic et al., 2021). Sleep quality in infants and toddlers was also improved with a pet in the household. Lastly, households, where parents practiced mindfulness techniques and had a schedule to facilitate good sleep hygiene showed improved overall sleep quality in infants and toddlers (Markovic et al., 2021).

Learning Environments

There were differences in sleep quality between children who returned to the classroom to learn versus those who learned remotely. Remote learners were also sub-categorized into synchronous and asynchronous learners. Children who stayed in a remote, synchronous learning environment had an overall increase in sleep quality and time compared to children who returned to school. They woke in a later circadian phase and reported a lower level of sleepiness, likely related to eliminating commute time to school (Stone et al., 2021). However, the later bedtime shift experienced during the COVID-19 pandemic increased morbidities (Burkhart et al., 2021). Medrano et al. (2021) also reported an increase in sleep time during the confinement period in Spain, with an overall decrease in physical activity and increase in total screen time for adolescents.

Children with synchronous learning environments were more likely to have physical education than children in asynchronous learning environments, and overall, there was less freedom to move around physically (no physical education classes, no walking to and from school or to and from classes, no sports practices or games, and no afterschool activities that had physical movement incorporated into the programming) (Stone et al., 2021).

Screen Time and Impact on Sleep Patterns

Children had an overall increased screen time use at the onset of the pandemic. Screen time is generally defined as the use of television, systems connected to television (such as gaming devices), smartphones, laptops, and tablets (Bani-Issa et al., 2023). Various research studies report increased use as high as 6.6–7.7 h/day outside of instructional time (Campbell et al., 2021; Nagata et al., 2022). Transition to remote learning, lockdown, decreased physical activity, increased stress, and overall loneliness were primary causes for increased screen time. Adolescents reported increased late-night screen time use, primarily on their smartphones to interact with peers, and this showed an increased association with sleep latency, sleep disturbance, and overall agitation based on PSQI scores (Bani-Issa et al., 2023). As the light wavelength for screen illumination is associated with suppressed melatonin release, these results are not surprising, and Bani-Issa et al. (2023) reported that almost half of the adolescents in their study did not achieve the recommended 8–10 h of sleep and the more screen time the adolescent used, the poorer the quality of sleep the adolescent received ($P < 0.001$). Quality sleep and overall sleep time are essential in brain maturation as adolescents make the transition from a more self-centered and "immediate gratification" thought process to the thought process of the young adult.

Barriers and Breakthroughs

Society has learned how to quickly pivot from an in-person school environment to a remote environment, and technology has allowed children to continue social interaction virtually, hoping that loneliness and anxiety can be decreased. However, many more barriers than breakthroughs remain.

Nutrition

Due to disruptions in supply chains, research and innovation led to breakthroughs in pandemic-related nutrition challenges. The pandemic increased demand for food assistance programs as well as the need for school meal delivery programs. Some innovative ways food pantries and school districts have distributed food to families in need include drive-through distribution, home deliveries, and mobile food pantries. Breastfeeding barriers during the pandemic included limited access to lactation education and skilled lactation support providers, poor access to human donor milk, inadequate paid family leave, and lack of lactation accommodations when returning to work (Asiodu, 2022).

Exercise

Mandated COVID-19 restrictions, school closures, and parental fear created barriers for youth to obtain the recommended amount of MTV exercise. The impact of decreased physical activity levels contributed to a decline in physical and mental health in children and adolescents.

Sleep

Radical schedule changes related to lockdown affected sleep quality from a day-to-day scheduling aspect, a mealtime schedule and quality of food ingested, a decrease in physical activity, and an increase in overall screen time use in all child age-groups.

Lessons Learned

We learned that the pandemic-related lockdown restrictions promoted significant weight gain. More significantly, we learned that obesity resulted in a higher risk of severe infection and increased risk of hospitalization. Weight gain was largely related to increased intake of hypercaloric and/or hyperglycemic foods along with reduced physical activity and altered sleep cycles. Urgent programmatic supports, policies, and direct patient education are needed to promote awareness of the impact of healthy lifestyle choices including nutrition, exercise, and sleep (LaFauci et al., 2022).

Nutrition

Lessons learned about childhood nutrition and the impact of the pandemic include the need for coordinated preparedness from all levels, local to global. Countries should prepare for global pandemics in advance. Ensure adequate food stocks and mechanisms are in place for immediate mobilization of food resources in their areas. Educate the public on the importance of nutrition-related personal health measures. The pandemic's stress led to children's and youth's detrimental and emotional eating habits at home. Current research has shown increased pandemic-related stress led to increased binge eating behaviors in adolescents and young adults, which causes a decrease in mental health well-being (Freizinger et al., 2022). Healthcare providers must remain cognizant of psychological distress, and the impact pandemic-related stress has on their pediatric patients.

Exercise

The COVID-19 pandemic highlighted the pre-existing exercise deficit in children and the impact of exercise on physical and mental health. The pediatric HCP's role in physical activity screening and exercise education is now more apparent as it is crucial in the journey to healthy physical activity levels in children and adolescents. Pediatric HCPs should regularly educate caregivers and parents about the importance of healthy physical activity levels and provide resources for physical activities and exercise programs outside of school-based physical education curricula. Caregiver and parent physical activity levels largely impact the importance placed on promoting exercise within the home setting for youth. Therefore, educating caregivers and parents about the impact exercise has on the physical and mental health of children and adolescents is a critical role for the pediatric HCP.

Sleep

For infants and toddlers, HCPs must be able to reach families and coach them on establishing routines in the home that facilitate sleep quantity and quality, such as promotion of regularly scheduled mealtimes, play times, and sleep times and decreased (or eliminated) use of screens with infants and toddlers. Increased exposure to screens suppresses melatonin release, and evening screen time use increases sleep latency, sleep disturbance, and agitation (Bani-Issa et al., 2023). Moving forward, as HCPs it will be essential to be able to coach families into consistent routines with an emphasis on mindfulness activities in the evenings to facilitate good sleep hygiene.

Calls to Action
- Coordinate preparedness from local, community, governmental, and global levels. There is a need for mechanisms for the immediate mobilization of food resources in times of crisis.
- Encourage and support breastfeeding (per AAP recommendations). Advocate for policies that address food insecurity, poverty, and increase funding for federal food assistance programs for children.
- Advocate at the national, state, and local levels for policies that ensure pediatric HCPs have immediate access to their patients through an online platform to provide quality well and acute care.
- Calls for HCPs to be reimbursed appropriately for telemedicine during a pandemic.

References

Abrams, S. A., & Duggan, C. P. (2022). Infant and child formula shortages: Now is the time to prevent recurrences. *The American Journal of Clinical Nutrition, 116*(2), 289–292. https://doi.org/10.1093/ajcn/nqac149

Altena, E., Baglioni, C., Espie, C. A., Ellis, J., Gavriloff, D., Holzinger, B., Schlarb, A., Frase, L., Jernelov, S., & Riemann, D. (2020). Dealing with sleep problems during home confinement due to the COVID-19 outbreak: Practical recommendations from a task force of the European CBT-I academy. *Journal of Sleep Research, 29*, e13052. https://doi.org/10.1111/jsr.13052

American Academy of Sleep Medicine. (2016). *Heath advisory: Child sleep duration.* https://aasm.org/wp-content/uploads/2017/10/child-sleep-duration-health-advisory.pdf

Arbour-Nicitopoulos, K., James, M. E., Moore, S. A., Sharma, R., & Martin Ginis, K. A. (2022). Movement behaviours and health of children and youth with disabilities: Impact of the 2020 COVID-19 pandemic. *Paediatrics & Child Health, 27*(Supplement_1), S66–S71. https://doi.org/10.1093/pch/pxac007

Armstrong, B., Hepworth, A. D., & Black, M. M. (2020). Hunger in the household: Food insecurity and associations with maternal eating and toddler feeding. *Pediatric Obesity, 15*(10), e12637. https://doi.org/10.1111/ijpo.12637

Asiodu, I. V. (2022). Infant formula shortage: This should not be our reality. *The Journal of Perinatal & Neonatal Nursing, 36*(4), 340–343. https://doi.org/10.1097/JPN.0000000000000690

Bani-Issa, W., Radwan, H., Saqan, R., Hijazi, H., Fakhry, R., Alameddine, M., Naja, F., Ibrahim, A., Lin, N., Naing, Y. T., & Awad, M. (2023). Association between quality of sleep and screen time during the COVID-19 outbreak among adolescents in the United Arab Emirates. *Journal of Sleep Research, 32*, e13666. https://doi.org/10.1111/jsr.13666

Bartle, N., & Harvey, K. (2017). Explaining infant feeding: The role of previous personal and vicarious experience on attitudes, subjective norms, self-efficacy, and breastfeeding outcomes. *British Journal of Health Psychology, 22*(4), 763–785. https://doi.org/10.1111/bjhp.12254

Bauer, L. (2020, May 6). The Covid-19 crisis has already left too many children hungry in America. *The Hamilton Project.* https://www.hamiltonproject.org/blog/the_covid_19_crisis_has_already_left_too_many_children_hungry_in_america

Becker, C., Middlemass, K., Taylor, B., Johnson, C., & Gomez, F. (2017). Food insecurity and eating disorder pathology. *The International Journal of Eating Disorders, 50*(9), 1031–1040. https://doi.org/10.1002/eat.22735

Bekelman, T., Knapp, E. A., Dong, Y., Dabelea, D., Bastain, T. M., Breton, C. V., Carroll, K. N., Camargo, C. A., Davis, A. M., Dunlop, A. L., Elliott, A. J., Ferrara, A., Fry, R. C., Ganiban, J. M., Gilbert-Diamond, D., Gilliland, F. D., Hedderson, M. M., Hipwell, A. E., Hockett, C. W., Huddleston, K. C., Karagas, M. R., Kelly, N., Lai, J. S., Lester, B. M., Lucchini, M., Melough, M. M., Mihalopoulos, N. L., O'Shea, T. M., Rundle, A. G., Stanford, J. B., Van Bronkhorst, S., Wright, R. J., Zhao, Q., & Sauder, K. A. (2023). Sociodemographic variation in Children's Health behaviors during the COVID-19 pandemic. *Childhood Obesity, 19*(4), 226–238. https://doi.org/10.1089/chi.2022.0085

Besedovsky, L., Lange, T., & Haack, M. (2019). The sleep-immune crosstalk in health and disease. *Physiological Reviews, 99*, 1325–1380.

Burkhart, S., Parker, H., Weaver, R. G., Beets, M. W., Jones, A., Adams, E. L., Chaput, J., & Armstrong, B. (2021). Impact of the covid pandemic on elementary schoolers' physical activity, sleep, screen time, and diet: A qualitative experimental interrupted time series study. *Pediatric Obesity, 17*(1), e12846. https://doi.org/10.1111/ijpo.12846

Calcaterra, V., Verduci, E., Vandoni, M., Rossi, V., Di Profio, E., Carnevale Pellino, V., Tranfaglia, V., Pascuzzi, M. C., Borsani, B., Bosetti, A., & Zuccotti, G. (2021). Telehealth: A useful tool for the management of nutrition and exercise programs in pediatric obesity in the COVID-19 era. Nutrients, 13(11), 3689-. https://doi.org/10.3390/nu13113689

Campbell, K., Weingart, R., Ashta, J., Cronin, T., & Gazmararian, J. (2021). COVID-19 knowl-
edge and behavior change among high school students in semi-rural Georgia. *The Journal of
School Health, 91*(7), 526–534.
Cassanello, P., Ruiz-Botia, I., Sala-Castellvi, P., Martin, J.C., Martinez-Sanchez, J.M., & Balaguer,
A. (2022). Comparing infant and toddler sleep patterns prior to and during the first wave of
home confinement due to COVID-19 in Spain. European Journal of Pediatrics, 181, 1719–1725.
Centers for Disease Control and Prevention. (2022, July 26). *Physical activity facts.* https://www.
cdc.gov/healthyschools/physicalactivity/facts.htm
Chaves, E., Reddy, S. D., Cadieux, A., Tomasula, J., & Reynolds, K. (2022). The continued impact
of the COVID-19 pandemic on pediatric obesity: A commentary on the return to a healthy new
"normal". *International Journal of Environmental Research and Public Health, 19*(9), 5597.
https://doi.org/10.3390/ijerph19095597
Coleman-Jensen, A., Rabbitt, M., Gregory, C., & Singh, A. (2022). Household food security in the
United States in 2021. *Amber Waves.*
Dayton, J., Ford, K., Carroll, S. J., Flynn, P. A., Kourtidou, S., & Holzer, R. J. (2021). The
deconditioning effect of the COVID-19 pandemic on unaffected healthy children. *Pediatric
Cardiology, 42*(3), 554–559. https://doi.org/10.1007/s00246-020-02513-w
Do, B., Kirkland, C., Besenyi, G. M., Smock, C., & Lanza, K. (2022). Youth physical activ-
ity and the COVID-19 pandemic: A systematic review. *Preventive Medical Reports, 29,*
101959–101959. https://doi.org/10.1016/j.pmedr.2022.101959
Freizinger, M., Jhe, G. B., Dahlberg, S. E., Pluhar, E., Raffoul, A., Slater, W., & Shrier, L. A. (2022).
Binge-eating behaviors in adolescents and young adults during the COVID-19 pandemic.
Journal of Eating Disorders, 10(1), 1–125. https://doi.org/10.1186/s40337-022-00650-6
Gitterman, B. A., Chilton, L. A., Cotton, W. H., Duffee, J. H., Flanagan, P., Keane, V. A., Krugman,
S. D., Kuo, A. A., Linton, J. M., McKelvey, C. D., Paz-Soldan, G. J., Daniels, S. R., Abrams,
S. A., Corkins, M. R., de Ferranti, S. D., Golden, N. H., Magge, S. N., & Schwarzenberg,
S. J. (2015). Promoting food security for all children. *Pediatrics, 136*(5), e1431–e1438. https://
doi.org/10.1542/peds.2015-3301
Hetrick, R. L., Rodrigo, O. D., & Bocchini, C. E. (2020). Addressing pandemic-intensified food
insecurity. *Pediatrics, 146*(4), e2020006924. https://doi.org/10.1542/peds.2020-006924
Imboden, A., Sobczak, B., & Kurilla, N. A. (2023). Impact of the infant formula shortage on breastfeeding rates. *Journal of Pediatric Health Care, 37*(3), 279–286. https://doi.org/10.1016/j.
pedhc.2022.11.006
Kakaei, H., Nourmoradi, H., Bakhtiyari, S., Jalilian, M., & Mirzaei, A. (2022). Effect of COVID-19
on food security, hunger, and food crisis. In *COVID-19 and the sustainable development goals*
(pp. 3–29). Elsevier. https://doi.org/10.1016/B978-0-323-91307-2.00005-5
Karpman, H. E., Frazier, J. A., & Broder-Fingert, S. (2023). State of emergency: A crisis in
children's mental health care. *Pediatrics, 151*(3), e2022058832. https://doi.org/10.1542/
peds.2022-058832
Khalil, A. M. S., & Elsayed, Z. E. H. (2020). Children dietary habits and quality of sleep during
COVID-19 pandemic. *International Journal of Nursing, 7*(2), 80–86. https://doi.org/10.15640/
ijn.v7n2a9
Kim-Mozeleski, J. E., Pike Moore, S. N., Trapl, E. S., Perzynski, A. T., Tsoh, J. Y., & Gunzler,
D. D. (2023). Food insecurity trajectories in the U.S. during the first year of the COVID-19
pandemic. *Preventing Chronic Disease, 20,* E03. https://doi.org/10.5888/pcd20.220212
LaFauci, G., Montalti, M., Di Valerio, Z., Gori, D., Salomoni, M. G., Salussolia, A., Solda, G.,
& Giaraldi, F. (2022). Obesity and COVID-19 in children and adolescents: Reciprocal detrimental influence-systematic literature review and meta-analysis. *International Journal
of Environmental Research and Public Health, 19*(13), 7603. https://doi.org/10.3390/
ijerph19137603
Markovic, A., Muhlematter, C., Beaugrand, M., Camos, V., & Kurth, S. (2021). Severe effects
of the Covid-19 confinement on young children's sleep: A longitudinal study identifying risk
and protective factors. Journal of Sleep Research, 30e13314. https://doi.org/10.1111/jsr.13314

Martinez-de-Quel, O., Suarez-Iglesias, D., Lopez-Flores, M., & Perez, C. A. (2021). Physical activity, dietary habits, and sleep before and during COVID-19 lockdown: A longitudinal study. *Appetite, 158*(1), 105019. https://doi.org/10.1016/j.appet.2020.105019

Mayurasakorn, K., Pinsawas, B., Mongkolsucharitkul, P., Sranacharoenpong, K., & Damapong, S. (2020). School closure, COVID-19 and lunch programme: Unprecedented undernutrition crisis in low-middle income countries. *Journal of Paediatrics and Child Health, 56*(7), 1013–1017. https://doi.org/10.1111/jpc.15018

Medrano, M., Cadenas-Sanchez, C., Oses, M., Arenaza, L., Amasene, M., & Labayen, I. (2021). Changes in lifestyle behaviours during the COVID-19 confinement in Spanish children: A longitudinal analysis from the MUGI project. *Pediatric Obesity, 16*(4), e12731. https://doi.org/10.1111/ijpo.12731

Meek, J. Y., & Noble, L. (2022). Policy statement: Breastfeeding and the use of human milk. *Pediatrics, 150*(1), e2022057988. https://doi.org/10.1542/peds.2022-057988

Nagata, J. M., Cortez, C. A., Cattle, C. J., Ganson, K. T., Iyer, P., Bibbins-Domingo, K., & Baker, F. C. (2022). Screen time use among U.S. adolescents during the COVID-19 pandemic: Findings from the adolescent brain cognitive development (ABCD) study. *JAMA Pediatrics, 176*(1), 94–96. https://doi.org/10.1001/jamapediatrics.2021.4334

National Center for Education in Maternal and Child Health (U.S.) & Story, M. (2002). *Bright futures in practice: Nutrition pocket guide*. National Center for Education in Maternal and Child Health.

Neville, R. D., Lakes, K. D., Hopkins, W. G., Tarantino, G., Draper, C. E., Beck, R., & Madigan, S. (2022). Global changes in child and adolescent physical activity during the COVID-19 pandemic: A systematic review and meta-analysis. *JAMA Pediatrics, 176*(9), 886–894. https://doi.org/10.1001/jamapediatrics.2022.2313

Paslakis, G., Dimitropoulos, G., & Katzman, D. K. (2021). A call to action to address COVID-19-induced global food insecurity to prevent hunger, malnutrition, and eating pathology. *Nutrition Reviews, 79*(1), 114–116. https://doi.org/10.1093/nutrit/nuaa069

Pavlovic, A., DeFina, L. F., Natale, B. L., Thiele, S. E., Walker, T. J., Craig, D. W., Vint, G. R., Leonard, D., Haskell, W. L., & Kohl, H. W. (2021). Keeping children healthy during and after COVID-19 pandemic: Meeting youth physical activity needs. *BMC Public Health, 21*(1), 485–485. https://doi.org/10.1186/s12889-021-10545-x

Plevinsky, J. M., Young, M. A., Carmody, J. K., Durkin, L. K., Gamwell, K. L., Klages, K. L., Ghosh, S., & Hommel, K. A. (2020). The impact of COVID-19 on pediatric adherence and self-management. *Journal of Pediatric Psychology, 45*(9), 977–982. https://doi.org/10.1093/jpepsy/jsaa079

Riazi, N., Wunderlich, K., Gierc, M., Brussoni, M., Moore, S. A., Tremblay, M. S., & Faulkner, G. (2021). "You Can't go to the park, you can't go here, you can't go there": Exploring parental experiences of COVID-19 and its impact on their children's movement behaviours. *Children (Basel), 8*(3), 219. https://doi.org/10.3390/children8030219

Schnitzer, P., Dykstra, H., & Collier, A. (2023). The COVID-19 pandemic and youth suicide: 2020–2021. *Pediatrics (Evanston), 151*(3), 1. https://doi.org/10.1542/peds.2022-058716

Sheldrick, M., Swindell, N. J., Richards, A. B., Fairclough, S. J., & Stratton, G. (2023). Correction: Homes became the "everything space" during COVID-19: Impact of changes to the home environment on children's physical activity and sitting (International Journal of Behavioral Nutrition and Physical Activity 2022;19(1):134, 10.1186/s12966-022-01346-5). *International Journal of Behavioral Nutrition and Physical Activity, 20*(1), 54. https://doi.org/10.1186/s12966-023-01409-1

Stone, J.E, Phillips, A.J.K., Chachos, E., Hand, A.J., Lu, S., Carskadon, M.A., Klerman, E.B., Lockley, S.W., Wiley, J.F., Bei, B., & Rajaratnam, S,M.W. (2021). In-person vs home schooling during the COVID-19 pandemic: Differences in sleep, circadian timing, and mood in early adolescence. Journal of Pineal Research, 71, e12757, 1–12.

Tan, W. (2021). School closures were over-weighted against the mitigation of COVID-19 transmission: A literature review on the impact of school closures in the United States. *Medicine (Baltimore), 100*(30), e26709–e26709. https://doi.org/10.1097/MD.0000000000026709

Thacker, N., Namazova-Baranova, L., Mestrovic, J., Carrasco-Sanz, A., Vural, M., Giardino, I., Indrio, F., Ferrara, P., & Pettoello-Mantovani, M. (2022). Child malnutrition during the coronavirus disease 2019 pandemic. *The Journal of Pediatrics, 244*, 257–258.e2. https://doi.org/10.1016/j.jpeds.2022.02.010

U. S. Food and Drug Administration. (2022, August 1). *FDA investigation of Cronobacter infections: Powdered infant formula* (February 2022). https://www.fda.gov/food/outbreaks-foodborne-illness/fda-investigation-cronobacter-infections-powdered-infant-formula-february-2022

Viner, R. M., Russell, S. J., Croker, H., Packer, J., Ward, J., Stansfield, C., Mytton, O., Bonell, C., & Booy, R. (2020). School closure and management practices during coronavirus outbreaks including COVID-19: A rapid systematic review. *Child Adolescent Health, 4*(5), 397–404. https://doi.org/10.1016/S2352-4642(20)30095-X

Wang, J., Wei, Z., Yao, N., Li, C., & Sun, L. (2023). Association between sunlight exposure and mental health: Evidence from a special population without sunlight in work. *Risk Management and Healthcare Policy, 16*, 1049–1057. https://doi.org/10.2147/RMHP.S420018

Wearick-Silva, L.E., Richter, S.A., Viola, T.W., & Nunes, L.M. (2022). Sleep quality among parents and their children during the COVID-19 pandemic. *Jornel de Pediatria, 98* (3), 248–255.

Wechsler, H., Devereaux, R. S., Davis, M., & Collins, J. (2000). Using the school environment to promote physical activity and healthy eating. *Preventive Medicine, 31*, S121–S137. https://doi.org/10.1006/pmed.2000.0649

Wickham, S., Amarsekara, N. A., Bartonicek, A., & Connor, T. S. (2020). The big three health behaviors and mental health and well-being among young adults: A cross-sectional investigation of sleep, exercise, and diet. *Frontline Psychology, 11*, 579205. https://doi.org/10.3389/fpsyg.2020.579205

World Health Organization [WHO]. (2019). *Guidelines on physical activity, sedentary behavior, and sleep for children under five years of age*. ISBN 978-92-4-155053-6.

World Health Organization [WHO]. (2022). *Physical activity.* https://www.who.int/news-room/fact-sheets/detail/physical-activity

World Health Organization [WHO]. (2023). *Sustainable development goals (SDG) 2030.* https://www.who.int/data/gho/data/themes/world-health-statistics#tab=tab_1

Xiang, M., Liu, Y., Yamamoto, S., Mizoue, T., & Kuwahara, K. (2022). Association of Changes of lifestyle behaviors before and during the COVID-19 pandemic with mental health: A longitudinal study in children and adolescents. *International Journal of Behavioral Nutrition and Physical Activity, 19*(1), 92. https://doi.org/10.1186/s12966-022-01327-8

Zahid, M. N., & Perna, S. (2021). Continent-wide analysis of COVID-19: Total cases, deaths, tests, socio-economic, and morbidity factors associated to the mortality rate and forecasting analysis in 2020-2021. *International Journal of Environmental Research and Public Health, 18*(10), 5350.

Zhang, J., Xu, D., Xie, B., Zhang, Y., Huang, H., Hongmei, L., Chen, H., Sun, Y., Shang, Y., Hashimoto, K., & Yuan, B. (2020). Poor sleep is associated with slow recovery from lymphopenia and an increased need for ICU care in hospitalized patients with COVID-19: A retrospective cohort study. *Brain, Behavior, and Immunity, 88*, 50–58.

Mental Health: Assessment of Risk, Clinical Manifestations, and Access to Care

Bernadette Melnyk and Rosie Zeno

> *Childhood is the foundation for the rest of adult life; investing in the mental health and well-being of our children and adolescents will reap a lifetime of benefits for them, their families, and our nation.*
>
> —Bernadette Mazurek Melnyk

Introduction and Background

Prior to the COVID-19 pandemic, there was a mental health epidemic in children and teens with one out of five children affected by a mental health disorder (Perou et al., 2013). During the pandemic, children and adolescents were faced with extraordinary challenges posed by sudden disruptions to their daily lives caused by implementation of mandated public health measures, including chronic social isolation, economic hardships, and loss of school and community supports. Following the pandemic, pediatric and adolescent mental health disorders skyrocketed, and there is now a youth mental health pandemic. The pandemic has had a profound adverse effect on the mental health of individuals worldwide; however, the impact on child and adolescent mental health is particularly alarming.

During the height of the COVID-19 public health emergency, healthcare claims for child and adolescent mental health conditions rose sharply. A FAIR Health White Paper (FAIR Health, 2021) analyzed changes in mental healthcare claims related to COVID-19 from 2019 to 2020 in young people aged 13–18 years. Findings from this database of 32 billion private healthcare claims containing all International Statistical Classification of Diseases and Related Health Problems-Clinical Modification, tenth revision (i.e., ICD-10-CM) diagnosis codes revealed that generalized anxiety disorder (GAD) increased by 93.6%, major depressive disorder (MDD) increased by 83.9%, and intentional self-harm increased by 90.7%. For late

B. Melnyk · R. Zeno (✉)
The Ohio State University College of Nursing, Columbus, OH, USA
e-mail: melnyk.15@osu.edu; zeno.7@osu.edu

© The Author(s), under exclusive license to Springer Nature Switzerland AG 2025
J. L. Peck (ed.), *COVID-19 Impacts on Child Health*,
https://doi.org/10.1007/978-3-031-80369-7_7

adolescents, those aged 19–22 years, GAD increased by 67.5%, MDD increased by 49.6%, and intentional self-harm increased by 16.4%. In another study on teen health during the pandemic, three in four parents reported that COVID-19 nega- tively impacted their teens' ability to interact with friends (C.S. Mott Children's Hospital, 2021). Further, in this same study, findings indicated that one in three teen girls and one in five teen boys experienced new or worsening anxiety. Another poll conducted with those aged 18–29 years during the COVID-19 pandemic found that one in two young adults reported feeling down, depressed, or hopeless (Harvard Kennedy School Institute of Politics, 2023). In addition, a national survey found that one out of four young adults considered suicide since the pandemic (Czeisler et al., 2020).

In a systematic review of pediatric mental health problems during the COVID-19 pandemic, findings revealed other adverse mental effects, including worry, helpless- ness, fear, nervousness, agitation, and aggressiveness (Oliveira et al., 2022). In addi- tion, some studies in this systematic review reported heightened emotional symptoms, conducted problems, hyperactivity-inattention, and peer problems, and decreased prosocial behaviors.

Although suicide is the second leading cause of death in 10- to 34-year-olds (Centers for Disease Control and Prevention, 2023), it rose to the number one cause of death in youth in the state of Colorado, resulting in a declaration of a public health emergency (Children's Hospital Colorado, 2021). As a result of these sky- rocketing mental health problems in children and youth, the office of the US sur- geon general issued a public health advisory in December of 2021, calling on the nation to take urgent action on the mental health crisis impacting children and youth. In this special report, it was pointed out that 44% of American high school students feel persistently sad or hopeless and that 11 years is the time gap between a child's first symptoms of a mental health issue and when they receive treatment (Office of the Surgeon General, 2021). Significant disparities also exist in the receipt of mental health services, with a disproportionate number of Black and Hispanic children affected (Ghandour et al., 2019; Marrast et al., 2016).

Points of Care

Assessment of Risk

Every visit to a healthcare provider (HCP) is an opportunity to screen for mental health problems in children and youth. Screening, assessment, and early detection as well as evidence-based intervention for mental health/behavioral problems are critical to prevent serious chronic adverse outcomes (Melnyk & Lusk, 2022). The three most common mental health disorders in children and adolescents are anxiety, depression, and attention-deficit/hyperactivity disorder. If pediatric providers can become highly skilled in assessing and intervening early for just these three mental health conditions, it would avert the current mental health crisis in children and youth. There are a number of risk factors for mental health disorders in children and youth, which should be assessed, including:

- Parents who have mental health problems, including use of substances
- Poor self-esteem
- Lack of developmental assets, such as poor coping skills and negative patterns of thinking
- Altered parenting (e.g., over-protective, controlling, rigid, permissive)
- Parent conflict, separation, divorce, or re-marriage
- Trauma, including death of a parent, guardian, or close family member
- An incarcerated parent
- Chronic illness or handicap in the child or family member
- Hospitalizations/life-threatening medical procedures
- Adverse childhood experiences (i.e., ACES)
- Presence of major life stressors
- Peers who engage in risk-taking behaviors
- Loneliness/social isolation
- Bullying by peers
- Difficult temperament
- Behavior issues
- Stressful home or school environment
- LGBTQ+
- Overweight/obesity
- Substance use (Melnyk & Lusk, 2022)

If risk factors are present, children and teens should be screened for mental health concerns. However, it is important to remember that screening only raises a red flag for a mental health condition and does not replace a developmentally sensitive and comprehensive clinical interview by a skilled pediatric HCP (Melnyk & Lusk, 2022). At every visit, parents should be asked if they have any concerns or worries about their children's mental/emotional health or their behaviors as well as whether there has been a change in usual temperament or behaviors at home or at school.

There are a variety of valid and reliable screening tools that can be used to determine whether a child or teen is at risk for mental health conditions (see Table 1). A comprehensive compilation of screening tools for all mental health conditions in children and youth along with guidance on diagnosis, management, and prevention is available in the book entitled *A Practical Guide to Child and Adolescent Mental Health Screening, Evidence-based Assessment, Intervention and Health Promotion*, third edition (Melnyk & Lusk, 2022).

Table 1 Common mental health screening tools

Screening tool	Age range	Items and format	Measure
Pediatric symptom checklist (Jellinek et al., 1988)	4–16 year	35 items Parent and youth ≥ age 11 Also available in a 17-item short form	Elicits symptoms of internalizing (e.g., depression, anxiety) and externalizing disorders (e.g., ADHD, conduct disorder, and oppositional defiant disorder)
Screen for child anxiety related disorders (SCARED) (Birmaher et al., 1999)	≥8 year	41 items Parent and youth	Elicits symptoms of anxiety-related disorders, including panic disorder, generalized anxiety disorder, separation anxiety, social anxiety disorder, and school avoidance
Generalized anxiety Disorder-7 (GAD-7) scale (Spitzer et al., 2006)	≥13 year	7 items	Screens for severity of generalized anxiety disorder symptoms
Patient Health Questionnaire-9 modified for teens (PHQ-9) (Johnson et al., 2002)	12–18 year	9 items Self-report adolescents Also available in a 2-item format	Screens for severity of symptoms in the domains of depression and suicidality
Center for Epidemiological Studies Depression Scale for Children (CES-DC) (Faulstich et al., 1986)	6–17 year	20 items	Screens for symptoms of depression
Ask suicide questions (ASQ) (Horowitz et al., 2012)	≥8 year	4 items	Elicits symptoms of suicidal ideations and behaviors to assess risk for suicide
National Initiative for Children's healthcare quality (NICHQ) Vanderbilt assessment scales (Wolraich et al., 2013)	6–12 year	55 items (parent) 43 items (teacher) 26-item parent/ teacher follow-up scales	Elicits symptoms in the domains of inattention, disruptive behavior, anxiety, depression, and a separate scale for functioning in the domain of school performance Follow-up scales include assessment of medication side effects
Swanson, Nolan, and Pelham (SNAP-IV) (Swanson et al., 2001).	6–18 year	90 items Parent and teacher Also available in a 26-item format	Screens for symptoms of hyperactivity-impulsiveness and inattention associated with ADHD and other comorbid disorders

Clinical Manifestations

Clinical manifestations of mental health disorders in children and teens can vary widely, but a change in typical emotions and behaviors in any child or adolescent should prompt a thorough screening and assessment. Further, any change in emotions or behaviors that interferes with a child or teen's usual functioning should always be a major red flag.

Children and youth who are suffering from an anxiety disorder typically display physical signs, such as restlessness and irritability, stomach aches, headaches, heart palpitations, muscle tension, hyperventilation, and difficulty sleeping. Behavioral signs of anxiety include escape behaviors, crying, clinging to caregivers, nail biting, thumb sucking, regression, and anger or irritability. Children and teens who have anxiety also tend to worry a lot and think something terrible will happen.

The most common feature of depressive disorders is the presence of a sad, empty, or irritable mood, which is associated with somatic (e.g., headaches and stomach aches) and cognitive changes that interfere with functioning at home, in school, and with peers (Melnyk et al., 2022). Young children less than 7 years of age who suffer from depression can be inattentive, impulsive, irritable, and hyperactive, often prompting people to think about ADHD instead of depression. Infants who are depressed typically have feeding and sleep problems, irritability, poor eye contact, or apathy. Toddlers and preschoolers usually exhibit behavior problems, temper tantrums, aggression, irritability, or regression (e.g., thumb sucking and wetting the bed). School-age children suffering from depression usually have sadness, irritability, crying spells, loss of pleasure or interest in activities, somatic complaints (e.g., headaches and stomach aches), and acting out behaviors. They will often complain that no one likes them. Adolescents with depression often exhibit sadness, hopelessness, anger, self-hatred, withdrawal, loss of interest or pleasure in activities, decrease or increase in sleep and appetite, and loss of concentration. Substance and alcohol use are common to self-regulate their symptoms, and co-morbidity with anxiety is common. To make a diagnosis of MDD, there must be either a depressed mood or loss of interest or pleasure in usual activities that is present every day, during most of the day, for at least 2 weeks.

Children with attention-deficit disorder (ADD) have difficulty sustaining attention and do not seem to listen or follow through on things. They typically have difficulty organizing tasks and activities and avoid things that required sustained mental efforts. In addition, they tend to be distracted, forgetful, and lose things. Children with attention-deficit hyperactivity disorder (ADHD) have symptoms of ADD in addition to hyperactivity and impulsivity. They are usually not able to sit still and leave their seat when being seated is expected. They also inappropriately run about or climb and are unable to be quiet. They tend to talk in excess, interrupt, are restless, and impatient.

Barriers and Breakthroughs

Access to Care

An appreciation of the ongoing barriers to care access is vital to shaping the future of pediatric mental health care in the post-pandemic era. By the end of 2021, the American Academy of Pediatrics, the American Academy of Child and Adolescent

Psychiatry, and the Children's Hospital Association had declared child and adolescent mental health to be a national emergency (Office of the Surgeon General, 2021). The rise in unmet needs for mental health care can be indirectly observed by the increasing numbers of youth seeking emergency and crisis care for mental health concerns. The average proportion of mental health-related ED visits and the average volume of calls, chats, and texts made to the 988 Suicide & Crisis Lifeline (formerly the National Suicide Prevention Lifeline) have continued to increase each year following the onset of the pandemic (Krass et al., 2021; Radhakrishnan et al., 2022; Substance Abuse and Mental Health Services Administration, 2023). The COVID-19 pandemic underscored escalating demand for accessible and affordable mental health services in the US barriers to pediatric mental health care can be attributed to several factors that have negatively impacted access to and delivery of mental health services during the pandemic.

A major barrier to addressing pediatric mental health needs during the pandemic is the ongoing deficit of available and accessible mental health services. The chronic shortage and geographic maldistribution of mental health professionals has been a key driver of the surge in unmet need for mental health care. Prior to the pandemic, just half of US children with a treatable mental health disorder received needed treatment or counseling (Whitney & Peterson, 2019). Most states have fewer than 40% of the mental health care professionals required to meet the needs of their population, leaving over 72% of the nation with unmet mental health care needs (Kaiser Family Foundation, 2022). Over 163 million individuals reside in a federally designated health professional shortage area for mental health care with rural populations experiencing the greatest disparity in access to HCPs for mental health prevention and treatment (Health Resources & Service Administration, 2023).

COVID-19 social distancing measures further hindered access to mental health prevention and treatment services. Many clinics, hospitals, and private practices reduced or suspended their services, worsening the scarcity of available HCPs. Moreover, schools often serve as important hubs for mental health services, including counseling and intervention programs (Ali et al., 2019). School closures disrupted these vital services leaving many children and adolescents without access to school-based mental health support during a time of critical need. Furthermore, children and adolescents were physically distanced from teachers and other school officials who are trained to identify signs of developmental, behavioral, and mental health concerns and serve as a point of referral or recognize signs of child maltreatment and neglect as mandated reporters.

Pandemic-related quarantine, lockdown, and stay-at-home restrictions catalyzed a massive shift to virtual healthcare to maintain critical access to services and alleviate the impact of unmet mental health care needs. Although in existence since the 1950s, telehealth technologies made a significant breakthrough in utilization with the onset of COVID-19. Post-pandemic telehealth usage has remained stable at 38 times greater than rates observed prior to the pandemic (Bestsennyy et al., 2021). The sizeable growth in telehealth usage was triggered by the crisis demand and facilitated by modifications in state and federal legislation that reduced barriers to healthcare practice and reimbursement (Shaver, 2022). Telehealth services helped many families to maintain continuity of their mental health care and improved access to care for individuals with barriers to in-person treatment. Although pediatric behavioral health subspecialty encounters decreased substantially during the pandemic, the proportion of visits conducted via telehealth increased to over 65% (Uscher-Pines et al., 2022).

While the expanded use of telehealth technologies can eliminate barriers to mental health services, digital accessibility issues still impede access for many. Transitioning to virtual care is challenging for families who may not be equipped with the requisite technology resources, digital literacy, or a secure and private space to engage in virtual mental health care (Chang et al., 2021; Cunningham, Ely, et al., 2021). Barriers to telehealth access disproportionately affect rural communities as well as those experiencing poverty, preventing these youth from receiving necessary mental health support and further exacerbating mental health disparities for these populations (National Academies of Sciences, Engineering, and Medicine, 2021).

A breakthrough in recent years that has provided access to evidence-based mental health care is the Creating Opportunities for Personal Empowerment (COPE) program. Developed by the first author of this chapter, COPE is a 7-weekly session evidence-based cognitive-behavioral skills building program that contains all key elements of cognitive-behavioral therapy. Over 20 studies have supported its efficacy in decreasing anxiety, depression, stress, and suicidal ideation as well as enhancing self-esteem and healthy lifestyle behaviors in children, teens, and young adults (Kozlowski et al., 2015; Lusk & Melnyk, 2013; Melnyk, 2020; Melnyk et al., 2013; Melnyk et al., 2015). The program is manualized in a workbook and can be delivered in 25–30-min individual sessions by non-mental health providers as well as mental health providers after a 4-h online training workshop. Thus, COPE has provided immediate access to tens of thousands of depressed and anxious children and youth who might not have otherwise received any treatment. Developmentally tailored versions of the COPE program are available for 7–11 year old children, 12–17 year old teens, and 18–24 year old young adults (see www.cope2thrive.com). A 15-session program (COPE Healthy Lifestyle TEEN [Thinking, Emotions, Exercise and Nutrition]) is also available and adds nutrition and exercise content to the seven cognitive-behavioral skills building sessions. This 15-session program is promoted by the National Institutes of Health as a research tested intervention program (RTIP) with the highest dissemination capacity as an adolescent obesity control program (see https://ebccp.cancercontrol.cancer.gov/viewProduct.do?viewMod e=preview&productId=25106526). The COPE program is being reimbursed in primary care across the country with the 99214 CPT code and is offered for telehealth delivery (Melnyk, 2020). A self-delivered online program is also available for adolescents. COPE can also be delivered in group and classroom settings in 45–50 min. Primary and secondary schools as well as universities across the country are delivering COPE as a preventive strategy to enhance mental resiliency and prevent mental health disorders (Hart Abney et al., 2019; Hoying et al., 2016; Hoying & Melnyk, 2016).

Lessons Learned

Amidst the unprecedented global challenges posed by the COVID-19 pandemic, pediatric HCPs found themselves at the forefront of a crisis that extended far beyond the physical morbidity of COVID-19 as child and adolescent mental health emerged as a critical concern. Although the pandemic's long-term impact on children and adolescents is not yet fully understood, we have gained invaluable insights into particular mental health risk factors that can inform evidence-based approaches aimed at safeguarding and nurturing pediatric mental health and well-being, especially during times of mass crisis.

Social Connection

Social connectedness is the conduit for optimal social-emotional development for children and adolescents. Limited social connection during key periods of growth and development has significant implications for youth mental health and well-being. Containment measures aimed at minimizing the risk of coronavirus transmission caused widespread disruptions to daily life. Children and adolescents were forced to navigate a new reality characterized by limited face-to-face interactions with peers and extended family during a time of extraordinary crisis and uncertainty. Children subjected to social isolation and quarantine orders have shown a fourfold rise in posttraumatic stress-related symptoms (Brooks et al., 2020; Loades et al., 2020). Prolonged experiences of loneliness and social isolation not only increase the risk of developing depression and anxiety but also the elevated risk may persist for up to 9 years following the initial experience (Loades et al., 2020). Social isolation, regardless of age or clinical severity, is the most significant and reliable predictor of suicidal ideation and fatal and non-fatal suicidal behaviors (Van Orden et al., 2010).

In 2023, a US Surgeon General Advisory called attention to the nation's epidemic of loneliness, isolation, and lack of social connection that is adversely impacting individual and societal well-being (Office of the Surgeon General, 2023). Healthcare professionals serve a crucial role in the early identification of developmental, behavioral, and mental health issues that impact youth and in preventing long-term consequences. Lessons learned from studying the impact of social isolation during the COVID-19 pandemic can inform preparedness for future crises or circumstances where social isolation becomes necessary. Potential life disruptions that trigger displacement or broken social connections with family, peers, and other community supports require readiness from pediatric HCPs to mitigate the loss of social connectedness and emotional support. Public health needs for social distancing should be weighed carefully against the fundamental need for social connection to support child growth and development and promote mental well-being.

Technology Use

Disease containment measures initiated in response to the COVID-19 pandemic caused a rapid and widespread reliance on digital technology for access to information, healthcare, education, and social connections. However, the benefits of virtual connectedness must be weighed in the context of emerging evidence of the link between mental health and digital media use in adolescents during the pandemic. Understanding these associations can inform risk assessments and guide interventions to promote the mental well-being of adolescents, especially during challenging times when greater social-emotional support is needed.

To alleviate the negative emotional experiences of social distancing, young people worldwide spent more time on digital devices during the pandemic. Adolescents reporting more time spent virtually connecting with friends reported less feelings of loneliness but significantly more depressive symptoms, with the association between reported pandemic-related stress and depression being strongest among adolescents reporting the highest social media use (Ellis et al., 2020). Several meta-analyses found statistically significant correlations between problematic digital media use and depression, anxiety, stress, and diminished well-being among adolescents and young adults (Cunningham, Hudson, & Harkness, 2021; Marciano et al., 2022; Shannon et al., 2022). Additionally, studies on excessive smartphone use in adolescents and young adults show an association with difficulty in cognitive-emotional regulation, impulsivity, impaired cognitive function, behavioral addiction to social media (i.e., problematic use), and low self-esteem (Wacks & Weinstein, 2021).

Not all technology use is detrimental to mental health, and some digital resources can even support mental and physical well-being, such as digital health and wellness apps for monitoring and managing depression and anxiety. A balanced approach is needed, and importantly, digital media use should not displace in-person relationships and other wellness routines like adequate sleep and exercise. A nuanced understanding of the potential impact of digital media use on youth mental health allows HCPs to tailor mental health promotion, identify at-risk individuals, and implement preventive strategies. Pediatric advocates should actively support future policies that prioritize pediatric mental well-being in the digital age.

Parental Well-being

The pandemic has provided the opportunity to recognize the critical connections between parental well-being and child well-being and to use these lessons to inform future responses to public health crises and policy for supporting families. COVID-19 profoundly impacted the family milieu due to the sheer volume of disruptions and challenges abruptly experienced by families worldwide. Parents faced a vast restructuring of daily routines and household income, increased burden of childcare during school closures, and concerns for their children's well-being.

Feelings of fear and uncertainty were heightened as families coped with grief and loss, adapted to limited social supports, and experienced decreased access to health-care and community resources. Many parents facing COVID-19-related challenges suffered traumatic stress, depression, or anxiety, as the numerous stressors experienced during the pandemic exacerbated existing vulnerabilities and triggered pervasive parental stress (Whaley & Pfefferbaum, 2023).

The pandemic catalyzed considerable interest in the emerging concept of *parental burnout*. Defined as a prolonged response to chronic and overwhelming parental stress, parental burnout is a consequence of persistently elevated levels of parenting-related stress caused by an imbalance between the demands of parenting and the available resources to cope with those demands (Mikolajczak et al., 2019). In a 2021 study, researchers found that 66% of working parents met criteria for parental burnout (Gawlik & Melnyk, 2022). Moreover, parental burnout was associated with depression, anxiety, increased alcohol consumption, and punitive parenting practices, as well as internalizing, externalizing, and attention symptoms in their children.

Approximately 7% of children aged 0–17 years have a parent with self-reported poor mental health, and these children are more likely to experience mental, emotional, or developmental disabilities, as well as adverse childhood experiences like violence exposure, family disruptions, or living in poverty (Wolicki et al., 2021). Furthermore, research shows that children can be affected by the posttraumatic mental health difficulties encountered by their parents, and these effects can persist over time (Hoven et al., 2009; Pfefferbaum et al., 2018). Lessons from the COVID-19 pandemic can inform and improve preparedness to identify and address the support needs of parents and caregivers who act in a parental role. Prioritizing the need for mental health services amidst persistent family stressors and addressing the identified barriers to accessing care can enhance family health and well-being during the post-pandemic recovery period and beyond.

Primary Care and Mental Health Integration

The COVID-19 pandemic highlighted the critical need for accessible and affordable mental health services in the United States, and traditional models of care have struggled to meet the demand. Within the current health care landscape, the need to integrate mental health services into the pediatric primary care setting has emerged as a national imperative. The National Association of Pediatric Nurse Practitioners *Position Statement on the Integration of Mental Health Care in Pediatric Primary Care Settings*, underscores the need for a transformative shift in healthcare delivery that acknowledges the interconnectedness between physical and mental well-being (Frye et al., 2020). Traditionally, physical and mental health care have been treated as separate domains, often leading to fragmented care and missed opportunities for early identification and intervention. Mental health integration seeks to bridge this gap.

Collaborative, interprofessional efforts are key to realizing a transformed health delivery system which embraces the synergetic physical-mental health connection. To expand access to care that routinely addresses the mental and behavioral health concerns faced by children and adolescents, primary care providers can collaborate with mental health specialists via telehealth, co-located services, and/or community partnerships (Walter et al., 2021). The integration of mental health services in primary care is bolstered by the roles of various mental health specialists, like psychologists, licensed social workers, psychiatrists, and/or psychiatric mental health nurse practitioners (PMHNPs). In this way, constructive interprofessional collaboration between primary care and mental health providers empowers care delivery in the primary care setting to comprehensively attend to the diverse needs of patients while ensuring that both the biological and psychosocial aspects of mental health are addressed.

Moreover, the American Academy of Pediatrics recommends that pediatric-focused HCPs be prepared to diagnose and manage mild-to-moderate mental health conditions in the primary care setting by incorporating mental health screenings, assessments, and evidence-based interventions as a standard part of their patient interactions (Wissow et al., 2016). NAPNAP has issued a resounding national call, through the *NAPNAP Cares* initiative, to address the pressing need for an increased number of pediatric-focused advanced practice registered nurses (APRNs) who are equipped to provide comprehensive mental health care. The NAPNAP Cares initiative advocates for specialized continuing education and training programs that empower pediatric-focused APRNs with the knowledge, skills, and competencies needed to provide effective mental health care that meets the growing need of children and their families in the primary care setting and beyond. The National Network of Child Psychiatry Access Program (NNCPAP) was established in 2011 to "support existing and emerging child psychiatry consultation programs and further national progress toward effective integration of the management of mental health… within primary care" (National Network of Child Psychiatry Access Programs [NNCPAP], 2023, para 1). This directory provides links to primary care providers in 46 states with free access to mental health specialist consultation to help increase access to mental health care.

Furthermore, the Pediatric Nursing Certification Board (PNCB) offers a Pediatric Mental Health Specialist (PMHS) subspecialty certification exam that validates the added knowledge, skills, and expertise of APRNs in the early identification, intervention, and collaboration of care for children and adolescents with mental and behavioral health concerns (Pediatric Nursing Certification Board, n.d.). A pediatric-focused APRN with PMHS certification is an APRN who specializes in providing comprehensive healthcare to children and adolescents, prepared with an enhanced focus on mental and behavioral health issues. Their role is holistically centered on the physical, emotional, and psychological well-being of pediatric patients. Their primary focus is on the assessment, diagnosis, treatment, and management of mental health conditions and psychiatric disorders. PMHNPs practice in a distinct but complimentary role. A PMHNP is a specialized APRN who focuses on providing mental health care to individuals across the lifespan, including children and adolescents. Currently approved pathways to PMHS certification include graduation from an accredited program as a pediatric primary care nurse practitioner (NP), a family NP, a psychiatric mental health NP, or a child and adolescent psychiatric mental health NP. In the wake of COVID-19, PNCB expanded alternative pathways to certification to be more inclusive of faculty persons and candidates who complete one of four approved specialty program pathways. Ideally, these adjuvant roles are professionally collaborative.

The KySS Mental Health Fellowship is a favored pathway among pediatric-focused APRNs seeking preparation for the PMHS certification exam. The KySS Mental Health Fellowship online continuing education program at the Ohio State University College of Nursing prepares HCPs in evidence-based screening, assessment, and intervention (see https://nursing.osu.edu/academics/continuing-education/kyss-mental-health-fellowship-child-and-adolescent-online). A key differentiator of this program is that it provides skills building and a seasoned mental health expert mentor.

COVID-19 catalyzed a national need for expanded access to affordable, quality mental health care that can no longer go unanswered. The integration of mental health care in the primary care setting is a vital priority as families continue to adapt to a post-pandemic era. Not only is mental health care an essential need in times of mass crisis, but longitudinally, it is also a proactive approach for normalizing mind-body connectedness and reducing stigma around mental health concerns that can cause family to be reluctant to seek care. Every pediatric health encounter must be an opportunity to screen for mental health concerns and provide families with the anticipatory guidance and resources they need to prevent the consequential impact of untreated mental health conditions on the developmental trajectories and the overall well-being of children and adolescents. By embracing this integrated approach, HCPs can forge a path toward better patient outcomes, reduced stigma surrounding mental health, and a more resilient and thriving society.

Three Calls to Action

Addressing the youth mental health crisis requires a multi-faceted approach involving policymakers, HCPs, educators, and communities. Increasing investment in mental health infrastructure, expanding the mental health workforce, and enhancing telehealth capabilities are critical steps to ensure more accessible and equitable mental health care for children and adolescents. As the world gradually recovers from the pandemic, there is an opportunity to prioritize pediatric mental health care and create a more resilient system that can better respond to future challenges. Integrating mental health support within educational settings, fostering community-based programs, and implementing innovative outreach and engagement strategies can promote early intervention and prevention. However, these efforts must be sustained and prioritized beyond the immediate crisis to ensure a lasting impact on pediatric mental health care. By prioritizing the mental well-being of our youth and

(continued)

fostering a supportive infrastructure, we can pave the way for a healthier and more resilient generation post-pandemic. The challenges brought to light during the COVID-19 pandemic serve as a call to action to improve pediatric mental health care in the United States.

- Equip all healthcare providers and students who care for children with the needed knowledge and evidence-based skills to prevent, screen, identify, and provide early interventions to children and youth at risk for mental health disorders through programs like the KySS Mental Health Fellowship.
- Provide all children, teens, and young adults with evidence-based skills (e.g., cognitive-behavioral skills and mindfulness) that are known to enhance mental resiliency and coping in order to deal with life's stressors and challenges as a strategy to prevent mental health disorders.
- Equip parents and teachers with the necessary knowledge and skills to prevent and identify mental health issues early to enhance management and child/adolescent outcomes.

Author Disclosure   Bernadette Melnyk has a company entitled COPE2Thrive, LLC that disseminates her COPE programs.

References

Ali, M. M., West, K., Teich, J. L., Lynch, S., Mutter, R., & Dubenitz, J. (2019). Utilization of mental health services in educational setting by adolescents in the United States. *The Journal of School Health, 89*(5), 393–401. https://doi.org/10.1111/josh.12753

Bestsennyy, O., Gilbert, G., Harris, A., & Rost, J. (2021). *Telehealth: A quarter-trillion-dollar post-covid-19 reality*. McKinsey & Company Healthcare Systems & Services. https://www.mckinsey.com/industries/healthcare/our-insights/telehealth-a-quarter-trillion-dollar-post-covid-19-reality#/

Birmaher, B., Brent, D. A., Chiappetta, L., Bridge, J., Monga, S., & Baugher, M. (1999). Psychometric properties of the screen for child anxiety related emotional disorders (SCARED): A replication study. *Journal of the American Academy of Child and Adolescent Psychiatry, 38*(10), 1230–1236. https://doi.org/10.1097/00004583-199910000-00011

Brooks, S. K., Webster, R. K., Smith, L. E., Woodland, L., Wessely, S., Greenberg, N., & Rubin, G. J. (2020). The psychological impact of quarantine and how to reduce it: Rapid review of the evidence. *Lancet, 395*(10227), 912–920. https://doi.org/10.1016/S0140-6736(20)30460-8

C.S. Mott Children's Hospital. (2021, March 15). *How the pandemic has impacted teen mental health* [Mott Poll Report, Volume 38, Issue 2]. https://mottpoll.org/reports/how-pandemic-has-impacted-teen-mental-health

Centers for Disease Control and Prevention. (2023, May 8). *Facts about suicide*. https://www.cdc.gov/suicide/facts

Chang, J. E., Lai, A. Y., Gupta, A., Nguyen, A. M., Berry, C. A., & Shelley, D. R. (2021). Rapid transition to telehealth and the digital divide: Implications for primary care access and equity in a post-COVID era. *The Milbank Quarterly, 99*(2), 340–368. https://doi.org/10.1111/1468-0009.12509

Children's Hospital Colorado. (2021, May 26). *Children's hospital Colorado declares a 'State of Emergency' for youth mental health.* https://www.childrenscolorado.org/about/news/2021/may-2021/youth-mental-health-state-of-emergency/

Cunningham, N. R., Ely, S. L., Barber Garcia, B. N., & Bowden, J. (2021). Addressing pediatric mental health using telehealth during coronavirus disease-2019 and beyond: A narrative review. *Academic Pediatrics, 21*(7), 1108–1117. https://doi.org/10.1016/j.acap.2021.06.002

Cunningham, S., Hudson, C. C., & Harkness, K. (2021). Social media and depression symptoms: A meta-analysis. *Research on Child and Adolescent Psychopathology, 49*(2), 241–253. https://doi.org/10.1007/s10802-020-00715-7

Czeisler, M. É., Lane, R. I., Petrosky, E., Wiley, J. F., Christensen, A., Njai, R., Weaver, M. D., Robbins, R., Facer-Childs, E. R., Barger, L. K., Czeisler, C. A., Howard, M. E., & Rajaratnam, S. M. W. (2020). Mental health, substance use, and suicidal ideation during the COVID-19 pandemic—United States, June 24–30, 2020. *Morbidity and Mortality Weekly Report, 69*(32), 1049–1057. https://doi.org/10.15585/mmwr.mm6932a1

Ellis, W. E., Dumas, T. M., & Forbes, L. M. (2020). Physically isolated but socially connected: Psychological adjustment and stress among adolescents during the initial COVID-19 crisis. *Canadian Journal of Behavioural Science, 52,* 177–187. https://doi.org/10.1037/cbs0000215

FAIR Health. (2021). *The impact of COVID-19 on pediatric mental health: A study of private healthcare claims* [White paper]. https://www.fairhealth.org/article/fair-health-releases-study-on-impact-of-covid-19-on-pediatric-mental-health

Faulstich, M. E., Carey, M. P., Ruggiero, L., Enyart, P., & Gresham, F. (1986). Assessment of depression in childhood and adolescence: An evaluation of the Center for Epidemiological Studies Depression Scale for children (CES-DC). *The American Journal of Psychiatry, 143*(8), 1024–1027. https://doi.org/10.1176/ajp.143.8.1024

Frye, L., Lusk, P., Van Cleve, S., Heighway, S., & Johnson-Smith, A. (2020). NAPNAP position statement on the integration of mental health in pediatric primary care settings. *Journal of Pediatric Health Care, 34,* 514–517. https://doi.org/10.1016/j.pedhc.2020.04.013

Gawlik, K., & Melnyk, B. M. (2022). *Pandemic parenting: Examining the epidemic of working parental burnout and strategies to help.* https://go.osu.edu/workingparentburnout

Ghandour, R. M., Sherman, L. J., Vladutiu, C. J., Ali, M. M., Lynch, S. E., Bitsko, R. H., & Blumberg, S. J. (2019). Prevalence and treatment of depression, anxiety, and conduct problems in US children. *The Journal of Pediatrics, 206,* 256–267.e3. https://doi.org/10.1016/j.jpeds.2018.09.021

Hart Abney, B. G., Lusk, P., Hovermale, R., & Melnyk, B. M. (2019). Decreasing depression and anxiety in college youth using the creating opportunities for personal empowerment program (COPE). *Journal of the American Psychiatric Nurses Association, 25*(2), 89–98. https://doi.org/10.1177/1078390318779205

Harvard Kennedy School Institute of Politics. (2023). *Harvard youth poll.* 45th ed. https://iop.harvard.edu/youth-poll/45th-edition-spring-2023

Health Resources & Service Administration. (2023). *Health workforce shortage areas.* https://data.hrsa.gov/topics/health-workforce/shortage-areas

Horowitz, L. M., Bridge, J. A., Teach, S. J., Ballard, E., Klima, J., Rosenstein, D. L., Wharff, E. A., Ginnis, K., Cannon, E., Joshi, P., & Pao, M. (2012). Ask suicide-screening questions (ASQ): A brief instrument for the pediatric emergency department. *Archives of Pediatrics & Adolescent Medicine, 166*(12), 1170–1176. https://doi.org/10.1001/archpediatrics.2012.1276

Hoven, C. W., Duarte, C. S., Wu, P., Doan, T., Singh, N., Mandell, D. J., Bin, F., Teichman, Y., Teichman, M., Wicks, J., Musa, G., & Cohen, P. (2009). Parental exposure to mass violence and child mental health: The first responder and WTC evacuee study. *Clinical Child and Family Psychology Review, 12*(2), 95–112. https://doi.org/10.1007/s10567-009-0047-2

Hoying, J., & Melnyk, B. M. (2016). COPE: A pilot study with urban-dwelling minority sixth grade youth to improve physical activity and mental health outcomes. *The Journal of School Nursing, 32*(5), 347–356. https://doi.org/10.1177/1059840516635713

Hoying, J., Melnyk, B. M., & Arcoleo, K. (2016). Effects of the COPE cognitive behavioral skills building TEEN program on the healthy lifestyle behaviors and mental health of Appalachian early adolescents. *Journal of Pediatric Health Care, 30*(1), 65–72. https://doi.org/10.1016/j.pedhc.2015.02.005

Jellinek, M. S., Murphy, J. M., Robinson, J., Feins, A., Lamb, S., & Fenton, T. (1988). Pediatric symptom checklist: Screening school-age children for psychosocial dysfunction. *The Journal of Pediatrics, 112*(2), 201–209. https://doi.org/10.1016/s0022-3476(88)80056-8

Johnson, J. G., Harris, E. S., Spitzer, R. L., & Williams, J. B. (2002). The patient health questionnaire for adolescents: Validation of an instrument for the assessment of mental disorders among adolescent primary care patients. *The Journal of Adolescent Health, 30*(3), 196–204. https://doi.org/10.1016/s1054-129x(01)00333-0

Kaiser Family Foundation. (2022). *State health facts. Mental health care health professional shortage areas (HPSAs) as of Sept. 30, 2022.* KFF. https://www.kff.org/other/state-indicator/mental-health-care-health-professional-shortage-areas-hpsas

Kozlowski, J., Lusk, P., & Melnyk, B. M. (2015). Pediatric nurse practitioner management of child anxiety in the rural primary care clinic with the evidence-based COPE. *Journal of Pediatric Health Care, 29*(3), 274–282. https://doi.org/10.1016/j.pedhc.2015.01.009

Krass, P., Dalton, E., Doupnik, S. K., & Esposito, J. (2021). US pediatric emergency department visits for mental health conditions during the COVID-19 pandemic. *JAMA Network Open, 4*(4), e218533. https://doi.org/10.1001/jamanetworkopen.2021.8533

Loades, M. E., Chatburn, E., Higson-Sweeney, N., Reynolds, S., Shafran, R., Brigden, A., Linney, C., McManus, M. N., Borwick, C., & Crawley, E. (2020). Rapid systematic review: The impact of social isolation and loneliness on the mental health of children and adolescents in the context of COVID-19. *Journal of the American Academy of Child and Adolescent Psychiatry, 59*(11), 1218–1239.e3. https://doi.org/10.1016/j.jaac.2020.05.009

Lusk, P., & Melnyk, B. M. (2013). COPE for depressed and anxious teens: A brief cognitive-behavioral skills building intervention to increase access to timely, evidence-based treatment. *Journal of Child and Adolescent Psychiatric Nursing, 26*(1), 23–31. https://doi.org/10.1111/jcap.12017

Marciano, L., Ostroumova, M., Schulz, P. J., & Camerini, A. L. (2022). Digital media use and adolescents' mental health during the Covid-19 pandemic: A systematic review and meta-analysis. *Frontiers in Public Health, 9*, 793868. https://doi.org/10.3389/fpubh.2021.793868

Marrast, L., Himmelstein, D. U., & Woolhandler, S. (2016). Racial and ethnic disparities in mental health care for children and young adults: A national study. *International Journal of Health Services: Planning, Administration, Evaluation, 46*(4), 810–824. https://doi.org/10.1177/0020731416662736

Melnyk, B. M. (2020). Reducing healthcare costs for mental health hospitalizations with the evidence-based COPE program for child and adolescent depression and anxiety: A cost analysis. *Journal of Pediatric Health Care, 34*(2), 117–121. https://doi.org/10.1016/j.pedhc.2019.08.002

Melnyk, B. M., Brown, H., & Lusk, P. (2022). Diagnosing, managing and preventing mental health disorders in children and adolescents. In B. M. Melnyk & P. Lusk (Eds.), *A practical guide to child and adolescent mental health screening, evidence-based assessment, intervention, and health promotion* (3rd ed.). Springer.

Melnyk, B. M., Jacobson, D., Kelly, S., Belyea, M., Shaibi, G., Small, L., O'Haver, J., & Marsiglia, F. F. (2013). Promoting healthy lifestyles in high school adolescents: A randomized controlled trial. *American Journal of Preventive Medicine, 45*(4), 407–415. https://doi.org/10.1016/j.amepre.2013.05.013

Melnyk, B. M., Jacobson, D., Kelly, S. A., Belyea, M. J., Shaibi, G. Q., Small, L., O'Haver, J. A., & Marsiglia, F. F. (2015). Twelve-month effects of the COPE healthy lifestyles teen program on overweight and depression in high school adolescents. *The Journal of School Health, 85*(12), 861–870.

Melnyk, B. M., & Lusk, P. (2022). *A practical guide to child and adolescent mental health screening, evidence-based assessment, intervention, and health promotion*. Springer. https://doi.org/10.1891/9780826167279

Mikolajczak, M., Gross, J. J., & Roskam, I. (2019). Parental burnout: What is it, and why does it matter? *Clinical Psychological Science: A Journal of the Association for Psychological Science, 7*(6), 1319–1329. https://doi.org/10.1177/2167702619858430

National Network of Child Psychiatry Access Programs [NNCPAP]. (2023). *Integrating physical and behavioral health care for every child*. https://www.nncpap.org/

Office of the Surgeon General. (2021). *Protecting youth mental health: The U.S. Surgeon General's Advisory*. U.S. Department of Health and Human Services. https://www.hhs.gov/sites/default/files/surgeon-general-youth-mental-health-advisory.pdf

Office of the Surgeon General. (2023). *Our epidemic of loneliness and isolation: The U.S. surgeon General's advisory on the healing effects of social connection and community*. U.S. Department of Health and Human Services. https://www.hhs.gov/sites/default/files/surgeon-general-social-connection-advisory.pdf

Oliveira, J. M. D., Butini, L., Pauletto, P., Lehmkuhl, K. M., Stefani, C. M., Bolan, M., Guerra, E., Dick, B., De Luca Canto, G., & Massignan, C. (2022). Mental health effects prevalence in children and adolescents during the COVID-19 pandemic: A systematic review. *Worldviews on Evidence-Based Nursing, 19*(2), 130–137. https://doi.org/10.1111/wvn.12566

Pediatric Nursing Certification Board. (n.d.). *Pediatric primary care mental health specialist (PMHS)*. Retrieved from https://www.pnch.org/pmhs

Perou, R., Bitsko, R. H., Blumberg, S. J., Pastor, P., Ghandour, R. M., Gfroerer, J. C., Hedden, S. L., Crosby, A. E., Visser, S. N., Schieve, L. A., Parks, S. E., Hall, J. E., Brody, D., Simile, C. M., Thompson, W. W., Baio, J., Avenevoli, S., Kogan, M. D., Huang, L. N., & Centers for Disease Control and Prevention (CDC). (2013). Mental health surveillance among children—United States, 2005–2011. *MMWR Supplements, 62*(2), 1–35.

Pfefferbaum, B., Simic, Z., & North, C. S. (2018). Parent-reported child reactions to the September 11, 2001, World Trade Center attacks in relation to parent post-disaster psychopathology three years after the event. *Prehospital and Disaster Medicine, 33*(5), 558–564. https://doi.org/10.1017/S1049023X18000869

Radhakrishnan, L., Leeb, R. T., Bitsko, R. H., Carey, K., Gates, A., Holland, K. M., Hartnett, K. P., Kite-Powell, A., DeVies, J., Smith, A. R., van Santen, K. L., Crossen, S., Sheppard, M., Wotiz, S., Lane, R. I., Njai, R., Johnson, A. G., Winn, A., Kirking, H. L., Rodgers, L., Thomas, C. W., Soetebier, K., Adjemian, J., & Anderson, K. N. (2022). Pediatric emergency department visits associated with mental health conditions before and during the COVID-19 pandemic—United States, January 2019–January 2022. *Morbidity and Mortality Weekly Report, 71*(8), 319–324. https://doi.org/10.15585/mmwr.mm7108e2

Shannon, H., Bush, K., Villeneuve, P. J., Hellemans, K. G., & Guimond, S. (2022). Problematic social media use in adolescents and young adults: Systematic review and meta-analysis. *JMIR Mental Health, 9*(4), e33450. https://doi.org/10.2196/33450

Shaver, J. (2022). The state of telehealth before and after the COVID-19 pandemic. *Primary Care, 49*(4), 517–530. https://doi.org/10.1016/j.pop.2022.04.002

Spitzer, R. L., Kroenke, K., Williams, J. B., & Löwe, B. (2006). A brief measure for assessing generalized anxiety disorder: The GAD-7. *Archives of Internal Medicine, 166*(10), 1092–1097. https://doi.org/10.1001/archinte.166.10.1092

Substance Abuse and Mental Health Services Administration. (2023). *988 lifeline performance metrics*. https://www.samhsa.gov/find-help/988/performance-metrics

Swanson, J. M., Kraemer, H. C., Hinshaw, S. P., Arnold, L. E., Conners, C. K., Abikoff, H. B., Clevenger, W., Davies, M., Elliott, G. R., Greenhill, L. L., Hechtman, L., Hoza, B., Jensen, P. S., March, J. S., Newcorn, J. H., Owens, E. B., Pelham, W. E., Schiller, E., Severe, J. B., Simpson, S., Simpson, S., Vitiello, B., Wells, K., Wigal, T., & Wu, M. (2001). Clinical relevance of the primary findings of the MTA: Success rates based on severity of ADHD and ODD symptoms at the end of treatment. *Journal of the American Academy of Child and Adolescent Psychiatry, 40*(2), 168–179. https://doi.org/10.1097/00004583-200102000-00011

Uscher-Pines, L., McCullough, C., Dworsky, M. S., Sousa, J., Predmore, Z., Ray, K., Magit, A., Rivanis, C., Lerner, C., Iwakoshi, J., Barkley, S., Marcin, J. P., McGuire, T., Browne, M. A., Swanson, C., Cleary, J. P., Kelly, E., Layton, K., & Schulson, L. (2022). Use of telehealth across pediatric subspecialties before and during the COVID-19 pandemic. *JAMA Network Open, 5*(3), e224759. https://doi.org/10.1001/jamanetworkopen.2022.4759

Van Orden, K. A., Witte, T. K., Cukrowicz, K. C., Braithwaite, S. R., Selby, E. A., & Joiner, T. E. (2010). The interpersonal theory of suicide. *Psychological Review, 117*(2), 575–600. https://doi.org/10.1037/a0018697

Wacks, Y., & Weinstein, A. M. (2021). Excessive smartphone use is associated with health problems in adolescents and young adults. *Frontiers in Psychiatry, 12*, 669042. https://doi.org/10.3389/fpsyt.2021.669042

Walter, H. J., Vernacchio, L., Correa, E. T., Bromberg, J., Goodman, E., Barton, J., Young, G. J., DeMaso, D. R., & Focht, G. (2021). Five-phase replication of behavioral health integration in pediatric primary care. *Pediatrics, 148*(2), e2020001073. https://doi.org/10.1542/peds.2020-001073

Whaley, G. L., & Pfefferbaum, B. (2023). Parental challenges during the COVID-19 pandemic: Psychological outcomes and risk and protective factors. *Current Psychiatry Reports, 25*(4), 165–174. https://doi.org/10.1007/s11920-023-01412-0

Whitney, D. G., & Peterson, M. (2019). US national and state-level prevalence of mental health disorders and disparities of mental health care use in children. *JAMA Pediatrics, 173*(4), 389–391. https://doi.org/10.1001/jamapediatrics.2018.5399

Wissow, L. S., van Ginneken, N., Chandna, J., & Rahman, A. (2016). Integrating children's mental health into primary care. *Pediatric Clinics of North America, 63*(1), 97–113. https://doi.org/10.1016/j.pcl.2015.08.005

Wolicki, S. B., Bitsko, R. H., Cree, R. A., Danielson, M. L., Ko, J. Y., Warner, L., & Robinson, L. R. (2021). Mental health of parents and primary caregivers by sex and associated child health indicators. *Adversity and Resilience Science, 2*(2), 125–139. https://doi.org/10.1007/s42844-021-00037-7

Wolraich, M. L., Bard, D. E., Neas, B., Doffing, M., & Beck, L. (2013). The psychometric properties of the Vanderbilt attention-deficit hyperactivity disorder diagnostic teacher rating scale in a community population. *Journal of Developmental and Behavioral Pediatrics, 34*(2), 83–93. https://doi.org/10.1097/DBP.0b013e31827d55c3

Loades, Elma E., Chatburn, E., Higson-Sweeney, N., Reynolds, S., Shafran, R., Brigden, A., Linney, C., McManus, M. N., Borwick, C., Crawley, E. (2020), Rapid Systematic Review: The Impact of Social Isolation and Loneliness on the Mental Health of Children and Adolescents in the Context of COVID-19. *Academy of Child and Adolescent Psychiatry*. doi: 10.1016/j.jaac.2020.05.009.

Mroczek, B., Kurpas, D., Gronowska, P. G., Kotwas, A., Karakiewicz, B. A., Jurczak, I. R. (2020), The Interpersonal Theory of Suicide. *Psychological Review*, 117(2), 575-600. doi: 10.1037/a0018697.

Wong, S. S., Wong, C. A. M. (2021), Intervention and telephone line to mental health problems in adolescents and young adults. *Psychiatry and Psychology*. C. *Mental Disorders* 2020, 256-265.

Vaccine-Preventable Diseases: COVID-19 and Global Impacts on Routine Immunization

Mary Koslap-Petraco

> *How wonderful it is that nobody wait a single moment before starting to improve the world.*
>
> —Anne Frank

Introduction and Background

If history is any predictor of the future, introduction of the COVID-19 vaccine was expected to be celebrated by the public as the harbinger of the end of the pandemic. In past communicable disease outbreaks, lines formed around the block with people eagerly awaiting vaccination. Most notably in recent memory is the introduction of the polio vaccine in 1955. In the 1940s and 1950s, polio caused approximately 3500 people per year to become disabled, most of them children. This era in American history largely occurred in the shadow of the presidency of a widely admired president, Franklin Delanore Roosevelt, who himself had been in a wheelchair after suffering the effects of polio. Shortly after introduction of the polio vaccine, a disaster at Cutter Laboratories resulted in an errantly activated polio vaccine being administered to nearly 200,000 children with 40,000 cases of polio ensuing and 200 children experiencing paralysis, and ten experiencing death. Despite the tragedy, public confidence in the vaccine did not waver, largely overshadowed by the tremendous threat of illness, disability, and death caused by the polio virus (Brink, 2021). Vaccines are widely acknowledged as the greatest medical miracle of modern medicine in the twentieth century with life-threatening diseases like smallpox being eradicated and many others eliminated in large part to public collectivism and cooperation. Vaccination success depends on a social contract for which the fabric is currently eroding in a broader context of anti-globalization, pro-nationalism, and popularity of populism. Vaccines can, as they have in the past, serve as a form of

M. Koslap-Petraco (✉)
Stony Brook University School of Nursing, Stony Brook, NY, USA
e-mail: mary.koslap-petraco@stonybrookunivesity.edu

J. L. Peck (ed.), *COVID-19 Impacts on Child Health*,
https://doi.org/10.1007/978-3-031-80369-7_8

diplomacy to keep a fundamental level of global and local cooperation alive and well (Gellin, 2020).

Immediately following the initial launch of the COVID-19 vaccination program, vaccine resistance and hesitancy increased dramatically, not only for the COVID-19 vaccine but also as a broader response to vaccination. Routine childhood vaccine rates dropped for a multitude of reasons. Not only were families missing routine child health visits because of disruption in physical and logistical service provisions related to altered office norms for mitigation of infectious disease spread, but some families were afraid to go to their healthcare provider (HCP) offices for fear of COVID-19 transmission. Increasingly, parents showed increasing hesitation for routine vaccines and with rising questions about vaccination in general (Santoli et al., 2020).

Vaccines are the most significant public health achievement of the twentieth century (Centers for Disease Control and Prevention, 1999). Vaccines save lives and have contributed to increasing life expectancy over the last century. Vaccination opportunity exists across the lifespan, with more opportunities for adult immunization in recent years with vaccines now available for shingles and pneumococcal disease. In some ways, vaccines have become victims of their own success as public fear of disease transmission diminishes in the face of rising fear of vaccine-related injury or illness. In the wake of the COVID-19 pandemic, life expectancy has decreased, with particularly concerning health disparities for communities of color (Andrasfay & Goldman, 2021). Prevention of morbidity and mortality related to vaccine-preventable disease will be a critical component of public health efforts moving forward.

Misinformation proliferates within online social networks, where neighborhood groups, wellness communities, and other virtual groups nurture connections for like-minded individuals. In these digital spaces, politicization occurs among implementation of public health measures, ranging from orderly discussions of personal rights to extreme conspiracy theories built on conjecture and mis- or disinformation. Emerging in the wake of COVID-19 is broadly increasing opposition to government implementation of public health measures, dismissing or denying morbidity and mortality associated with the COVID-19 pandemic, and growing hesitation to adopt vaccine recommendations issued by governmental and health organizations (Wilson & Wiysonge, 2020).

Understanding the threat posed by anti-vaccination efforts on social media is critically important. Some organized campaigns have been traced to foreign pseudo-state actors promoting anti-vaccination content on social media from abroad. Within the United States, the use of social media to organize offline action often promotes the message that vaccinations are inherently unsafe, with such beliefs mounting as more formal organization occurs on social media. Foreign disinformation campaigns online are associated with a drop in mean vaccination coverage over time and increased negative discussion of vaccines on social media. A one-point shift upwards in the five-point disinformation scale is associated with a two-percentage point drop in mean vaccination coverage year over year and a 15% increase in negative social media posts on certain platforms about vaccines. The need for discussion surrounding ethical procedures for coordinated action removing vaccine disinformation from social media platforms and moderating vaccine misinformation while also fostering open and transparent communication is imperative. Coordinated action against the sources of intentional anti-vaccination disinformation campaigns abroad must be addressed in light of the substantial relationship between foreign disinformation campaigns and declining vaccination coverage (Rauhala, 2020).

Personal decision-making surrounding vaccines is often emotional, encompassing a wide range of feelings such as fear, anxiety, confusion, confidence, optimism, satisfaction, and passion. Vaccine hesitancy is not a symptom of public ignorance, but often of mistrust—a lesson that applies to the challenges of vaccination for COVID-19 as well as other vaccines. Fear is the neglected dimension of health in terms of actually characterizing it, studying it, and recognizing how it can help inform not just communication efforts but how engagement and interaction between HCPs with patients and their families are better served from a perspective of empathy. Fear is not an emotion to be "righted" in a clinical sense. Providers need to share credible information in the context of therapeutic communication (Hall, 2021).

All healthcare professions have an important role in vaccination efforts. By virtue of the nature of their profession, nurses have an advantage in vaccine advocacy for themselves, their patients, and their communities. Nursing is consistently ranked as the most trusted of all professions (Saad, 2020). The public generally trusts education provided by nurses, who are skilled in therapeutic communication delivered with respect and empathy. They are also the largest healthcare workforce in the world and generally have the most face-to-face time in patient encounters. Nurses have a professional capacity to clarify misinformation about vaccines, counter disinformation with credible sources of information, provide evidence-based education, and help families understand the risks and benefits to make informed decisions with reputable recommendations on vaccination as their guide to optimize the health and longevity of their families (Koslap-Petraco, 2022).

Points of Care

Historical Perspective of Anti-vaccine Sentiments

Although vaccine hesitancy may seem like a newly emerging topic for some, fear of vaccines dates back to at least the eighteenth century. Vaccines were previously seen as an attempt to oppose God's punishments upon man for his sins. Early arguments against vaccination included philosophical and moral opposition to derivation from animal sources. There was growing mistrust of the medical establishment, and public perceptions of violations against personal liberty because of governmental entities enacting mandatory vaccinations. Recent history recounts opposition to smallpox vaccination in the United States with false claims of vaccination causing syphilis, typhoid, and tuberculosis. Smallpox existed as one of the most deadly communicable diseases, with eighteenth century outbreaks in cities like Boston infecting half the population and killing close to one in five persons. Opponents characterized smallpox vaccination as unethical exploitation of the poor rather than an effort in alleviating the suffering and death of thousands. However, mass vaccination efforts continued and by 1972 smallpox vaccination was ended after the disease was successfully eradicated in the United States and by 1980 it was eradicated from the world with no naturally occurring infections occurring since (Durbach, 2000; Wolfe & Sharpe, 2002). In 1998, former British physician Andrew Wakefield recommended further investigation of a possible relationship between bowel disease, autism, and the Measles-Mumps-Rubella (MMR) vaccine. Although the study was widely and rapidly discredited, retracted by the Lancet after publication, and renounced by the other study authors after serious ethical misconduct was credibly brought to light and resulted in Wakefield's license being revoked, the damage was done. Measles vaccination rates in England plummeted in the aftermath. The United States even experienced a 2% decline in measles, mumps, and rubella vaccination from 1999 to 2000. Despite reams of credible research to the contrary involving millions of children, public perceptions and fears about vaccines and autism remain with persisting impacts in vaccination rates (Deer, 2011; Hussain et al., 2018).

As opposition to COVID-19 vaccination began to emerge, popular public citations included a pamphlet originally published by Canadian physician to voice opposition to vaccination in the midst of the deadly smallpox epidemic of 1885 in Montreal. In the first 5 weeks of that particular outbreak nearly 1400 Canadians died of smallpox, with about 90% of those victims being children under the age of 10 years old. Old arguments were recycled to counter new public health threats associated with COVID-19. Vaccination was met with public skepticism over the potential for pharmaceutical company profits. However, prominent anti-vaccine activists and organizations face similar accusations of exploiting the public for financial profit (Larson, 2020; Vincent, 2022; Zadrozny, 2022). The reports of anti-vaccine advocate funding success underscores how lucrative the pandemic may have been for a handful of individuals and groups facing allegations of spreading health misinformation and undermining public faith in vaccines (Zadrozny, 2022).

Other communities in both the United States and around the world have been affected by the deliberate introduction of false information (disinformation, see chapter "Disinfodemic: Responding to Rising Misinformation") into the community, often resulting in outbreaks of vaccine-preventable diseases. In Minnesota, child vaccination rates for MMR in a Somalian community plummeted from 92% in 2004 to 42% in 2014 amid fears that Somali children had inequitably high rates of autism. These concerns attracted the attention of anti-vaccine activists, who held several meetings with Somali community groups in Minnesota in 2010–2011 (Dyer, 2017). In another instance, a handbook was anonymously authored by a group called Parents Educating and Advocating for Children's Health (PEACH) with an intended audience of ultra-Orthodox Jews, whose expanding and insular community was at the epicenter of one of the largest measles outbreaks in the United States in decades in Brooklyn and Rockland County, just outside New York City beginning in 2018. The PEACH book claimed vaccines contain monkey, rat, and pig DNA as well as cow-serum blood, all of which are forbidden for consumption according to kosher dietary law. Vaccines are often grown in a broth of animal cells, but the final product is highly purified. Although the PEACH book cited a few very well-known rabbis who expressed vaccine opposition, most prominent ultra-Orthodox rabbis view vaccines as kosher and urge observant Jews to be immunized (Page, 2019).

The parents of 24,000 children in northern Pakistan refused to allow health workers to administer polio vaccinations in 2007, with fears stemming from rumors that the vaccine was an American plot to sterilize innocent Muslim children (Polio cases jump in Pakistan as clerics declare vaccination an American plot, 2007). Female polio workers and a police officer were killed in Pakistan and Afghanistan, leading to a decrease in the number of women who are willing to work in vaccination programs (Gunmen, 2022; UN condemns, 2022). Russian internet bots and trolls spread malware and unsolicited content to disseminate antivaccine messages that promoted discord. Accounts masquerading as legitimate users created false equivalency, eroding public consensus on vaccination (Broniatowski et al., 2018). These are just a few examples of the many cases of anti-vaccine sentiment and occurrence, which have untold impacts of child morbidity and mortality.

Development of COVID-19 Vaccines

Vaccine development has always been a years' long process from inception to final approval and implementation. Polio virus was successfully cultivated in human tissue in 1949, leading to the development of the first successful polio vaccine created by US physician Jonas Salk. Dr. Salk tested his experimental killed-virus vaccine on himself and his family in 1953, and 1 year later on 1.6 million children in Canada, Finland, and the United States. The encouraging results were announced on April 12, 1955, and Salk's inactivated polio vaccine (IPV) was licensed on the same day. There was a span of 7 years between the cultivation of the polio virus to the licensing of the vaccine (World Health Organization, 2023).

The dramatic effects of the COVID-19 pandemic and the horrific loss of life and dire effects on the population not just in America but throughout the entire world raised the issue of how fast a safe and effective vaccine could be responsibly produced. The Biomedical Advanced Research and Development Authority (BARDA), the World Health Organization (WHO), and the Gates Foundation gave billions of dollars toward developing a safe and effective COVID-19 vaccine faster than the world ever thought possible. The US government diminished business risks associated with vaccine development for the pharmaceutical industry by financing phase 3 trials and mass production of the vaccine. The project became known as "Operation Warp Speed." COVID-19 vaccines still needed to go through three distinct trial phases, just as had occurred with previous vaccine development. Phase 1 begins with 20–100 healthy volunteers. This phase looks for safety, effectiveness, serious side effects, and dose-related side effects. If Phase 1 trials are successful, the vaccine is subjected to Phase 2 trials in which several hundred volunteers are enrolled. Phase 2 looks for the most common short-term side effects and how the volunteers' immune systems react to the vaccine. If Phase 2 trials are successful, then the vaccine moves to Phase 3, which requires thousands of participants. In the case of COVID-19 vaccine, roughly 30,000 participants were enrolled in Phase 3 trials (Offit, 2019a). In the case of COVID-19 vaccination, for the first time, these three trial phases were staggered and overlapped each other rather than occurring separately and distinctly, with one phase ending before the next phase commenced. In December of 2020, just 1 year after the pandemic onset, the Federal Drug Administration (FDA) issued an emergency use authorization (EUA) after verifying the vaccine met statutory clearance criterion encompassing both safety and efficacy (Food and Drug Administration [FDA], 2021). The Advisory Committee for Immunization Practices (ACIP) is a group of medical and public health experts who make recommendations for vaccine administration to the CDC and the Secretary of Health and Human Services. Each year, this guidance culminates in annual updates to the CDC vaccine schedule, which is then reviewed by professional organizations including the American Academy of Pediatrics (AAP), American Academy of Family Practitioners (FAAP), National Association of Pediatric Nurse Practitioners (NAPNAP), and the American College of Nurse Midwives (ACNM), among others, who independently review the CDC schedule and determine organizational endorsement that the vaccine benefits outweigh risks and should be administered in selected populations, dosing, and schedule as recommended (Offit, 2019b). Parents and patients can feel confident in the rigorous process to develop, test, and license vaccines that are recommended in the United States. In the case of COVID-19 vaccination, expedited clinical trials resulted in the same three phases of pre-licensure studies, followed by FDA vaccine licensure, ACIP recommendations, and organizational endorsement and/or affirmation before arriving at the point of administration to the general public. However, public skepticism on the speed of vaccine development and perceptions of cutting corners and sacrificing safety resounded in the public square with many entities lamenting in hindsight naming the project "Operation Warp Speed." Rather than being received by the public as a monumental scientific achievement, the name instead fueled public perception of pursuing speed over safety and scientific rigor, particularly in light of public unfamiliarity with mRNA vaccine technology (Hutto, 2024).

Vaccine Safety

Vaccines must be considered both safe and effective to justify recommendations for widespread public administration. The United States has a vigorous program to regulate and monitor vaccine safety.

Vaccine safety monitoring programs in the United States include the following:

- Vaccine Adverse Event Reporting System (VAERS): a national safety surveillance program that serves an early warning system to monitor vaccine safety post-FDA authorization and licensure; co-managed by the CDC and FDA; anyone can make a report; reports do not prove causation; patterns of events or serious singular events warrant initiate further investigation.

- Vaccine Safety Datalink (VSD): a collaboration between the CDC and 13 healthcare organizations that act as data-providing sites or subject matter expertise; uses electronic health data to monitor vaccine safety, conducts research and safety studies based on alerts emerging from VAERS.
- V-safe: a safety monitoring system operated by the CDC that allows vaccine recipients to share their post-vaccine experience with personalized, confidential health check-ins; started in December 2020 for COVID vaccination, expanded to include mpox and RSV; >10 million participants contributing >151 million health surveys since launch.
- Clinical Immunization Safety Assessment (CISA) Project: started in 2001 in response to unmet vaccine safety clinical research needs; nationwide collaborative network of vaccine safety experts from the CDC, research centers, and other partners; objective to improve understanding of post-immunization adverse events; HCPs can request consultation from CDC COVIDvax for complex COVID-19 safety questions by calling 800-CDC-INFO.
- COVID-19 Vaccine Pregnancy Registry: a smartphone-based system that uses text messages and personalized health surveys to monitor V-safe participants who reported pregnancy at the time of COVID-19 vaccination or shortly thereafter; closed to new participants in May 2023.
- National Vaccine Injury Compensation Program (NVICP): created by the National Childhood Vaccine Injury Act of 1986; a no-fault alternative to the traditional legal system pathways to provide resolution for vaccine injury petitions; any individual may file a petition within the statute of limitations; not all vaccines are covered.

Misinformation about VAERS in particular has been a point of contention among individuals and communities expressing vaccine concerns. VAERS accepts and analyzes reports of adverse events after a person has received a vaccination. Anyone can report an adverse event to VAERS. Healthcare professionals are required to report certain adverse events, and vaccine manufacturers are required to report all adverse events that come to their attention. VAERS is a passive reporting system, meaning it relies on individuals to send in reports of their experiences to the CDC and the FDA. VAERS is not designed to determine if a vaccine caused a health problem but is especially useful for detecting unusual or unexpected patterns of adverse event reporting that might indicate a possible safety problem with a vaccine. This way, VAERS can provide CDC and FDA with valuable information that additional work and evaluation are necessary to further assess a possible safety concern (Vaccine Adverse Event Reporting System, n.d.). However, VAERS data is often informally cited equating inclusion of unverified reports to actual incidence and prevalence.

The available evidence supports overall safety of the routine childhood vaccination schedule. Existing federal vaccine safety surveillance systems are robust and responsive to concerns expressed by parents of young children. The 2013 Institute of Medicine (IOM) Report on the immunization schedule suggested a new field of study to examine cumulative, repeated exposures to vaccines and vaccine ingredients and long-term health outcomes. At the time of IOM Report, few studies of the safety of the schedule "as a whole" had been published. Over time, the evidence accumulated around specific testable hypotheses, which can be communicated to parents by HCPs. The general benefits of vaccination strongly outweigh known and potential risks (Daly, 2023).

In recent years, parental concern about the growing number of recommended vaccines has increased with fears that simultaneous administration of multiple vaccines could overwhelm or weaken the immune system or be dangerous in some way. Rigorous, peer-reviewed scientific research concludes that there is no significant difference in cumulative vaccine antigen exposure and the likelihood of Emergency Department (ED) or inpatient encounters for infections not covered by routine vaccination. This same review also noted that there is no evidence that the current schedule as recommended by the CDC "overwhelms" the immune system (Glanz et al., 2018). Still other studies found that vaccines were not associated with an increased risk of Type I diabetes mellitus (DMI). An interesting finding actually noted a decreased risk of DMI with higher vaccine aluminum exposure, but the investigators believe that more study is needed to refute or replicate this finding (Alessandrini et al., 2020; Goullé et al., 2020; Hogenesch, 2012; Sastry et al., 2017).

Because there is a considerable amount of public interest in aluminum as a preservative in vaccines, another large study looked at children with and without eczema and a positive correlation was noted on primary analysis, but a secondary review noted positive associations in some but not all cases. This study had more strengths. It was a large sample with a deliberate process and extensive feedback using Vaccine Safety Datalink (VSD) data with sophisticated analyses. The study did have limitations. There were no data on dietary/environmental aluminum exposure (although little to none of ingested aluminum is absorbed according to a recent AAP report). There were also no data on social determinants of health, unmeasured confounding, or antigen effects (Daley et al., 2023). A new larger cohort study in the VSD was conducted with a longer follow-up time. Aluminum exposure before 12 months of age was noted in the subjects, and eczema was included as a covariate. The outcome indicated that asthma was diagnosed at a later age (60 through 84 months of age). Asthma diagnosed earlier may represent viral-induced wheezing (not asthma). Other data sources could help assess the relationship between vaccine aluminum exposure and subsequent asthma risk. While recognizing the small effect sizes identified and the potential for residual confounding, additional investigation of this hypothesis appears warranted (Daley et al., 2023).

Vaccine Hesitancy

Vaccine hesitancy, fueled in part by misinformation, has resulted in a steady decrease in regular childhood vaccinations in young children throughout the United States. During the 2020–2021 school year, national coverage with state-required vaccines among kindergarten students declined from 95% to approximately 94%. During the 2021–2022 school year, coverage decreased again to approximately 93% for all state-required vaccines. Although 2.6% of kindergartners had an exemption for at least one vaccine, an additional 4.4% who did not have an exemption were not up-to-date with MMR vaccination (Erratum, 2023; Seither et al., 2023). These data are alarming. Herd immunity against measles requires about 95% of a population to be vaccinated. Although a one-point percentage drop may seem small, with approximately 72 million children in the United States, these statistics represent a substantial number and concern for future outbreak is real (World Health Organization (WHO), 2020).

Coinciding with the COVID-19 outbreak, an upsurge of social movements gave outlet for Americans to question authority and traditional sources of expertise. Women pushed back against patriarchy. Environmentalists pushed back against industry. Patients pushed back against HCPs. Rally cries for social justice causes emerged for issues like climate change, gender and reproductive rights, influx of refugee and migrant populations, gun violence, food insecurity, homelessness, poverty, and police violence. Some well-organized movements became well-recognized including the #MeToo Movement and Black Lives Matter. As the vaccine schedule and its enforcement expanded, a growing number of parents amid other social movements of the day pushed back against required vaccines and joined a growing anti-vax movement (Conis, 2023).

There is a difference between vaccine hesitancy and vaccine resistance. Vaccine hesitancy refers to delay in acceptance or refusal of vaccination despite availability of vaccination services. Vaccine hesitancy is complex and context specific, varying across time, place, and vaccines. It is influenced by factors referred to as the 3C's: complacency, convenience, and confidence (MacDonald, Noni E, and SAGE Working Group on Vaccine Hesitancy, 2015). Vaccine hesitant parents or individuals often have many questions and if those questions are addressed in a respectful manner, the parent or individual is more likely to choose vaccination and to feel confident about their decision-making. Persons who refuse vaccines, also sometimes referred to as vaccine resistors in the United States, do not share a singular unifying outlook or ideology and refuse for a wide variety of reasons but are most commonly grouped in one of four categories: (1) religious reasons; (2) personal beliefs or philosophical reasons, (3) safety concerns, and/or (4) dissatisfaction with current questions being answered (McKeem & Bohannon, 2016). One commonality, however, is that most parents and families are subject to a confusing mix of sometimes contradictory information and misinformation about vaccines and vaccine safety (Larson & Mnookin, 2016). Vaccine resistant individuals will continue to refuse vaccines despite best efforts of HCPs. However, HCPs should continue to respectfully bring up a discussion of vaccines at each medical encounter to ensure families have fully informed consent on their decisions.

Addressing vaccine hesitancy is a key strategy for increasing vaccination rates and reducing health care disparities. Healthcare providers are well equipped to build trust with patients and communities, provide culturally responsive care, and address concerns and misinformation about vaccines (Olson et al., 2020). While HCPs who do not support vaccines are often singularly featured in news stories, data indicate that as a group nurses overwhelmingly support vaccines. Data from a 2021 survey of more than 4500 nurses nationwide conducted by the American Nurses Association (ANA) in conjunction with the COVID Vaccine Facts for Nurses campaign highlights that the majority of nurses support the science of COVID-19 vaccines. According to the survey findings, most nurses (90%) are vaccinated against COVID-19 or plan to get vaccinated and say they are comfortable recommending COVID-19 vaccines (91%) (ANA. NEW SURVEY DATA, 2021). A meta-analysis of 51 studies ($n = 41,098$ nurses) from 36 countries indicated a rate of 20.7% (95% CI = 16.5–27%) COVID-19 vaccine refusal rate. The rates of vaccination refusal were higher from March 2020 to December 2020 compared to the rates from January 2021 to May 2021. The major reasons for COVID-19 vaccine refusal were concerns about vaccine safety, side effects, and efficacy; misinformation and lack of knowledge; and mistrust in experts, authorities, or pharmaceutical companies. The major factors associated with acceptance of the vaccines were male gender, older age, and flu vaccination history. The decrease in refusal rate from 2020 to 2021 indicates that nurses' reasons for refusal were being adequately addressed (Khubchandani et al., 2022). The best way for healthcare leaders to encourage their colleagues to be vaccinated against COVID-19 is to operate from a place of compassion and kindness, conveying sincerely held recommendations emerging not from a place of legal obligation or mandate but of personal care.

Nurses and other HCPs did raise concerns about COVID-19 vaccines, including but not limited to: the research was done too quickly; it wasn't fully FDA-approved (at first); and HCPs already have antibodies from working the front lines of the pandemic or perhaps from getting the virus already. Many were concerned about how the vaccine affects fertility after unfounded conjecture fueled rapidly spreading rumors. In many of these cases, misinformation was shared widely and HCPs are not immune to the detrimental effects. Some HCPs had limited exposure to immunization content in their medical training programs, and some HCPs received their training long before the wave of new vaccine developments and recommendations emerging over the last decade, leaving them feeling ill-prepared to navigate the avalanche of emerging recommendations and evidence (Shivaram, 2021). In some states, high-ranking medical officials, including physicians, issued health guidance recommendations that conflicted with national recommendations. This public conflict likely undermined public trust in public health guidance and recommendations (Tahir, 2022).

Black, indigenous, and other people of color (BIPOC) communities have been disproportionately impacted by health disparities associated with COVID-19 vaccination (Racial and ethnic disparities are discussed in greater detail in chapter "Racism: Assessment of the Impact on Pediatric Holistic Health"). Within the Black community, painful memories of Tuskegee, Henrietta Lacks, and other similar government-sponsored research conducted unethically foster lingering mistrust. Black Americans represent an alarmingly disproportionate number of positive cases and deaths due to COVID-19 with an estimate that 97.9 of every 100,000 died from COVID-19 from March through September of 2020. This mortality rate was one-third higher than Latino populations and more than double for White and Asian populations (Reyes, 2020). Although there was widespread initial mistrust of COVID-19 vaccination recommendations, Black individuals demonstrated larger increases in vaccination intention than White individuals relative to baseline in March 2021. Beliefs that the vaccines are safe and effective were positively associated with vaccination intention. Effective strategies that increased community trust include information that appeared on trusted community platforms, messaging that was authentic and based on ethnic and cultural shared experiences, and experts who looked like members of their own community (Black Doctors Organization, 2020).

Celebrities have historically served as influencers in vaccine efforts. During the polio vaccine campaign, Elvis Presley, "the King of Rock and Roll," publicly received his polio vaccination on national television. The rates among American youth skyrocketed to 80% after just 6 months following this event. Elvis's public act contained three crucial ingredients inherent to many of the most effective behavioral change campaigns: social influence, social norms, and vivid examples. In 2020, stardom and influence are not nearly as concentrated as they were when the King of Rock n' Roll reigned supreme more than 60 years ago (Hershfield & Brody, 2021). However, modern celebrities across multiple media domains were engaged by various commercial and governmental entities as influencers in the COVID-19 vaccine efforts. Empirical analysis demonstrates that influencers do play a significant role in swaying the opinions of their followers, with interactivity and information content being the primary factors. Generating the perception of public demand for vaccines seems to be more efficient and effective than efforts concentrated on generating trust (Wei et al., 2022). More research is needed to study the ethics and impacts of engaging media influence to direct public health behaviors.

Barriers and Breakthroughs

Barriers to successful implementation of immunization programs include the inordinate amount of misinformation circulation, especially through unregulated channels of social media. The overwhelm of information sources generates confusion among the layperson public as well as HCPs. Vaccine hesitancy cannot be underestimated in its influence on vaccine acceptance. Social media has given many people the opportunity to speak their opinions without repercussions while creating coalitions of like-minded people. Over the past two decades, anti-vaccine activism in the United States has evolved from a fringe subculture into an increasingly well-organized and well-financed networked movement with important repercussions for public health. The COVID-19 pandemic exacerbated this evolution and magnified the reach of vaccine misinformation. Anti-vaccine activists, who for many years spoke primarily to niche communities hesitant about childhood vaccinations, have harnessed traditional and social media to amplify vaccine-related mistruths about COVID-19 vaccines while also targeting historically marginalized racial and ethnic communities. These efforts contributed to COVID-19 vaccine hesitancy and expanded the movement, with early indications suggesting this hesitancy could now also be increasing hesitancy that existed pre-pandemic toward other vaccines (Carpiano et al., 2023).

In the years preceding the COVID-19 pandemic, anti-vaccine activism became more visible in the United States. Pre-pandemic, anti-vaccine activists adeptly leveraged social media to shape opinion, gain allies, influence policy, and galvanize political partisanship. Reflecting broader, growing trends in anti-intellectual or anti-science populist discourse, clinicians and other HCPs who were publicly involved in pro-vaccine policy or commentary in advance of the pandemic were subject to harassment, physical threats, and violence by anti-vaccine activists (Carpiano et al., 2023). Although anti-vaccine activism was already increasing in the United States and internationally, the 2020 emergence of COVID-19 served as an accelerant, helping turn a niche movement into a more powerful force. Whereas earlier anti-vaccine activism focused primarily on parents and school immunization requirements, the universal nature of the COVID-19 pandemic provided anti-vaccine activists with concerned audiences that were far larger and broader. As the pandemic unfolded, anti-vaccine activists capitalized on discontent over pandemic measures such as physical distancing, school closures, and vaccine and mask mandates, joining politically affiliated groups, elected officials, and even religious leaders in opposing public health interventions via appeals to health liberty, and downplaying the severity of COVID-19 (Bergengruen, 2022; McWhinney, 2022).

Lack of financial resources may not be the primary barrier, as previously perceived, especially since the implementation of the Vaccines for Children (VFC) program established in 1994. VFC was established to provide vaccines to children whose parents or guardians are not be able to afford them. Vaccines available through the VFC Program are those recommended by the Advisory Committee on Immunization Practices. Inadequate access to healthcare (including inconvenient and limited clinic hours), lack of reliable transportation and childcare, inability to get time off from work to have children immunized, language barriers, and the absence of a reminder system for missed vaccinations all are current contributors to disparities in childhood vaccination (Kulkarni et al., 2021).

The other challenges noted previously mainly involve availability of vaccines. Vaccine hesitancy, however, is a matter of attitudes. Hesitancy toward vaccines creates reluctance toward or refusal of vaccines, even when available, as the result of complacency, inconvenience, or doubt about their effectiveness. This issue was one of the World Health Organization's top 10 threats to global health in 2019. The choice not to vaccinate may seem small, but it can have big implications on global health. Between 2016 and 2019, cases of measles increased by over 200% globally. This includes countries where the disease was close to elimination, partially as the result of hesitancy (Alexander, 2020). In the first quarter of 2024, at least 125 cases of measles across 17 states had been reported, more cases than were reported in all of 2022 (the most current prior year with measles outbreaks in the United States). The number of measles cases globally doubled from 2022 to 2023 to more than

320,000 cases. This poses a real and current threat to the previously acquired elimination status, a shocking step backward from such a momentous and historic public health achievement (Tin, 2024).

Distance from an urban health center or living in a rural area is not the only challenge for children accessing vaccination. An increasing number of children in urban areas is unable to access vaccines. Limited or nonexistent public services can prevent people in these communities from accessing vaccines in the context of political and social neglect. Fragility also poses a challenge to vaccination. In areas where people face displacement due to conflict, natural disasters, or humanitarian crises, providing vaccination becomes even more difficult. This is especially troubling when considering that fragility can make diseases more prevalent. In areas where health systems are nonexistent or difficult to access, it is more difficult for people to receive any sort of medical care, let alone vaccines (Alexander, 2020). Supply must be sufficient for demand. Vaccine shortages have waxed and waned over the last several decades. Even when there is adequate vaccine supply, making sure that other resources are in place to effectively store and transport them is also a challenge, which was particularly relevant to the specialized freezer capacity and storage needs for COVID-19 vaccines, especially when transported, prepared, and administered in mass vaccination sites often occurring in public parks and other spaces ill-equipped for specialized storage (Alexander, 2020).

Breakthroughs must be innovative to ensure that all children everywhere are offered the opportunity to be fully protected from vaccine-preventable disease-related morbidity and mortality. Building a network of trusted community health workers is essential to combatting hesitancy. When community health workers are available with credible information, communities are more receptive to listening to what they perceive as a credible source in vaccine decision-making. Vaccines deliver an unrivalled return on investment; and every dollar spent on vaccination delivers a return on investment of US $26. Innovative financing solutions are a key catalyst for this step change and offer essential opportunities to maximize returns and pursue new and diversified sources of funding (Alexander, 2020).

A total of 67 million children missed out on vaccinations between 2019 and 2021, with vaccination coverage down in 112 countries. The alarming data on global immunization is part of a slate of urgent issues highlighted in *The State of the World's Children 2023: For Every Child, Vaccination*, released by UNICEF. The report highlights the largest sustained backslide in childhood immunization coverage in 30 years—fueled by the COVID-19 pandemic—and presents a clear agenda of concrete recommendations to ensure every child, everywhere has access to care to be vaccinated and to strengthen global primary health care systems for present and future challenges. The use of new technologies and modern approaches for timelier, more granular data, as well as a range of innovations in high-quality and fit-for-purpose data for targeted action can help identify unimmunized and under-immunized children (Alexander, 2020).

Meeting vaccination challenges in conflict, emergency, and fragile settings requires focus and investment in innovative and inventive solutions—from vaccines with longer shelf-lives to logistical breakthroughs in drone deliveries with digital and mobile money systems for supporting and paying HCPs. For the long-term, smart, sustainable innovations are key to systems that are both future-friendly and future-proof—ensuring resilience and responsiveness to new outbreaks, as well as the unfolding challenges of conflict, crisis, and climate change. Novel technologies such as solar-powered cold chains, heat-resistant vaccines, and micro-array patches can ensure vaccine access for communities in the toughest settings, and digitalization of data for stock management and supply chains can protect and strengthen supply chains at local, regional, and global levels (Alexander, 2020).

Public perception and confidence in the importance of vaccines for children declined during the pandemic. Innovative, people-centered approaches in social listening, community engagement, and caregiver support—especially with a lens considerate of gender gaps, barriers, and roles—are fundamental to understanding and shaping attitudes on immunization and health services. The Office of Innovation, together with UNICEF Innocentia and the Regional Office for Europe and Central Asia, is collaborating on the innovative use of behavioral insights (BI) to identify, understand, and tackle vaccine hesitancy and immunization uptake for a range of preventable diseases (Alexander, 2020).

Lessons Learned

A look back at the beginning of the COVID-19 pandemic provides the opportunity to learn from past efforts. The effects of social media have caused incalculable harm to the credibility of immunizations and the Public Health System yet also present great opportunity to be effectively leveraged by the healthcare community. Although most HCPs are reticent to engage on social media, it is what the public is demanding and the absence of credible presence leaves opportunity for ill-informed or ill-intended influencers and entrepreneurs to fill the gap. The best constructed vaccine administration programs are useless without public confidence. As the most trusted profession, the largest healthcare workforce in the world, and the clinical discipline with the most face-to-face interaction with patients for vaccine administration, nurses in particular are well-equipped to address the questions of the public. Nurses' voices need to be adequately represented across all levels of healthcare organization and government when it comes to vaccine communication. Evidence-based strategies need to be implemented in healthcare systems worldwide to increase the uptake of vaccines among HCPs and their patients to ensure the nurses' safety and the safety of their patients and community members (Koslap-Petraco, 2022).

Calls to Action

1. All HCPs need to seek education, resources, and professional development opportunities to increase knowledge and expertise while conducting patient encounters with empathy and respect. (One such resource is the CDC's *Epidemiology and Prevention of Vaccine-Preventable Diseases* course, known as the "Pink Book Course") (Koslap-Petraco, 2022).

2. Develop networked communities capable of reaching the public at the right time, at the right place, and with the right messenger about vaccine-related information—especially to pre-empt well-funded and amplified messages fueled by mis- and disinformation. Solicit input from outside the usual public health agencies to effectively counter the array of expanded efforts by anti-vaccine activists and groups or individuals who influence or monetize disinformation efforts, which necessitates a wide breadth of expertise. Networked and coordinated credible communities need to be leveraged to counter relevant trends in anti-vaccine efforts. This action includes mitigating anti-vaccine activist harassment of public health communicators (Carpiano et al., 2023).

3. Routine primary care visits and back-to-school appointments are an opportune time for HCPs to recommend routine vaccination for children and adolescents, which can provide protection against infectious diseases within childcare or school systems and communities (CDC, 2022). However, every healthcare encounter should be leveraged as an opportunity to provide immunization education and check for any current vaccine recommendations.

References

Alessandrini, F., et al. (2020). Mimicking antigen-driven asthma in rodent models-how close can we get? *Frontiers in Immunology, 11*, 575936.

Alexander, A. (2020, March 3). *Five vaccine challenges you need to know*. ONE Blog. Retrieved July 01, 2023, from https://www.one.org/international/blog/5-vaccination-challenges/

ANA. NEW SURVEY DATA. (2021, August 18). *Nurses recommend COVID-19 vaccines and support mandates and boosters if recommended*. Retrieved May 26, 2023, from https://www.nursingworld.org/news/news-releases/2021/ew-survey-data%2D%2Dnurses-recommend-covid-19-vaccines/

Andrasfay, T., & Goldman, N. (2021). Reductions in 2020 US life expectancy due to COVID-19 and the disproportionate impact on the black and Latino populations. *Proceedings of the National Academy of Sciences of the United States of America, 118*(5), e2014746118. https://doi.org/10.1073/pnas.2014746118

Bergengruen, V. (2022, January 26). *How the anti-vax movement is taking over the right*. Time. Retrieved July 01, 2023, from https://time.com/6141699/anti-vaccine-mandate-movement-rally/

Black Doctors Organization. (2020, August 18). *BDO survey: 58% of African Americans say they won't take COVID-19 vaccine*. Retrieved June 30, 2023, from https://www.prnews-wire.com/news-releases/bdo-survey-58-of-african-americans-say-they-wont-take-covid-19-vaccine-301113496.html

Brink, S. (2021, May 3). *Can't help falling in love with a vaccine: How polio campaign beat vaccine hesitancy*. NPR. https://www.npr.org/sections/health-shots/2021/05/03/988756973/cant-help-falling-in-love-with-a-vaccine-how-polio-campaign-beat-vaccine-hesitan

Broniatowski, D. A., et al. (2018). Weaponized health communication: Twitter bots and Russian trolls amplify the vaccine debate. *American Journal of Public Health, 108*(10), 1378–1384. https://doi.org/10.2105/AJPH.2018.304567

Carpiano, R. M., et al. (2023). Confronting the evolution and expansion of anti-vaccine activism in the USA in the COVID-19 era. *Lancet (London, England), 401*(10380), 967–970. https://doi.org/10.1016/S0140-6736(23)00136-8

CDC. (2022, November 29) *12 COVID-19 vaccination strategies for your community*. Retrieved May 26, 2023, from https://www.cdc.gov/vaccines/covid-19/vaccinate-with-confidence/community.htm

Centers for Disease Control and Prevention. (1999). Ten Great Public Health Achievements—United States, 1900–1999. *Morbidity and Mortality Weekly Report, 48*(12), 241–243. https://www.cdc.gov/mmwr/pdf/wk/mm4812.pdf. Accessed 22 May 2023

Conis, E. (2023). *Vaccination resistance in historical perspective*. The American Historian. Retrieved June 30, 2023, from https://www.oah.org/tah/issues/2015/august/vaccination-resistance/

Daley, M. F., et al. (2023). Association between aluminum exposure from vaccines before age 24 months and persistent asthma at age 24 to 59 months. *Academic Pediatrics, 23*(1), 37–46. https://doi.org/10.1016/j.acap.2022.08.006

Daly, M. (2023, June 23). *The childhood immunization schedule and safety: Studies in the vaccine safety datalink*. Report to Advisory Committee on Immunization Practices (ACIP). Retrieved June 26, 2023, from https://www.cdc.gov/vaccines/acip/meetings/downloads/slides-2023-06-21-23/02-VaxSafety-Daley-508.pdf

Deer, B. (2011). How the vaccine was meant to make money. *BMJ, 342*, c5258. www.bmj.com/content/342/bmj.c5258

Durbach, N. (2000). They might as well brand us: Working class resistance to compulsory vaccination in Victorian England. *The Society for the Social History of Medicine, 13*, 45–62. Retrieved May 22, 2023, from academic.oup.com/shm/article/13/1/45/1628528

Dyer, O. (2017). Measles outbreak in Somali American community follows anti-vaccine talks. *BMJ, 357*, j2378. https://www.bmj.com/content/357/bmj.j2378.full. Accessed 25 June 2023

Erratum: Vol. 72, No. 2. MMWR Morb Mortal Wkly Rep 2023;72:268. https://doi.org/10.15585/mmwr.mm7210a5.

Food and Drug Administration [FDA]. (2021). https://www.fda.gov/news-events/press-announcements/fda-takes-key-action-fight-against-covid-19-issuing-emergency-use-authorization-first-covid-19

Gellin, B. (2020). Why vaccine rumours stick—and getting them unstuck. *Lancet, 396*(10247), 303–304. https://doi.org/10.1016/S0140-6736(20)31640-8

Glanz, M. F., et al. (2018). Association between estimated cumulative vaccine antigen exposure through the first 23 months of life and non-vaccine-targeted infections from 24 through 47 months of age. *JAMA, 319*(9), 906–913.

Goullé, J. P., et al. (2020). Aluminum and vaccines: Current state of knowledge. *Médecine et Maladies Infectieuses, 50*, 16–21.

Gunmen in northwest Pakistan kill polio worker, two policemen. (2022, June 28). *Al Jazeera*. https://www.aljazeera.com/news/2022/6/28/gunmen-in-northwest-pakistan-kill-polio-worker-two-policemen

Hall, C. (2021, October 4). *Vaccine hesitancy expert says fear and emotion are neglected dimension of health*. Keck School of Medicine USC Department of Population and Public Health Sciences. Grand Rounds. Retrieved May 22, 2023, from https://pphs.usc.edu/vaccine-hesitancy-expert-says-fear-and-emotion-are-neglected-dimension-of-health/

Hershfield, H., & Brody, I.. (2021, January 18). *How Elvis got Americans to accept the polio vaccine*. Scientific American. Retrieved June 30, 2023, from https://www.scientificamerican.com/article/how-elvis-got-americans-to-accept-the-polio-vaccine/

Hogenesch, H. (2012). *Frontiers in Immunology, 3*, 406.

Hussain, A., Ali, S., Ahmed, M., et al. (2018). The anti-vaccination movement: A regression in modern medicine. *Cureus, 10*(7), e2919. https://doi.org/10.7759/cureus.2919

Hutto, E. (2024). *Was the name 'operation warp speed misleading'?*. https://www.medpagetoday.com/publichealthpolicy/fdageneral/108179

Khubchandani, J., et al. (2022). COVID-19 vaccine refusal among nurses worldwide: Review of trends and predictors. *Vaccine, 10*(2), 230. https://doi.org/10.3390/vaccines10020230

Koslap-Petraco, M. (Spring 2022). *Be a vaccine champion: With kindness and respect we can help others choose to be vaccinated AFT Health Care*. Retrieved May 22, 2023, from https://www.aft.org/hc/spring2022/koslap-petraco

Kulkarni, A., Desai, R., Alcalá, H., & Balkrishnan, R. (2021). Persistent disparities in immunization rates for the seven-vaccine series among infants 19–35 months in the United States. *Health Equity, 5*(1), 135–139. https://doi.org/10.1089/heq.2020.0127. Retrieved July 01, 2023, from https://www.liebertpub.com/doi/pdf/10.1089/heq.2020.0127

Larson, P. (2020, October 4) *COVID-19 anti-vaxxers use the same arguments from 135 years ago*. The Conversation-Academic Rigor-Journalistic Flair. Retrieved May 24, 2023, from https://theconversation.com/covid-19-anti-vaxxers-use-the-same-arguments-from-135-years-ago-145592?emci=13788ce8-1907-eb11-96f5-00155d03affc&emdi=daf4976d-1b07-eb11-96f5-00155d03affc&ceid=4111873

Larson, H., & Mnookin, S. (2016). Trust and confidence in vaccines: Tales of three vaccines, lessons for others. *The Vaccine Book*. 2nd edition. Retrieved June 30, 2023, from https://www.sciencedirect.com/topics/medicine-and-dentistry/vaccination-refusal

MacDonald, Noni E, and SAGE Working Group on Vaccine Hesitancy. (2015). Vaccine hesitancy: Definition, scope and determinants. *Vaccine, 33*(34), 4161–4164. https://doi.org/10.1016/j.vaccine.2015.04.036

McKeem, C., & Bohannon, K. (2016). Exploring the reasons behind parental refusal of vaccines. *Journal of Pediatric Pharmacology and Therapeutics, 21*(2), 104–109. https://www.ncbi.nlm.nih.gov/pmc/articles/PMC4869767/

McWhinney, J. (2022, May 16). *How a San Diego church became a nexus of anti-vaccine, anti-COVID lockdown and right-wing political organizing*. Voice of San Diego News. Retrieved July 01, 2023, from https://voiceofsandiego.org/2022/05/16/how-a-san-diego-church-became-a-nexus-of-anti-vaccine-anti-covid-lockdown-and-right-wing-political-organizing/

Offit, P. (2019a, October 19). *Childrens' Hospital of Philadelphia Vaccine Education Center. Making vaccines: Process of vaccine development*. Retrieved May 25, 2023, from https://www.chop.edu/centers-programs/vaccine-education-center/making-vaccines/process-vaccine-development

Offit, P. (2019b, October 09). *Childrens' Hospital of Philadelphia Vaccine Education Center. Making vaccines: Licensure, recommendations and requirements*. https://www.chop.edu/centers-programs/vaccine-education-center/making-vaccines/licensure-recommendations-and-requirements

Olson, O., Berry, C., & Kumar, N. (2020). Addressing parental vaccine hesitancy towards childhood vaccines in the United States: A systematic literature review of communication interventions and strategies. *Vaccines (Basel), 8*(4), 590. Published 2020 Oct 8. https://doi.org/10.3390/vaccines8040590

Page, T. (2019, April 9). Vaccines are often grown in a broth of animal cells, but the final product is highly purified. Most prominent ultra-orthodox rabbis agree that vaccines are kosher, and urge observant Jews to be immunized. *New York Times*. Retrieved May 25, 2023, from https://www.nytimes.com/2019/04/09/nyregion/jews-measles-vaccination.html

Polio cases jump in Pakistan as clerics declare vaccination an American plot. (2007, February 14). *The Guardian*. Retrieved May 25, 2023, from https://www.theguardian.com/world/2007/feb/15/pakistan.topstories3

Rauhala, E. (2020, October 07) The pandemic is amplifying the U.S. anti-vaccine move-ment—and globalizing it. *The Washington Post*. Retrieved May 30, 2023, from https://www.washingtonpost.com/world/coronaviurs-antivax-conspiracies/2020/10/06/96dd d2c2-028e-11eb-b92e-029676f9ebec_story.html?emci=cca22c4e-7309-eb11-96f5-00155d 03affc&emdi=9907e93f-7409-eb11-96f5-00155d03affc&ceid=4111873

Reyes, M. (2020). The disproportional impact of COVID-19 on African Americans. *Health and Human Rights, 22*(2), 299–307. https://www.ncbi.nlm.nih.gov/pmc/articles/PMC776290 8/#:~:text=Approximately%2097.9%20out%20of%20every,Asians%20(40.4%20per%20 100%2C000)

Saad, L. (2020, December 2). *U.S. ethics ratings rise for medical workers and teachers*. Gallup. Retrieved May 22, 2023, from https://news.gallup.com/poll/328136/ethics-ratings-rise-medical-workers-teachers.aspx

Santoli, J. M., Lindley, M. C., DeSilva, M. B., et al. (2020). Effects of the COVID-19 pandemic on routine pediatric vaccine ordering and administration—United States, 2020. *MMWR. Morbidity and Mortality Weekly Report, 69*, 591–593. https://doi.org/10.15585/mmwr.mm6919e2

Sastry, M., et al. (2017). Adjuvants and the vaccine response to the DS-Cav1-stabilized fusion glycoprotein of respiratory syncytial virus. *PLoS One, 12*, e0186854.

Seither, R., Calhoun, K., Yusuf, O. B., et al. (2023). Vaccination coverage with selected vaccines and exemption rates among children in kindergarten—United States, 2021–22 school year. *MMWR. Morbidity and Mortality Weekly Report, 72*, 26–32. https://doi.org/10.15585/mmwr. mm7202a2

Shivaram, D. (2021, September 18). *In the fight against COVID, health workers aren't immune to vaccine misinformation*. NPR. Retrieved June 29, 2023, from https://www.npr. org/2021/09/18/1037975289/unvaccinated-covid-19-vaccine-refuse-nurses-heath-care-workers

Tahir, D. (2022, February 1). *Medical boards get pushback as they try to punish doctors for Covid misinformation*. Politico. Retrieved June 30, 2023, from https://www.politico.com/ news/2022/02/01/covid-misinfo-docs-vaccines-00003383

Tin, A. (2024). https://www.cbsnews.com/news/measles-cases-reach-125-2024-topping-2022-outbreaks/

UN condemns brutal killing of eight polio workers in Afghanistan. (2022, February 24). Retrieved May 25, 2023, from https://news.un.org/en/story/2022/02/1112612

Vaccine Adverse Event Reporting System. (n.d.). *About VAERS*. Retrieved June 30, from https:// vaers.hhs.gov/about.html

Vincent, I. (2022, February 02). Robert F. Kennedy Jr. is making millions off his anti-vax crusade. *New York Post*. Retrieved June 23, 2023, from https://nypost.com/2022/02/02/ robert-f-kennedy-jr-anti-vax-crusade-is-making-him-millions/

Wei, J., Zhoa, M., Meng, F., Chen, J., & Xu, Y. (2022). Influence of internet celebrity medical experts on COVID-19 vaccination intention of young adults: An empirical study from China. *Frontiers in Public Health, 10*, 887913. https://www.ncbi.nlm.nih.gov/pmc/articles/ PMC9062698/

Wilson, S. L., & Wiysonge, C. (2020). Social media and vaccine hesitancy. *BMJ Global Health, 5*, e004206. https://doi.org/10.1136/bmjgh-2020-004206

Wolfe, R. M., & Sharpe, L. K. (2002). Anti-vaccinationists past and present. *BMJ, 325*, 430. https://doi.org/10.1136/bmj.325.7361.430

World Health Organization. (2023). *History of polio vaccination*. Retrieved May 25, 2023, from https://www.who.int/news-room/spotlight/history-of-vaccination/history-of-polio-vaccination

World Health Organization (WHO). (2020, December 31). *Coronavirus disease (COVID-19): Herd immunity, lockdowns and COVID-19*. Retrieved June 29, 2013, from https://www.who. int/news-room/questions-and-answers/item/herd-immunity-lockdowns-and-covid-19

Zadrozny, B. (2022, February 03). Once struggling, anti-vaccination groups have enjoyed a pan-demic windfall. *NBC News*. Retrieved June 28, 2023, from https://www.nbcnews.com/tech/ internet/struggling-anti-vaccination-groups-enjoyed-pandemic-windfall-rcna14402

Pharmacotherapy: Traditional Medication and Complementary Alternative Therapies

Andrea Archer and Mili Vakharia

It is easy to get a thousand prescriptions, but hard to get one single remedy.

—A Chinese Proverb

Introduction and Background

Historically, respiratory viruses are among the leading causes of morbidity and mortality among children in the United States and worldwide (Schuster & Williams, 2018). COVID-19 is now recognized as a leading respiratory cause of death in the pediatric population, with significantly greater mortality than any other vaccine-preventable disease considered since the twentieth century and subsequent emergence of modern vaccines (Flaxman et al., 2023). The first reported case of severe acute respiratory distress syndrome coronavirus type 2 (SARS-CoV-2), now known as coronavirus disease 2019 or COVID-19, was reported in December 2019 in Wuhan, China (De Los Santos et al., 2022). COVID-19 has similar genomic characteristics as a previous respiratory virus (severe acute respiratory distress syndrome coronavirus CoV [SARS –CoV]), discovered in Guangdong, China in 2002 (Caldaria et al., 2020). Despite similar genomic characteristics, COVID-19 presented with a higher transmission rate and mortality rate. On March 11, 2020, the World Health Organization declared COVID-19 a pandemic.

Although children are less likely to contract or transmit COVID-19 than adults and their symptoms are usually less severe, pediatric patients still account for

A. Archer
Louise Herrington School of Nursing, Baylor University, Waco, TX, USA
e-mail: andrea_archer@baylor.edu

M. Vakharia (✉)
Baylor College of Medicine, Pediatric Diabetes and Endocrinology,
Texas Children's Hospital, Houston, TX, USA
e-mail: mili.vakharia@bcm.edu

© The Author(s), under exclusive license to Springer Nature
Switzerland AG 2025
J. L. Peck (ed.), *COVID-19 Impacts on Child Health*,
https://doi.org/10.1007/978-3-031-80369-7_9

approximately 17.9% of reported COVID-19 cases (American Academy of Pediatrics, 2023). As of May 2023, approximately 15.6 million children had tested positive for COVID-19 since the beginning of the pandemic (American Academy of Pediatrics, 2023). Children who test positive are less likely to be hospitalized than their adult counterparts. One hypothesized reason for the decrease in severity of illness in children is their overall general good health (Reardon, 2021). Children are less likely to have co-morbidities such as diabetes, heart disease, obesity, and existing chronic respiratory illnesses which are known to contribute to the potential severity of COVID-19 (Reardon, 2021). This pandemic's escalation of occurrence and varying severity demanded rapid identification and development of effective therapies and leveraging existing traditional and alternative medicinal remedies to treat COVID-19 in both adults and children.

Perspective from Past Therapy Approaches

Primary methods of prevention include handwashing, limiting exposure to illness, promoting optimal sleep and nutrition, and other well-established health protection measures that are non-pharmaceutical in nature. Illness prevention decreases the need for medication therapy of symptoms and sequelae. Prophylaxis for RSV, such as palivizumab, a monoclonal antibody, is indicated for specified high-risk infants who are particularly susceptible to contracting RSV and requiring escalated medical care. Palivizumab is not useful for the treatment of RSV and should only be used prophylactically (Rogovik et al., 2010). In 2023, nirsevimab was granted approval from the Food and Drug Administration (FDA) as a longer acting monoclonal antibody for the prevention of RSV, with more universal administration recommendations for all infants aged 8 months or younger born during or entering into their first RSV season. Additional dosing parameters are given for certain high-risk circumstances. Other vaccinations are critical in respiratory disease prevention for illnesses such as whooping cough and are discussed in further detail in this chapter.

Common childhood respiratory illnesses such as RSV, asthma, and pneumonia are treated using extensively reviewed clinical guidelines often endorsed by reputable professional organizations or governmental health entities, with specific recommendations for pharmaceutical interventions and vaccines for prevention of illness and/or illness severity when appropriate. For example, bronchiolitis (including respiratory syncytial virus [RSV] etiology) is typically treated with evidence-based therapies such as supplemental oxygen as needed, rest, oral and intravenous fluids, and a high-humidity environment. Medications such as beta2-adrenergic agonists, antibiotics (if infection is present), bronchodilators, supplemental oxygen, inhaled steroids, and anti-inflammatory drugs are traditionally used to treat other common childhood respiratory illnesses with a high degree of clinician confidence and an established profile of safety and efficacy. However, the development of COVID-19 presented a challenge to healthcare providers (HCPs), particularly those serving pediatric populations. Internationally, scientists urgently studied effective treatments for this emerging, highly contagious, and life-threatening virus but safe science moves slowly and clinical trials involving children were quick to emerge.

Initially, COVID-19 was generally treated with supportive measures including supplemental oxygen, mechanical ventilation, and anti-inflammatory agents such as corticosteroids (Inocian et al., 2022). Children with COVID-19 present similarly to adults and have symptoms along a continuum of severity from those that mimic the common cold to severe pneumonia and even fatal acute respiratory distress syndrome (ARDS). The severity of COVID-19 illness in adults was profound, especially in adult patients with preexisting risk factors or co-morbidities such as renal disease, obesity, smoking, cardiac disease, hypertension, and diabetes mellitus (Sobu et al., 2021). There is limited information about known risk factors for the pediatric population; however, preexisting conditions likely also put children at risk for more serious complications from COVID-19 infection (De Los Santos et al., 2022). One study found obesity to be a risk factor for older children (>6 years); however, the risk was significantly lower than it was for adults (Shekerdemian et al., 2020).

Considerations of Pathophysiology

After almost 4 years of studying COVID-19, including its origins, methods of transmission, incubation times, severity, and subsequent variants of the disease, it is obvious the immune system and the inflammatory response of both adult and pediatric patients play a vital role in how a patient will present clinically and direct the course of disease progression (Costagliola et al., 2021). Inflammation has a particularly relevant role when considering the severity of COVID-19, especially in children. After being exposed to COVID-19, the immune system reacts by releasing a group of signaling proteins called cytokines. Cytokines play a significant role in normal immune responses, but large amounts released in the body simultaneously can be harmful (Cleveland Clinic, 2023). Cytokines stimulate, recruit, and proliferate immune cells in response to threatening viruses or pathogens. Cytokines are classified into the following groups: interleukins (IL), chemokines, interferons, and tumor necrosis factors (TNFs). This process is crucial for organizing cell-mediated immune responses and has a key role in controlling immune response (Cleveland Clinic, 2023). Patients who have severe cases of COVID-19 that are accompanied by additional respiratory complications such as ARDS or septic shock have elevated levels of proinflammatory cytokines that may cause a condition referred to as "cytokine storm" (Costagliola et al., 2021). This phenomenon is a severe immune reaction in which the body releases too many cytokines into the blood too quickly. This reaction may also occur after receiving immunotherapy. Symptoms of cytokine storms include nausea, fatigue, and body aches and vary in severity (Cleveland Clinic, 2023).

Management for cytokine storm depends on the severity of inflammation and specific needs of the patient. Medications used in treatment are intended to target and reduce inflammation in efforts to reduce symptoms and severity of the illness and prevent further tissue damage that may result from prolonged, severe inflammation. Classes of drugs used to achieve this include corticosteroids and anti-inflammatories. Other drugs, such as monoclonal antibodies, are used to target specific cytokines. These drugs include tocilizumab, a monoclonal antibody that binds to IL-6, anakinra (Kineret), an IL-1 blocker, and canakinumab, a monoclonal antibody that selectively blocks IL-1B (Rangappa, 2021).

In addition to traditional pharmaceutical anti-inflammatory medications, there is emerging research about the role of proper nutrition and corresponding vitamin levels in the treatment of COVID-19 in both adult and pediatric populations (Aslan et al., 2020; Cereda et al., 2021; Sobu et al., 2021; Szarpak et al., 2021). Diseases identified as risk factors for COVID-19, such as diabetes and obesity, deprive the body of essential elements that reduce inflammation; therefore, patients with these conditions can present with far more severe case presentations (Cheriyedath, 2021). Not only do vitamin and mineral deficiency intensify the severity of COVID-19 infection, but recent research suggests that including vitamin and mineral supplementation could improve the function of the innate and adaptive immune systems (Beigmohammadi et al., 2021). Vitamins and minerals also have anti-inflammatory benefits due to their function of regulating the immune system via the epigenetic regulation of physiologic pathways controlling the inflammatory and immune systems. Vitamin D reduces proinflammatory cytokines that play a role in COVID-19. The AAP states that many children and adolescents in the United States are deficient in Vitamin D, contributing to a decrease in immunity (Porto, 2022). In a study involving 212 adult patients, there was a statistically meaningful relation between vitamin D levels and severity of COVID-19 infection (Aslan et al., 2020). In children, Vitamin D is recognized for promoting optimal bone health. More recent findings suggest both antimicrobial and anti-inflammatory actions and reduce production of proinflammatory cytokines. Prior research demonstrates a link between Vitamin D deficiency, as is the case in rickets, and higher incidence of respiratory infections. Vitamin D levels may have a protective role against tuberculosis, otitis media, bronchiolitis, and viral wheezing as well as atopic conditions like asthma, food allergies, and eczema (Peroni et al., 2024). However, there is a paucity of research in related supplementation considerations for children and little-to-no formal guidance on pediatric vitamin supplementation outside of standard iron and vitamin D recommendations for infants until 12 months of age with a dose of 400 IU daily. Beyond 1 year of age, there is no consensus among the health professional community or through professional guidelines to standardize recommendations for older children although most guidelines recommend prophylaxis in the presence of risk factors not modifiable by environmental interventions (Peroni et al., 2024). Current guidelines from the American Academy of Pediatrics state that children with a well-balanced diet do not need vitamin supplementation above the recommended daily allowance (RDA). With some parents clamoring for vitamin therapies at times during the COVID-19 pandemic, HCPs could find it challenging to make evidence-based recommendations that were supported by robust research data and established clinical practice guidelines.

Points of Care

Pharmacologic Management Strategies in Pediatrics

Vaccination remains one of the most important and effective tools in preventing COVID-19 infection and sequelae of hospitalization in children and adolescents, including critical illness in adolescents (American Academy of Pediatrics, 2023; Centers for Disease Control and Prevention, 2023). The clinical presentation of COVID-19 varies on a spectrum from asymptomatic infection to mild respiratory tract symptoms to severe pneumonia with ARDS and multisystem inflammatory syndrome (MIS-C) or multiorgan dysfunction.

According to the Infectious Disease Society of America, the general approach to COVID-19 pharmacotherapy consists of assessing a patient's severity of COVID-19, timing of onset of symptoms, risk factors for disease progression, end-organ involvement, age, and pregnancy status. COVID-19 viral load is elevated during the early phase of infection. Thus, antiviral treatment options including nirmatrelvir/ritonavir and remdesivir are most likely to be efficacious within 5–7 days of symptom onset. As disease severity progresses and there is hyperinflammatory response, anti-inflammatory therapy such as corticosteroids, interleukin-6 inhibitors, or JAK inhibitors can be effective. Factors that warrant caution or prohibit treating with COVID-19 therapies include patients presenting with elevated liver function studies, low glomerular filtration rate, sexually active with childbearing potential, and/or pregnant status (Infectious Diseases Society of America, 2023).

As such, it is crucial for frontline HCPs to be familiar with management strategies provided by expert task force groups in various organizations including the World Health Organization, the United States Centers for Disease Control and Prevention, the Infectious Disease Society of America, the American Academy of Pediatrics, the American College of Cardiology, the American College of Rheumatology, and others (Centers for Disease Control and Prevention, 2023).

Chronic Non-hospitalized Setting

There is paucity of pediatric data regarding the use of oral SARS-COV-2 antiviral therapies for children and adolescents in the context of safety, efficacy, or pharmacokinetics (American Academy of Pediatrics, 2023). Given that randomized clinical trials typically consist of adult populations, there are general therapeutic adult-specific recommendations provided by the National Institute of Health (NIH) COVID-19 Treatment Guideline Panel (COVID-19 Treatment Guidelines Panel, 2019) that includes systematic assessment of risk progression to severe disease based on the patient's underlying medical condition, vaccination status, illness severity, and age. As such, clinical management of COVID-19 in pediatrics is loosely extrapolated from adult treatment guidelines. Additionally, qualification for outpatient COVID-19 treatments in children and adolescents is dependent on "high risk" status and disease severity (American Academy of Pediatrics, 2023). Patients with progressing disease severity must be closely monitored for hemodynamic instability and the need for respiratory support (Waleed et al., 2021). During the acute phase of COVID-19, management is like any other infectious disease processes including following sepsis guidelines as well as preventing further transmission of the disease and secondary infection (National Institutes of Health, 2023).

Children and adolescents deemed with elevated risk for severe COVID-19 include (American Academy of Pediatrics, 2023):

- Obesity, defined as BMI >95th percentile for age and sex based on CDC growth charts
- Immunocompromised state, including having received immunosuppressive agents
- Neurodevelopmental disorders such as cerebral palsy and trisomy 21 that may result in impaired airway clearance
- Complex medical conditions including technological dependences such as tracheostomy, continuous positive airway pressure (CPAP), and gastrostomy
- Severe congenital or acquired heart disease
- Severe chronic lung disease including asthma or other chronic respiratory conditions
- Pregnancy

The following conditions have moderate association with progression to severe COVID-19 in pediatric patients (American Academy of Pediatrics, 2023):

- Sickle cell disease
- Uncontrolled diabetes mellitus
- Chronic renal disease
- Chronic liver disease (including cirrhosis and autoimmune hepatitis)
- Non-severe cardiac, neurologic, or metabolic disease
- Infants less than 1 year of age

Children with the following conditions have lower risk of progression to severe COVID-19 (American Academy of Pediatrics, 2023).

- Mild asthma
- Overweight
- Well-controlled diabetes

Antiviral therapies are not usually recommended for children and adolescents with minimal risk of COVID-19 disease severity and/or hospitalization. Due to lack of efficacy and concerns for harmful effects in light of limited research, systemic corticosteroids are not recommended to treat patients with mild-to-moderate COVID-19 who do not require supplemental oxygen (National Institutes of Health, 2023).

As of December 2021, the FDA issued an Emergency Use Authorization (EUA) for early antiviral therapy, Pfizer's Paxlovid for treating mild-to-moderate COVID-19 in non-hospitalized, high-risk adults and pediatric patients 12 years of age and older, weighing at least 40 kg, and evaluated in outpatient settings. Paxlovid, consisting of nirmatrelvir and ritonavir, inhibits a SARS-CoV-2 protein to stop the virus from replicating and slows the breakdown of nirmatrelvir so that it remains in the body for longer duration at higher concentrations, respectively (U.S. Food & Drug Administration, 2021). It should be administered within 5 days of symptom onset as three tablets (two tablets of nirmatrelvir and one tablet of ritonavir) taken together orally twice daily for 5 days, for 30 tablets. Of note, Paxlovid is not authorized for usage lasting greater than five consecutive days. Patients must be counseled on side effects including impaired sense of taste, diarrhea, high blood pressure, and muscle aches. Additionally, it is not recommended for use in patients with severe renal and liver impairments. Those with moderate renal disease may use Paxlovid at a reduced dose (U.S. Food & Drug Administration, 2021).

Acute Inpatient Setting

In late April 2020, there were worldwide reports of children exposed to SARS-CoV-2 presenting with hyperinflammatory shock syndrome that mimicked Kawasaki disease and toxic shock syndrome (Cheung et al., 2020; Riphagen et al., 2020; Toubiana et al., 2020). Children and adolescents presenting with MIS-C should be cared for at centers with access to multidisciplinary pediatric specialists including cardiology, hematology, infectious disease, intensivists, and rheumatology (National Institutes of Health, 2023). MIS-C case definition listed below includes patients aged <21 years and those with absence of a more likely alternative diagnosis (Centers for Disease Control and Prevention, 2020a):

- Fever (temperature > 38.0 °C)
- Severe clinical status requiring hospitalization
- C-reactive protein >3.0 mg/dl
- Onset of symptoms in >2 following organ systems:
  - Cardiac: coronary artery dilation/aneurysm, left ventricular ejection fraction <55% or troponin elevated above normal
  - Shock
  - Dermatology: rash, oral mucosal inflammation, conjunctivitis/conjunctival injection, or extremity findings (erythema, edema)
  - Gastrointestinal: abdominal pain, vomiting, or diarrhea
  - Hematologic: platelet count <150,000/µl, absolute lymphocyte count <1000/µl.

MIS-C usually takes place 2–6 weeks following an acute SARS-COV-2 infection. Children typically present critically ill with fever, multisystem organ involvement, and elevated laboratory markers of inflammation. Of note, diagnosis can be difficult because the presentation of MIS-C is like other conditions such as Kawasaki disease, toxic shock syndrome, and severe acute COVID-19 (Centers for Disease Control and Prevention, 2023).

According to the American College of Rheumatology, intravenous immunoglobulin (IVIG) and glucocorticoids are mainstay immunomodulatory medications that should be utilized in treating children with MIS-C. Data from various non-randomized studies suggests that first-line IVIG in conjunction with glucocorticoids leads to lower likelihood of treatment failure, faster recovery of cardiac function, and shorter intensive care unit stay as well as decreased need for additional treatment such as adjunctive immunomodulators including anakinra, infliximab, or high-dose glucocorticoids. Isolated IVIG is reserved for children with glucocorticoid contraindication. IVIG is weight-based at the dose of 2 g/kg with a maximum dose of 100 grams (about 3.53 oz). It is essential for clinicians to monitor cardiac function and fluid status during the infusion (Henderson et al., 2021).

Systemic glucocorticoids such as methylprednisolone (Medrol) or alternative agents at an equivalent dose of 1–2 mg/kg/day can be utilized as a low-to-moderate dose if clinically indicated. As the child improves clinically with indicators such as afebrile status, end-organ dysfunction resolution, and downward trending inflammatory markers, then steroids can be tapered if previously administered in high doses for a period of more than 2 weeks. This is to avoid rebound inflammation and is often patient-specific, dependent on clinical status. In general, corticosteroids are used to reduce host inflammatory response within the lungs, preventing acute lung injury and acute respiratory distress syndrome.

Clinicians must carefully outweigh the risk–benefit ratio of prescriptive therapies, given risk of delayed viral clearance and increased secondary infections (Henderson et al., 2021). There are several adverse effects of glucocorticoid treatments depending on the duration of therapy including obesity, development of diabetes mellitus, hypertension, sarcopenia, osteoporosis, atherosclerosis, cardiovascular disease, and thromboembolism (Alexaki & Henneicke, 2021). Given the greater benefit of anti-inflammatory response, literature suggests the use of glucocorticoids to treat ARDS and other critical infections associated with COVID-19 (Alexaki & Henneicke, 2021).

Corticosteroids such as low-dose dexamethasone (Decadron) are effective in lowering mortality in adult patients with severe or critical COVID-19 disease (Horby et al., 2020). Dexamethasone (Decadron) is generally reserved for hospitalized pediatric patients with SARS-COV-2 RT-PCR who require increased respiratory support such as high flow nasal cannula, mechanical ventilation, or other positive pressure support (Horby et al., 2020; Sterne et al., 2020). For patients with progressive respiratory disease, a combination therapy of remdesivir and dexamethasone (Decadron) should be considered (National Institutes of Health, 2023).

In children with refractory MIS-C and those who do not improve within 24 h of initial immunomodulatory therapy, it is recommended to intensify therapy using anakinra (Kineret), high-dose glucocorticoids, or infliximab. It is important that anakinra and infliximab are not used in combination to avoid potential adverse effects. Methylprednisolone (Medrol) is a high-dose glucocorticoid therapy dosed at 10–30 mg/kg/day given intravenously over 1–3 days with subsequent moderate dose of 1–2 mg/kg/day. Second doses of IVIG are not recommended due to risk of IVIG resistance with rapid rate of disease escalation as well as potential for fluid overload in patients with MIS-C. In the event multiple immunomodulatory agents are administered, exceptional care must be taken to monitor the risk of infection (Deville et al., 2023).

The most utilized biologic medication for treatment of MIS-C in the United States is Anakinra (Kineret) because of adequate safety and efficacy in pediatric patients with other hyper inflammatory syndromes. These include systemic juvenile idiopathic arthritis, Kawasaki disease, and macrophage activation syndrome. It has been particularly useful in successfully treating IVIG resistant Kawasaki disease. It has a shorter half-life of 4–6 h, adding to the benefit of being able discontinue quickly in comparison to tapering as is required with other longer acting immuno-modulators. High-dose anakinra of 5-to −0 mg/kg/day has better efficacy in treating macrophage activation syndrome. The duration of therapy varies from 1 to 2 weeks (Henderson et al., 2021).

Infliximab (Remicade) is an FDA-approved medicine to treat inflammatory bowel disease and juvenile idiopathic arthritis. It can also be utilized for IVIG resistant Kawasaki disease. In patients with MIS-C, it can be administered as single dose of 5–10 mg/kg/day as intensification therapy. Cole et al. (2021) report that patients who receive combination of infliximab and IVIG have shorter hospital admission to the intensive care unit, less cardiac dysfunction and are less likely to need additional therapy after 24 h. The effects of infliximab (Remicade) can last for several weeks, allowing for steroid-sparing effect in MIS-C patients.

Other monoclonal antibodies such as tocilizumab (Actemra), an IL-6 receptor antagonist, are FDA approved to treat rheumatoid arthritis in children and adults. It is also used and approved for treatment of COVID-19 in hospitalized adult patients receiving systemic glucocorticoids or needing supplemental oxygenation (Sanders et al., 2020). Tocilizumab (Actemra) is administered as single 60-min intravenous infusion with a dose of 8–12 mg/kg. Patients must be closely monitored for infusion reaction, and it is contraindicated for those with absolute neutrophil count <1000 cells/μL, platelet counts <50,000/μL, alanine aminotransferase >five times the normal, or higher risk of gastrointestinal perforation (Deville et al., 2023).

Intravenous remdesivir (Veklury), FDA approved in April 2022, became the first and only antiviral medication to be authorized for use in young children, specifically ≥28-days-old children, weighing ≥3 kg, who are either hospitalized or non-hospitalized, showing a high risk for progression to severe COVID-19 (prone to hospitalization or death). Of note, it should be prescribed within 7 days of symptom onset. Maximum benefit is achieved when it is administered early in the course of disease, given the broad-spectrum activity (Elsawah et al., 2020). The dose depends on age and weight, including 5 mg/kg on day one, followed by 2.5 mg/kg once daily on day two and three for patients 3–40 kg. For those greater than 12 years old and above 40 kg, remdesivir 200 mg daily is prescribed followed by 100 mg, IV daily on days two and three. Side effects include headache, nausea, and cough. Patients are monitored during and for at least 1 h after the dose for possible infusion-related reactions. Clinicians must consider operational and reimbursement challenges that remdesivir can bring with its need for inpatient infusion. Remdesivir carries risk of adverse effects and drug interactions including liver inflammation, worsening respiratory failure, constipation, and nausea. As such, during the infusion, the patients' liver function, partial thromboplastin time, and renal function are monitored closely along with any sign or symptoms of infusion reaction (Deville et al., 2023; Goldman et al., 2020).

Antithrombotic Treatment for MIS-C

The American College of Rheumatology (2020) recommends that patients presenting with MIS-C associated with COVID-19 infection and without risk factors for bleeding should receive low-dose prophylactic anticoagulation using aspirin. This guidance was extrapolated based on data from children with Kawasaki disease and their greater likelihood of developing analogous platelet activation with endothelial dysfunction due to MIS-C. According to the American Heart Association guidelines for Kawasaki disease, patients with MIS-C presenting with large coronary artery aneurysm should receive therapeutic anticoagulation. This also includes children with left ventricular dysfunction and elevated D-dimer levels who are at risk for intracardiac thrombosis (National Institutes of Health, 2023). However, there is no clear consensus on using either prophylactic or therapeutic anticoagulation in patients with MIS-C who do not have large coronary aneurysm and/or moderate to severe left ventricular dysfunction.

Of note, consensus guidelines formulated by the American Society of Hematology also recommend anticoagulation prophylaxis for thromboembolism for all hospitalized adults greater than 18 years of age (American Society of Hematology, 2021). For those less than 18 years of age and with primary COVID-19 or MIS-C admitted to intensive care unit or presenting with risk factors such as elevated D-dimer >2 UG/ml, active cancer, presence of central line, obesity, history of thrombosis, thrombocytopenia, elevated PT, or fibrinogen levels, then prophylactic anticoagulation may be considered (American Society of Hematology, 2021; Loi et al., 2020; Loomba et al., 2021). It is not warranted to start anticoagulant prophylaxis in hospitalized children without MIS-C or other pro-thrombotic risk (Del Borrello et al., 2021).

A pediatric study of patients with acute COVID-19 and MIS-C found indwelling catheters, age >12 years, malignancy, admission to ICU, and elevated D-dimer levels to be independent risk factors for thrombosis (Whitworth et al., 2021). Twice a day low-dose and low-molecular weight heparin subcutaneous injections have also been suggested as anticoagulation thromboprophylaxis for hospitalized children with COVID-19 related illness including MIS-C and known elevated D-dimer levels (Goldenberg et al., 2020). There are also reports of major bleeding events in MIS-C patients undergoing treatment for anticoagulation (Whitworth et al., 2021). With uncertain benefits, anticoagulation should be highly individualized based on risk factors for thrombosis (National Institutes of Health, 2023).

Antibiotics and Other Off-label Agents

Ivermectin (stromectol) is approved by the FDA to treat a multitude of tropical para-sitic diseases such as malaria, onchocerciasis, helminthiases, and scabies. However, the FDA and CDC have disapproved of its use for routine treatment of COVID-19. Though at a cellular level, ivermectin has demonstrated the ability to inhibit replica-tion of SARS-CoV-2, experimental usage of ivermectin could lead to severe toxicity including severe post-ivermectin encephalopathies and death as it requires 100-fold higher dose than approved for use (Caly et al., 2020; Farah et al., 2022; Deville et al., 2023). Additionally, synergistic effects of hydroxychloroquine combined with azithromycin was also widely publicized during the pandemic for potential use in treating COVID-19 while preventing secondary infections.

One pediatric multi-center study reported that their cohort of patients also fre-quently received hydroxychloroquine either alone or as combination therapy with azithromycin, remdesivir, interleukin 6, and tocilizumab that was like adult patient data (Shekerdemian et al., 2020). However, the efficacy for hydroxychloroquine has been questioned due to concerns for severe cardiac adverse events, especially QT prolongation (Chaccour et al., 2020; Deng et al., 2021). Data from randomized control trials suggests that single or routine dose of azithromycin is ineffective in clearing symptoms of SARS-CoV-2 and reducing time to recovery nor risk of hos-pitalization (Oldenburg et al., 2021; PRINCIPLE Trial Collaborative Group, 2021). In fact, the authors recommended antibiotic stewardship efforts to reduce the misuse of antibiotics during the pandemic (PRINCIPLE Trial Collaborative Group, 2021). During the early pandemic, the Infectious Disease Society of America recom-mended against the use of such therapies in the absence of clinical trials due to inadequate data on efficacy and risk of adverse effects (Infectious Diseases Society of America, 2023).

Barriers and Breakthroughs

The unexpected emergence of the COVID-19 virus left HCPs in the United States and worldwide rushing to meet public demand to identify treatments, vaccines, and effective methods of virus prevention. Four years later, researchers, scientists, and HCPs are reflecting on previously used treatments and looking forward to the future to improve treatment and spread of infection.

One barrier to treating and learning new therapies is the limitations of past research regarding initial practices in management of COVID-19, especially regard-ing pediatric populations. Children critically ill and hospitalized with COVID-19 were treated primarily with prescribed medications indicated for recognized and significantly researched viral and respiratory illnesses. Among these medications, the most frequently prescribed and used were remdesivir and/or steroids (Szarpak et al., 2021; Costagliola et al., 2021). Medications were used off label in the pediatric population and with no compelling data for use in children. Looking to the future, the development of structured, supported, credible pediatric-specific networks may expedite inclusion of children in clinical trials to facilitate opportune, quality data to support treatment.

The research surrounding therapeutic use of vitamin D and micronutrients is also limited. It is known that pathology surrounding COVID-19 involves a cytokine storm, a proinflammatory process (Cheriyedath, 2021). Vitamin D reduces proinflammatory cytokines in autoimmune inflammatory processes; however, research is limited in its effectiveness in COVID-19, particularly in the pediatric population. There has been research investigating supplementation of vitamin D, as well as vitamins A, B, C, and E (Aslan et al., 2020). Adult patients who were treated with these supplements or presented with normal values of these vitamins were less likely to be hospitalized for a prolonged period (Beigmohammadi et al., 2021). Favorable results have been achieved using vitamin therapies with "traditional" anti-inflammatory drugs. For example, vitamin C combined with hydrocortisone and thiamine significantly decreases mortality and prevents organ failure in patients with systemic inflammatory conditions, such as sepsis (Song, 2020). Again, studies are not specific to COVID-19, especially in the pediatric population; however, addressing the issue of widespread inflammation and potentially transferring knowledge to the known cytokine storm that occurs in the presence of COVID-19 should be considered for future research. Nutritional supplements such as fish oils, probiotics, iron, selenium, and zinc can optimize immunity and prevent COVID-19 infection although there are no official recommendations for pediatric supplementation (Beigmohammadi et al., 2021; Cheriyedath, 2021).

One of the noteworthy breakthroughs of the COVID-19 pandemic is evidence that supports necessity of maintaining optimal health, especially in the absence of disease to prevent contracting the COVID-19 virus and if it is contracted, optimal health may lessen the severity. Currently, existing research involving co-morbidities such as obesity, diabetes, coronary artery disease, and respiratory diseases comprises adult populations. There is little evidence that includes pediatric populations; however, pediatric clinicians have contributed to literature encouraging optimal health by eating a diet rich with antiviral properties (Cheriyedath, 2021) such as coconut oil, ginger, kimchi, and fermented foods that contain probiotics. Additionally, pediatric HCPs should encourage caregivers to have their children "eat the rainbow" (meaning eating foods with different colors representing different antioxidant and other nutrition properties). This includes fruits and vegetables that are full of antioxidants which have historically been valuable in destroying free radicals that may weaken immunity (Song, 2020).

In addition to stressing the importance of optimizing child health with adequate nutrition, pediatric HCPs also emphasize the necessity for adequate hydration, recommending water, coconut water, herbal teas, and foods that have immune supporting properties such as bone broth for age and situation-specific indications (Song,

Table 1 Sleep recommendations for children by age

Ages	Hours of sleep
1–2 years	11–14
3–5 years	10–13
6–12 years	9–12
13–18 years	8–10

2020). General recommendations also include avoiding processed foods and simple sugars. Blood samples suggest lowered immune system just 30 min after eating a simple sugar. This contributes to a reduction in the body's ability to leverage white blood cell production to kill germs and fight further infection. This effect is present up to 5 h after ingestion of simple sugars. Maintaining healthy, optimal blood sugar is essential for immune health (Song, 2020).

Continuing the recent emphasis of supporting good health includes daily exercise and obtaining adequate sleep and minimizing stress. Daily exercise boosts production of macrophages; however, high intensity exercises may reduce the body's ability to fight infection, so moderate exercise is recommended. With respect to adequate sleep, it is necessary to increase white blood cell production. Consequently, lack of sleep will promote inflammation throughout the body and will increase susceptibility to catching an illness and increase the severity of illness (Bland, 2022). Johns Hopkins All Children's Hospital (Johns Hopkins All Childrens Hospital, 2023) sleep recommendations for children are listed in Table 1. Finally, stress lowers the immune defenses and makes individuals, even children, more likely to become ill (Song, 2020).

While there have been tremendous breakthroughs in research and literature regarding the origins of COVID-19, transmission of the disease, who is at risk and who will be most severely affected, there is much research needed to effectively prevent, treat, and potentially cure COVID-19. Specifically, there are limited studies considering the importance of micronutrients and their role in the prevention and treatment of COVID-19. Some emerging research supports the role of optimal vitamin levels in reducing inflammation as they relate to other inflammatory and autoimmune disorders, especially in adult populations, but evidence is severely limited in pediatric populations, resulting in a lack of formal recommendations from traditional authoritative sources in pediatrics (Cereda et al., 2021).

Lessons Learned

Direct clinical trials that evaluated treatments for COVID-19 in pediatric patients remain scarce. Much of the data is applied from adult literature, leading to its own unique challenges with paucity of pediatric-specific data regarding medication safety and efficacy. It is essential to note that many pediatric patients experience mild illness with COVID-19 infection compared to adults who have much greater mortality and need for hospitalization (Centers for Disease Control and Prevention, 2020b). Therefore, HCPs must carefully outweigh risk-versus-benefit for pharmacologic therapies in children with COVID-19 depending on disease severity. There is a larger consensus for lesser need and a lower prescribing threshold for pharmacologic agents in otherwise healthy children infected with COVID-19. Intravenous infusion of gamma globulin and immunomodulators could be considered for severe and critical pediatric cases (see Chap. 1).

Mainstays of therapy in pediatric patients include symptomatic and supportive treatment through hand hygiene, masking or social distancing for certain children in certain circumstances, rest, hydration, electrolyte balance, stabilizing internal temperature, and monitoring closely for oxygen saturation as well as blood pressure. If a patient deteriorates to anoxic dyspnea, oxygen therapy using non-invasive or invasive ventilation is recommended. Patients progressing to ARDS may require extracorporeal membrane oxygenation (ECMO). Biologic agents such as anakinra or high-dose glucocorticoid therapy should be considered in refractory MIS-C associated with COVID-19. Children who require intravenous IVIG, corticosteroids, antiviral, and/or immunomodulators must be cared at a center with access to multiple specialties to closely monitor for potential adverse effects.

Antiviral therapies have not been well studied in pediatric patients with COVD-19 and MIS-C. There is no clear treatment benefit given that MIS-C is an immune-mediated phenomenon occurring weeks after primary SARS-COV-2 infection. As such, it is not recommended to use remdesivir for patients with MIS-C. Outside of primary prevention with vaccination, there is no COVID-19 monoclonal antibody or antiviral agent authorized for use as pre- or post-exposure prophylaxis. However, FDA approved or over-the counter-medications including vitamins and electrolyte supplements given with appropriate provider recommendation can be useful to overcome post-COVID symptoms such as headache, fatigue, etc.

It has been well and long established that optimal nutrition plays a critical role in enhancing immunity and reducing risk of infections. Individuals with improper nutrition are at greater risk of developing bacterial, viral, and other infections. Although there is limited specific data on nutrition and immunomodulatory action on COVID-19, there is emerging data regarding intake of nutrients such as Vitamin D, C, and zinc in relation to other infections (Ali et al., 2021). For instance, zinc supplementation could bolster one's ability to generate an adequate immune response (Costagliola et al., 2021). Vitamin C, a co-factor for many enzymes, facilitates antioxidation and limits inflammation and tissue damage associated with immune responses (Ali et al., 2021). Adequate Vitamin D levels could help lower the risk of developing acute respiratory infections associated with viral infection by 12 to 75%. Researching the use of homeopathic treatments as supplemental therapy to manage inflammation is a subject in need of greater study. In concluding, it is important to note that pharmacotherapies are rapidly evolving in the context of COVID-19 treatment response. This chapter reflects information current at the time of the writing, but readers should verify current guidelines and recommendations to guide prescriptive practices while understanding historical context and scientific rationales for revisions in therapy regimens to help guide patient understanding.

Calls to Action

1. Nutrition:

   - Good nutrition practices could positively impact immune and metabolic function and reduce the risk of severe COVID-19 disease and associated pulmonary symptoms. All HCPs should recognize the role of a proper diet, appropriate vitamin supplementation, and the potential impacts of vitamin/nutritional deficiencies.
   - The importance of maintaining optimal health through a proper diet and individualized vitamin supplementation recommendations should be communicated to parents and caregivers. This education should be included during well visit examinations as outlined in Bright Futures, a national health promotion and prevention initiative led by the American Academy of Pediatrics.

2. Pediatric research:

   - There is a greater need for pediatric-focused studies evaluating the safety and efficacy of pharmacologic and non-pharmacologic therapies in children with COVID-19.
   - To effectively advance pediatric clinical research, formulation of collaborative partnerships is essential, particularly through the NIH and CDC. Nurse-led COVID-19 research is limited in general and has a greater potential for growth (Castro-Sánchez et al., 2021). Health leaders at the university level should advocate for systematic inclusion of COVID-19 related research into their academic agendas and funding procurement efforts.

3. Access to care:

   - Ensuring multi-specialty access to care must be prioritized for underserved populations. It is essential to recognize limited access to antiviral therapies for patients who may experience greater social vulnerability and are less likely to receive anti-SARS-CoV-2 antibody medications (Wiltz et al., 2022). More advocacy efforts are needed in federal legislation to allow patients and families to receive quality healthcare in a timely manner (AANP, 2022).
   - Advance practice providers are in high demand and can bridge gap to healthcare services in today's era of sub-specialty provider shortages across the United States. The Improving Care and Access to Nurses (ICAN) Act as introduced in the 118th and 119th sessions of the US Congress would help ameliorate this access to care in underserved areas through expanding the scope of practice for advanced practice registered nurses.

References

Alexaki, V. I., & Henneicke, H. (2021). The role of glucocorticoids in the management of COVID-19. *Hormone and Metabolic Research, 53*(1), 9–15. https://doi.org/10.1055/a-1300-2550

Ali, Z., Jatoi, M. A., Al-Wraikat, M., Ahmed, N., & Li, J. (2021). Time to enhance immunity via functional foods and supplements: Hope for SARS-CoV-2 outbreak. *Alternative Therapies in Health and Medicine, 27*(S1), 30–44.

American Academy of Pediatrics. (2023). *Management strategies in children and adolescents with mild to moderate COVID-19.* Available at www.aap.org/en/pages/2019-novel-coronavirus-covid-19-infections/clinical-guidance/outpatient-covid-19-management-strategies-in-children-and-adolescents/

American Association of Nurse Practitioners. (2022, September 13). *AANP applauds U.S. House legislation strengthening patient access to health care.* News release. Retrieved September 13, 2022 from https://www.aanp.org/new-feed/aanp-applaud-us-house-legislation-strengthening-patient-access-to-health-care. https://www.aanp.org/news-feed/aanp-applauds-us-house-legislation-strengthening-patient-access-to-health-care

American Society of Hematology. (2021). *COVID—19 and VTE/Anticoagulation: Frequently asked questions.* Available at https://www.hematology.org/covid-19/covid-19-and-vte-anticoagulation

Aslan MT, Aslan İÖ, Özdemir Ö. Letter to the Editor: Is Vitamin D One of the Key Elements in COVID-19 Days? J Nutr Health Aging. 2020;24(9):1038-1039. https://doi.org/10.1007/s12603-020-1413-5. PMID: 33155635; PMCID: PMC7597430.

Beigmohammadi, M. T., Bitarafan, S., Hoseindokht, A., et al. (2021). The effect of supplementation with vitamins A, B, C, D, and E on disease severity and inflammatory responses in patients with COVID-19: A randomized clinical trial. *Trials, 22,* 802. https://doi.org/10.1186/s13063-021-05795-4

Bland, J. S. (2022). Clinical understanding of the sleep-immune connection. *Integrative Medicine (Encinitas), 21*(1), 12–14.

Caldaria, A., Conforti, C., Di Meo, N., Dianzani, C., Lotti, T., Zalaudek, I., & Giuffrida, R. (2020). *Dermatologic therapy.* Available at Retrieved July 07, 2023 from wileyonlinelibrary.com/journal/dth. https://doi.org/10.1111/dth.13395.

Caly, L., Druce, J. D., Catton, M. G., Jans, D. A., & Wagstaff, K. M. (2020). The FDA-approved drug ivermectin inhibits the replication of SARS-CoV-2 in vitro. *Antiviral Research, 178,* 104787. https://doi.org/10.1016/j.antiviral.2020.104787

Castro-Sánchez, E., Russell, A. M., Dolman, L., & Wells, M. (2021). What place does nurse-led research have in the COVID-19 pandemic? *International Nursing Review, 68*(2), 214–218. https://doi.org/10.1111/inr.12660

Centers for Disease Control and Prevention. (2020a). *Multisystem inflammatory syndrome in children (MIS-C) associated with coronavirus disease 2019 (COVID 19).* Available at https://emergency.cdc.gov/han/2020/han00432.asp

Centers for Disease Control and Prevention. (2020b). Coronavirus disease 2019 in children—United States, February 12–April 2, 2020. *MMWR. Morbidity and Mortality Weekly Report,* (69), 422–426. https://doi.org/10.15585/mmwr.mm6914e4

Centers for Disease Control and Prevention. (2023). *Information for pediatric healthcare providers.* Available at www.cdc.gov/coronavirus/2019-ncov/hcp/pediatric-hcp.html

Cereda, E., Bogliolo, L., Klersy, C., Lobascio, F., Masi, S., Crotti, S., DeStefano, L., Bruno, R., Corsico, A. G., Di Sabatino, A., Perlini, S., Montecucco, C., & Caccialanza, R. (2021). Vitamin D 25OH deficiency in COVID-19 patients admitted to a tertiary referral hospital. *Clinical Nutrition, 40,* 2469–2472. https://doi.org/10.1016/j.clnu.2020.10.055

Chaccour, C., Hammann, F., Ramón-García, S., & Rabinovich, N. R. (2020). Ivermectin and COVID-19: Keeping rigor in times of urgency. *The American Journal of Tropical Medicine and Hygiene, 102*(6), 1156–1157. https://doi.org/10.4269/ajtmh.20-0271

Cheriyedath, S. (2021, June 18). *Which vitamins and minerals help with COVID?* https://www.news-medical.net/news/20210618/Which-vitamins-and-minerals-help-with-COVID.aspx

Cheung, E. W., Zachariah, P., Gorelik, M., Boneparth, A., Kernie, S. G., Orange, J. S., & Milner, J. D. (2020). Multisystem inflammatory syndrome related to COVID-19 in previously healthy children and adolescents in New York City. *JAMA, 324*(3), 294–296. https://doi.org/10.1001/jama.2020.10374

Cleveland Clinic. (2023). *Cytokine Release Syndrome (CRS)*. available at: https://my.clevelandclinic.org/health/diseases/22700-cytokine-release-syndrome

Cole, L. D., Osborne, C. M., Silveira, L. J., et al. (2021). IVIG compared to IVIG plus infliximab in multisystem inflammatory syndrome in children. *Pediatrics, 148*(6), e2021053702. https://doi.org/10.1542/peds.2021-052702

Costagliola, G., Spada, E., Comberiati, P., & Peroni, D. G. (2021). Could nutritional supplements act as therapeutic adjuvants in COVID - 19? *Italian Journal of Pediatrics, 47*, 32. https://doi.org/10.1186/s13052-021-00990-0

COVID-19 Treatment Guidelines Panel. (2019). *Coronavirus disease 2019 (COVID-19) treatment guidelines*. National Institutes of Health. Available at Retrieved July 21, 2023 from https://www.covid19treatmentguidelines.nih.gov/

De Los Santos, J., Bhisitkul, D., Carman, M., Wilson, K., Hasara, S., Homa, K., Reyes, P., Bugajski, A., & Barbera, A. (2022). The use of monoclonal antibody therapy in pediatric patients with COVID—19: A retrospective case series. International. *The Journal of Emergency Medicine, 15*(9), 9. https://doi.org/10.1186/s12245-022-00414-8

Del Borrello, G., Giraudo, I., Bondone, C., Denina, M., Garazzino, S., Linari, C., Mignone, F., Pruccoli, G., Scolfaro, C., Spadea, M., Pollio, B., & Saracco, P. (2021). SARS-COV-2-associated coagulopathy and thromboembolism prophylaxis in children: A single-center observational study. *Journal of Thrombosis and Haemostasis, 19*(2), 522–530. https://doi.org/10.1111/jth.15216

Deng, J., Zhou, F., Heybati, K., Ali, S., Zuo, Q. K., Hou, W., Dhivagaran, T., Ramaraju, H. B., Chang, O., Wong, C. Y., & Silver, Z. (2021). Efficacy of chloroquine and hydroxychloroquine for the treatment of hospitalized COVID-19 patients: A meta-analysis. *Future Virology*. https://doi.org/10.2217/fvl-2021-0119

Deville, J., Song, E., & Quellette, C. P. (2023). Remdesivir: Pediatric drug information. *Up to Date*. Available at www.uptodate.com/contents/remdesivir-pediatric-drug-information/print

Elsawah, H., Elsokary, M., Abdallah, M., & Elshafie, A. (2020). Efficacy and safety of remdesivir in hospitalized COVID-19 patients: Systematic review and meta-analysis including network meta-analysis. *Reviews in Medical Virology*, e2187. https://doi.org/10.1002/rmv.2187

Farah, R., Kazzi, Z., Brent, J., Burkhart, K., Wax, P., Aldy, K., & Toxicology Investigators Consortium FACT Study Group. (2022). Ivermectin associated adverse events in the treatment and prevention of COVID-19 reported to the FACT pharmacovigilance project. *Clinical Toxicology (Philadelphia, PA), 60*(8), 942–946. https://doi.org/10.1080/15563650.2022.2070187

Flaxman, S., Wittaker, C., Semenova, E., Rashid, T., Parks, R. M., Blenkinsop, A., Unwin, H. J. T., Mishra, S., Bhatt, S., Gurdasani, D., & Ratmann, O. (2023). Assessment of COVID—19 as the underlying cause of death among children and young people aged 0 to 19 years in the US. *Journal of the American Medical Association, 6*(1), e2253590. https://doi.org/10.1001/jamanetworkopen.2022.53590

Goldenberg, N. A., Sochet, A., Albisetti, M., Biss, T., Bonduel, M., Jaffray, J., MacLaren, G., Monagle, P., O'Brien, S., Raffini, L., Revel-Vilk, S., Sirachainan, N., Williams, S., Zia, A., Male, C., & Pediatric/Neonatal Hemostasis and Thrombosis Subcommittee of the ISTH SSC. (2020). Consensus-based clinical recommendations and research priorities for anticoagulant thromboprophylaxis in children hospitalized for COVID-19-related illness. *Journal of Thrombosis and Haemostasis, 18*(11), 3099–3105. https://doi.org/10.1111/jth.15073

Goldman, J., Lye, D., Hui, D., Marks, D., Bruno, R., et al. (2020). Remdesivir for 5 or 10 days in patients with severe COVID-19. *The New England Journal of Medicine, 383*(19), 1827–1837. https://doi.org/10.1056/NEJMoa2015301

Henderson, L. A., Canna, S. W., Friedman, K. G., Gorelik, M., Lapidus, S. K., Bassiri, H., Behrens, E. M., Ferris, A., Kernan, K. F., Schulert, G. S., Seo, P., Son, M. B. F., Tremoulet, A. H., Yeung, R. S. M., Mudano, A. S., Turner, A. S., Karp, D. R., & Mehta, J. J. (2021). American College of

Rheumatology Clinical Guidance for multisystem inflammatory syndrome in children associated with SARS-CoV-2 and Hyperinflammation in pediatric COVID-19: Version 2. *Arthritis Rheumatology (Hoboken, NJ), 73*(4), e13–e29. https://doi.org/10.1002/art.41616

Horby, P., Lim, W., Emberson, J., Mafham, M., Bell, J., Linsell, L., et al. (2020). Dexamethasone in hospitalized patients with COVID-19: Preliminary reports (recovery trial). *The New England Journal of Medicine, 384*(8), 693–704. https://doi.org/10.1056/NEJMoa2021436

Infectious Diseases Society of America. (2023). *Infectious Diseases Society of America guidelines on the treatment and management of patients with COVID-19*. Retrieved September 22, 2023 from https://www.idsociety.org/practice-guideline/covid-19-guideline-treatment-and-management/

Inocian, E. P., Incian, I. H., Pandann, I. N., & Reynaldo, R. F. D. (2022). Pharmacotherapeutics and vaccines for COVID—19. *Medsurg Nursing, 31*(3), 188–192.

Johns Hopkins All Childrens Hospital. (2023). *The importance of sleep for kids*. Available at: https://www.hopkinsallchildrens.org/ACH-News/General-News/The-importance-of-sleep-for-kids

Loi, M., Branchford, B., Kim, J., Self, C., & Nuss, R. (2020). COVID-19 anticoagulation recommendations in children. *Pediatric Blood & Cancer, 67*(9), e28485. https://doi.org/10.1002/pbc.28485

Loomba, R. S., Aggarwal, G., Villarreal, E. G., Farias, J. S., Flores, S., Lavie, C. J., & Aggarwal, S. (2021). Factors associated with deep venous thrombosis in patients infected with coronavirus disease 2019: A meta-analysis. *Blood Coagulation & Fibrinolysis, 32*(1), 23–28. https://doi.org/10.1097/MBC.0000000000000974

National Institutes of Health. (2023). *Coronavirus disease 2019 (COVID-19) treatment guidelines*. https://files.covid19treatmentguidelines.nih.gov/guidelines/covid19treatmentguidelines.pdf

Oldenburg, C. E., Pinsky, B. A., Brogdon, J., et al. (2021). Effect of oral azithromycin vs placebo on COVID-19 symptoms in outpatients with SARS-CoV-2 infection: A randomized clinical trial. *JAMA, 326*(6), 490–498. https://doi.org/10.1001/jama.2021.11517

Peroni et al. (2024). https://www.sciencedirect.com/science/article/pii/S2667009723000660

Porto, A. (2022). *Vitamin D for babies, children, and adolescents*. Health. Children.org. Available at: https://www.healthychildren.org/English/healthy-living/nutrition/Pages/vitamin-d-on-the-double.aspx?_gl=1*1ew6aa7*_ga*MTE4MzcwOTIxMS4xNjk1MzEzNDg4*_ga_FD9D3XZVQQ*MTY5NTMxMzQ4Ny4xLjEuMTY5NTMxMzc1NC4wLjAuMA

PRINCIPLE Trial Collaborative Group. (2021). Azithromycin for community treatment of suspected COVID-19 in people at increased risk of an adverse clinical course in the UK (PRINCIPLE): A randomized, controlled, open-label, adaptive platform trial. *Lancet (London, England), 397*(10279), 1063–1074. https://doi.org/10.1016/S0140-6736(21)00461-X

Rangappa, P. (2021). Cytokine storm and immunomodulation in COVID-19. *Indian Journal of Critical Care Medicine, 25*(11), 1288–1291. https://doi.org/10.5005/jp-journals-10071-24029

Reardon, S. (2021). Why don't kids tend to get as sick from COVID-19? *The Smithsonian Magazine*, 2021. Available at https://www.smithsonianmag.com/science-nature/why-dont-kids-tend-get-sick-covid-19-180978639/

Riphagen, S., Gomez, X., Gonzalez-Martinez, C., Wilkinson, N., & Theocharis, P. (2020). Hyperinflammatory shock in children during COVID-19 pandemic. *Lancet, 395*(10237), 1607–1608. https://doi.org/10.1016/S0140-6736(20)31094-1. Epub 2020 May 7.

Rogovik, A. L., Carleton, B., Solimano, A., & Goldman, R. D. (2010). Palivizumab for the prevention of respiratory syncytial virus infection. *Canadian Family Physician, 56*(8), 769–772.

Sanders, J. M., Monogue, M. L., Jodlowski, T. Z., & Cutrell, J. B. (2020). Pharmacologic treatments for coronavirus disease 2019 (COVID-19): A review. *JAMA, 323*(18), 1824–1836. https://doi.org/10.1001/jama.2020.6019

Schuster, J. E., & Williams, J. V. (2018). Emerging respiratory viruses in children. *Infectious Disease Clinics of North America, 32*, 65–74. https://doi.org/10.1016/j.idc.2017.10.001

Shekerdemian, L. S., Mahmood, N. R., Wolfe, K. K., et al. (2020). Characteristics and outcomes of children with coronavirus disease 2019 (COVID-19) infection admitted to US and Canadian pediatric intensive care units. *JAMA Pediatrics, 174*(9), 868–873. https://doi.org/10.1001/jamapediatrics.2020.1948

Sobu, E., Karaasian, A., Cetin, C., & Akin, Y. (2021). Vitamin D levels of COVID -19 positive symptomatic pediatric cases. *The Journal of Current Pediatrics, 19*, 9–14.

Song, E. (2020). Coronavirus (COVID-19): What a pediatrician wants you to know. *Integrative Medicine, 19*(2), 28–36. http://www.uptodate.com/contents/remdesivir-pediatric-drug-information/print

Sterne, J., Murthy, S., Diaz, J., Slutsky, A., Villar, J., Angus, D., et al. (2020). Association between administration of systemic corticosteroids and mortality among critically ill patients with COVID 19: A meta-analysis. *JAMA, 324*(16), 1330–1341. https://doi.org/10.1001/jama.2020.17023

Szarpak, L., Rafique, Z., Gasecka, A., Chirico, F., Gawel, W., Hernik, J., Kaminska, H., Filipiak, K. J., & Jaguszewski, M. J. (2021). A systemic review and meta-analysis of the effect of vitamin d levels on the incidence of COVID—19. *Cardiology Journal, 28*(5), 647–654. https://doi.org/10.5603/CJ.a2021.0072

Toubiana, J., Poirault, C., Corsia, A., Bajolle, F., Fourgeaud, J., Angoulvant, F., Debray, A., Basmaci, R., Salvador, E., Biscardi, S., Frange, P., Chalumeau, M., Casanova, J. L., Cohen, J. F., & Allali, S. (2020). Kawasaki-like multisystem inflammatory syndrome in children during the covid-19 pandemic in Paris, France: Prospective observational study. *BMJ (Clinical Research Ed), 369*, m2094. https://doi.org/10.1136/bmj.m2094

U.S. Food & Drug Administration. (2021). *Coronavirus (COVID-19) Update: FDA authorizes first oral antiviral for treatment of COVID-19.* Available at www.fda.gov/news-events/press-announcements/coronavirus-covid-19-update-fda-authorizes-first-oral-antiviral-treatment-covid-19

Waleed, A., Evans, L., Fayez, A., Moller, M., Marlies, O., Prescott, H., et al. (2021). Surviving sepsis campaign guidelines on the management of adult with coronavirus disease 2019 (COVID-19) in the ICU: First update. *Critical Care Medicine, 49*(3), e219–e234. https://doi.org/10.1097/CCM.0000000000004899

Whitworth, H., Sartain, S. E., Kumar, R., Armstrong, K., Ballester, L., Betensky, M., Cohen, C. T., Diaz, R., Diorio, C., Goldenberg, N. A., Jaffray, J., Keegan, J., Malone, K., Randolph, A. G., Rifkin-Zenenberg, S., Leung, W. S., Sochet, A., Srivaths, L., Zia, A., & Raffini, L. (2021). Rate of thrombosis in children and adolescents hospitalized with COVID-19 or MIS-C. *Blood, 138*(2), 190–198. https://doi.org/10.1182/blood.2020010218

Wiltz, J. L., Feehan, A. K., Molinari, N. M., Ladva, C. N., Truman, B. I., Hall, J., Block, J. P., Rasmussen, S. A., Denson, J. L., Trick, W. E., Weiner, M. G., Koumans, E., Gundlapalli, A., Carton, T. W., & Boehmer, T. K. (2022). Racial and ethnic disparities in receipt of medications for treatment of COVID-19—United States, March 2020–August 2021. *MMWR. Morbidity and Mortality Weekly Report, 71*(3), 96–102. https://doi.org/10.15585/mmwr.mm7103e1

Long COVID: Identification, Management, and Holistic Support

Tomika S. Harris

After climbing a great hill, one only finds that there are many more hills to climb.

—Nelson Mandela

Introduction and Background

Shortly after the beginning of the pandemic, anecdotal reports from adult patients experiencing persistent symptoms after being infected with SARS-CoV2, the virus that causes COVID-19, began to emerge (Callard & Perego, 2021). These patients formed support groups and began to refer to themselves as "Long Haulers" and coined the term "long COVID" (Callard & Perego, 2021; Department of Health and Human Services, Office of the Assistant Secretary for Health, 2022). Two of these members completed a survey and informal map of associated patients in the United States and in the United Kingdom and in May 2020 published the first landmark survey detailing symptoms experienced by people with long COVID (Patient Led Research Collaborative, 2020). This early identification by the patient community generated substantial interest among professional research circles and within a short period, resulted in advances in defining and understanding long COVID (Department of Health and Human Services, Office of the Assistant Secretary for Health, 2022). Long COVID has been referred to by several names, including post-COVID conditions, long-haul COVID, post-acute COVID-19, chronic COVID, and post-acute sequelae of SARS CoV-2 infection (PASC) (Centers for Disease Control and Prevention, n.d.-a). For this text, the term long COVID will be used as it highlights the ongoing effects of COVID-19 rather than implying complete resolution or recovery.

T. S. Harris (✉)
McGovern Medical School, UT Health Houston, High Risk Children's Clinic, Houston, TX, USA
e-mail: Tomika.S.Harris@uth.tmc.edu

© The Author(s), under exclusive license to Springer Nature Switzerland AG 2025
J. L. Peck (ed.), *COVID-19 Impacts on Child Health*,
https://doi.org/10.1007/978-3-031-80369-7_10

Much of the early long COVID research involved definitions of long COVID for adults. In October 2021, the World Health Organization published a clinical case definition of post-COVID-19 condition. Post COVID-19 occurs in (1) individuals with a history of probable or confirmed SARS CoV-2 infection, (2) with symptoms persisting 3 months or more after the onset of COVID-19, and (3) symptoms that last for at least 2 months and cannot be explained by an alternative diagnosis. Symptoms generally have an impact on everyday functioning, may persist or develop after the initial infection, and may fluctuate or relapse over time (WHO, 2021).

Children infected with SARS-CoV2 are generally asymptomatic or have mild symptoms that resolve within a few weeks of onset (Waghmare & Hijano, 2023). Reports of lingering symptoms in children after acute SARS-CoV2 began to emerge in the months after the start of the pandemic (Pellegrino et al., 2022). Increasing numbers of children experiencing symptoms of long COVID highlighted the need for guidance specific to children. To further define long COVID in children and adolescents, the World Health Organization (WHO) developed a clinical case definition for post-COVID-19 condition in children and adolescents. Post-COVID-19 condition occurs in (1) youth with a history of confirmed or probable SARS-CoV-2 infection, (2) with symptoms persisting for at least 2 months, and (3) initially occurred within 3 months of acute COVID-19. The symptoms have an impact on everyday functioning, may continue or develop after SARS-CoV-2 infection, and may fluctuate or relapse over time (WHO, 2023). It is important to note that long COVID in children and adolescents is distinct from multisystem inflammatory syndrome in children (MIS-C), also known as pediatric inflammatory multisystem syndrome temporally associated with SARS-CoV-2. MIS-C is a rare but serious complication of SARS-CoV-2 infection in children and adolescents generally occurs 2–6 weeks after SARS-CoV-2 infection (Carter et al., 2021; Feldstein et al., 2020).

Children of all ages are affected by long COVID (Davis et al., 2023). The reported prevalence of long COVID in children varies significantly from 1.6% to 70% (Baptista de Lima et al., 2023; Lopez-Leon et al., 2022; Pellegrino et al., 2022; Zimmermann et al., 2022). In addition, there is considerable variation in the frequency and types of symptoms reported. Common symptoms reported in children and adolescents include fatigue, mood disorders, sleep disorders, headaches, and respiratory symptoms (Baptista de Lima et al., 2023; Kumar & Jat, 2023; Lopez-Leon et al., 2022; Pellegrino et al., 2022; Rao et al., 2022; Zimmermann et al., 2022). There is limited data on the epidemiology of and risk factors for long COVID in children and adolescents. Some studies cite older age, ICU admission, and history of allergic disease as possible risk factors for long COVID in children (Asadi-Pooya et al., 2021; Osmanov et al., 2022). The pathogenesis of long COVID is unknown; however, there is emerging evidence suggesting latency of SARS-CoV2, reactivation of herpes viruses, abnormal immune response, and chronic endotheliitis as potential causes (Morello et al., 2023).

Guidelines for the identification and management of long COVID in children and adolescents are limited. Treatment guidelines for adults cannot be systematically applied to children as there are unique factors including age and developmental level that must be considered when approaching children with symptoms of long COVID (Malone et al., 2022). It is important to take a comprehensive, holistic approach in the assessment and management of this condition in children as symptoms can present in clusters that overlap and affect multiple body symptoms (Malone et al., 2022; Morello et al., 2023). In 2022, the American Academy of Physical Medicine and Rehabilitation (AAPM&R) Multidisciplinary PASC Collaborative (PASC Collaborative) published a consensus guidance statement on the assessment and treatment of long COVID in children and adolescents (Malone et al., 2022). This guide was developed to assist primary care and specialists with evaluations for children and adolescents with long COVID and will be used as an essential reference point throughout this chapter.

Points of Care

Initial Evaluation

The initial point of healthcare contact for children and adolescents with long COVID symptoms is likely to be their primary care provider. For those with more complex needs, referral to a multidisciplinary pediatric long COVID clinic may be necessary (Morrow et al., 2021; Vance et al., 2021). In the spring of 2020, multidisciplinary clinics designed to treat patients with long COVID opened (Malone et al., 2022). However, the numbers of pediatric-focused long COVID clinics are limited, and this much needed care may not be readily available to all, with limitations including distance, availability of trained healthcare providers (HCPs), and lack of insurance coverage or other financial means (Cirruzzo, n.d.). In such cases, the primary care provider will play an essential role in the management and care and will be responsible for coordinating diagnostic testing and specialty evaluations (Malone et al., 2022). Goals for the initial visit are to identify symptoms and the resulting impact on daily function, determine which additional evaluations are needed, identify symptoms that warrant urgent testing and/or referrals, and differentiate symptoms from preexisting or new conditions (Malone et al., 2022).

The diagnosis of long COVID can be supported by prior laboratory confirmed SARS-CoV2 infection. However, negative testing need not exclude diagnosis of the condition. Some children with long COVID will not have a positive test for SARS-CoV2 because of lack of timely testing, decreased antibody levels, or false-negative testing (Breuer et al., 2021; Buonsenso et al., 2023; Centers for Disease Control and Prevention, n.d.-b; WHO, 2023). Additionally, children with SARS-CoV2 infection are generally asymptomatic or have mild symptoms that are not recognized but can still result in development of long COVID (Lopez-Leon et al., 2022; Pellegrino et al., 2022; WHO, 2023; Zimmermann et al., 2022). The initial evaluation should include a detailed history and review of systems followed by a complete and systematic physical examination. Labs and diagnostic testing may be indicated based on symptoms reported (Malone et al., 2022).

A comprehensive initial assessment allows HCPs to identify persistent symptoms, both physical and psychological, and determine the severity and extent of impairment. Long COVID may have on daily activities, academic performance, and overall quality of life. Information obtained during the assessment aids healthcare professionals in the creation of individualized treatment plans that may involve a multidisciplinary approach, including medical, rehabilitative, psychological, and educational interventions. The initial assessment also establishes a baseline against which the child's progress can be measured over time. Routine follow-up is necessary to determine if interventions are successful or if adjustments to the treatment plan are needed (Malone et al., 2022).

Components of the Initial Assessment

The initial assessment for a child with long COVID should include the following (Malone et al., 2022):

1. Description of the acute SARS-CoV2 infection including symptoms, severity, duration, complications, and treatments.
2. Description of current symptoms: Onset, duration, timing, triggers, and treatments that lead to improvement or worsening should be noted.
3. Functional evaluation: Assess level of functional activity limitations. Compare current level of function to baseline, including impact on physical activity and mobility, academic performance, sports, hobbies.
4. Past medical history: Preexisting conditions, surgeries, hospitalizations, and vaccination status.
5. Family history: Family members with history of COVID-19 and/or long COVID, autoimmune/inflammatory disorders, genetic conditions, cognitive issues, and mental and/or behavioral health issues.
6. Social history: Review of school attendance and academic performance, extracurricular activities, family structure, family stressors, and support networks.
7. Review of current medications, supplements, and allergies.
8. Vital signs: Temperature, blood pressure, oxygen saturation, respiratory rate, heart rate, height and weight.
9. Comprehensive physical examination.
10. Psychological evaluation: This includes assessing for mental and behavioral health issues such as anxiety, depression, and other psychological issues that may result from long COVID.
11. Cognitive assessment: Assess for cognitive impairments, such as difficulties with memory, attention, or executive functions.

12. Assessment: Clinical syndromes or disorders in addition to long COVID may be diagnosed based on history, physical exam, and diagnostic testing.
13. Labs/radiology: Obtain pertinent labs and diagnostic tests based on history and presenting symptoms.
14. Follow-up plan and referrals.

Management by System

Systemic/Constitutional

Easy fatigability is a commonly reported symptom in children and adolescents with long COVID (Lopez-Leon et al., 2022; Waghmare & Hijano, 2023; Zimmermann et al., 2022). Activity and post-exertional malaise have also been reported. A consistent daily routine can be beneficial to combat these symptoms. Recommendations for physical activity should be individualized, goal-oriented, and encourage a progressive increase in activity (American Academy of Pediatrics, n.d.-a). Myalgic encephalomyelitis/chronic fatigue syndrome (ME/CFS) should be considered in patients with fatigue occurring for 6 months or more with significant impairment of daily functioning (American Academy of Pediatrics, n.d.-a). Additional characteristics of ME/CFS include post-exertional fatigue, unrefreshing sleep, impaired cognition, and orthostatic intolerance (Komaroff & Lipkin, 2023). Patients who report profound post-exertional fatigue or "crashing" after a period of physical or cognitive activity may benefit from a referral to physical therapy or physical medicine and rehabilitation (American Academy of Pediatrics, n.d.-a; Malone et al., 2022).

Sleep difficulties, including insomnia or excessive daytime sleepiness, have been reported in children and adolescents with long COVID (Lopez-Leon et al., 2022; Morello et al., 2023; Tyack et al., 2022; Waghmare & Hijano, 2023). Adequate sleep is essential for overall physical health and growth. Lack of sleep or poor-quality sleep can lead to fatigue, inability to concentrate, irritability, and decreased immune response (American Academy of Sleep Medicine, n.d.; Malone et al., 2022). Good sleep hygiene, consistent sleep schedule, and limited screen time before bed should be encouraged (Malone et al., 2022).

Mental and Behavioral Health

Mental and behavioral health concerns emerging in children and adolescents with long COVID have been increasingly reported (American Academy of Pediatrics, n.d.-a). Youth battling the long-term effects of COVID-19 may experience various psychiatric symptoms, ranging from mild to severe. These symptoms can manifest in various ways, including but not limited to anxiety, depression, cognitive difficulties, and behavioral changes (Avittan & Kustovs, 2023; Mat Hassan et al., 2023).

Anxiety may present as excessive worry, restlessness, irritability, and difficulty concentrating. Symptoms of depression may surface as persistent sadness, lack of interest in previously enjoyed activities, feelings of worthlessness, or changes in appetite and sleep patterns (Gleason & Thompson, 2022). Behavioral changes seen in youth with long COVID include behavioral or academic regression, mood swings, and aggression (Gupta et al., 2022; Mat Hassan et al., 2023). Mental and behavioral health symptoms can have a profound impact on academic progress, social interactions, and overall well-being.

Given the potential seriousness of these symptoms, an interdisciplinary approach that includes mental health professionals, educators, and HCPs is essential (Gupta et al., 2022). A complete mental and behavioral health screen should be included in all evaluations of children and adolescents after COVID-19 infection at 1 month and again at 3 to 4 months, ensuring that any emerging concerns are identified and addressed promptly (Mat Hassan et al., 2023). Early identification and intervention through comprehensive assessments and individualized treatment plans will be instrumental in mitigating long-term sequelae and supporting the child as they recover. Furthermore, caregivers and parents play a vital role in recognizing these symptoms and seeking appropriate care for their children. Open communication, education, and support mechanisms should be readily available to parents, equipping them with the necessary tools to understand and address the mental and behavioral health challenges encountered by their child (American Academy of Pediatrics, n.d.-b).

Autonomic Dysfunction and Orthostatic

Orthostatic symptoms, including lightheadedness, dizziness, syncope, and palpitations have been reported in children and adolescents with long COVID (Morrow et al., 2022). Patients with these symptoms, when combined with significant orthostatic tachycardia, may meet criteria for a diagnosis of postural tachycardia syndrome (POTS). POTS is a chronic disorder of the autonomic nervous system that primarily affects females between the ages of 12 and 50 and can be triggered by infection, pregnancy, fever, or trauma (Vernino et al., 2021). The diagnosis of POTS requires (1) heart rate increase of at least 30 beats/min (bpm), (40 bpm for 12–19 years old) within 10 min of standing up, (2) absence of orthostatic hypotension, (3) additional orthostatic symptoms, (4) symptoms for at least 3 months, (5) not explained by other symptoms or conditions (Raj et al., 2021; Vernino et al., 2021). These symptoms can dramatically impact quality of life.

While the exact mechanisms linking long COVID and the development of POTS are unknown, multiple hypotheses have been proposed. One hypothesis suggests that the initial COVID-19 infection triggers an autoimmune response, leading to autonomic dysfunction. Another hypothesis proposes that viral-induced inflammation affects blood vessels, disrupting normal cardiovascular regulation (Ormiston et al., 2022). These hypotheses underscore the complexity and diverse nature of long COVID and its associated complications. Accurate diagnosis is essential to develop an appropriate management plan suitable for children and adolescents with long COVID POTS. Tilt table testing, which assesses heart rate and blood pressure responses to positional changes, may aid in the diagnosis of POTS (Cheshire Jr & Goldstein, 2019). Until further evidence is available regarding the differentiation in the treatment of Postural Orthostatic Tachycardia Syndrome (POTS) between individuals with and without COVID-19, it is recommended to adhere to the current guidelines for POTS management (Ormiston et al., 2022).

The current guidelines for treating POTS focus on a multidisciplinary team approach that includes lifestyle modifications, non-pharmacological interventions, and medication options. The effectiveness of treatment may vary among patients, but overall, a combination of strategies is usually employed to manage symptoms effectively (Cheshire Jr & Goldstein, 2019; Ormiston et al., 2022; Zhang et al., 2020). Lifestyle modifications and non-pharmacological strategies, including physical therapy, progressive exercise programs, and adequate fluid and salt intake, have shown promising outcomes in symptom management (Cheshire Jr & Goldstein, 2019; Ormiston et al., 2022; Zhang et al., 2020). Medications such as beta-blockers may be prescribed to alleviate symptoms and regulate heart rate (Malone et al., 2022; Zhang et al., 2020). For those children and adolescents with orthostatic symptoms who do not meet the diagnostic criteria for POTS, lifestyle modifications and non-pharmacological interventions should still be discussed, and medications can be considered to manage symptoms (Malone et al., 2022). Finally, it is important to screen for mental health concerns as POTS symptoms may present similarly to symptoms of anxiety and depression (Malone et al., 2022).

Neurological

A range of cognitive symptoms have been observed in children with long COVID. These include difficulties with attention and concentration, impaired memory and recall, diminished executive functioning, and reduced processing speed (Avittan & Kustovs, 2023; Buonsenso et al., 2021; Davis et al., 2023). These challenges may lead to academic regression, affecting a child's learning potential and educational progress, necessitating additional support and accommodations.

Healthcare providers, educators, and caregivers play an essential role in monitoring the child's cognitive functioning and ensuring appropriate interventions are provided. Early identification and intervention are crucial to prevent poor outcomes. Neuropsychological testing is recommended for children who have persistent cognitive symptoms with functional impairments to inform therapeutic interventions and the development of an individualized treatment plan (Malone et al., 2022). Educational accommodations such as a 504 plan should also be discussed (Tyack et al., 2022).

Headaches are commonly reported in children with long COVD (Davis et al., 2023; Zheng et al., 2023) The evaluation and management of headache in a child with long COVID are the same as any child presenting with headache. Neuroimaging should be obtained for patients with abnormal neurological exam or concerning history (Szperka, 2021). Headache in children and adolescents with long COVID may be related to medications, sleep disturbances, dehydration, poor nutrition, and other stressors (Tyack et al., 2022). Treatment may involve a combination of non-pharmacological interventions and pharmacological interventions. Non-pharmacological measures such as maintaining a regular sleep pattern, stress reduction techniques, and ensuring proper hydration and nutrition are the mainstay of treatment and can significantly contribute to headache management (Malone et al., 2022; Szperka, 2021; Tyack et al., 2022). If headaches do not improve with lifestyle changes or are severe, pharmacological options should be carefully selected, considering the child's age, severity of symptoms, and any additional comorbidities (Szperka, 2021).

Respiratory

Persistent respiratory symptoms following acute COVID-19 infection are common. Symptoms reported in children and adolescents include exertional dyspnea, cough, and exercise intolerance (Leftin Dobkin et al., 2021; Sansone et al., 2023). Respiratory evaluation should include pulse oximetry, chest X-ray, spirometry, and evaluation by a pulmonologist if available. If symptoms are persistent or if there are abnormal findings on the exam or initial workup, additional tests may be indicated (Malone et al., 2022).

One of the predominant respiratory symptoms seen in children with long COVID is a persistent or prolonged cough. The cough may linger for weeks or even months following the initial infection and often presents as a dry cough that can be trouble-some, both at night and during the day (Song et al., 2021). Adequate hydration, supportive measures, and monitoring for any worsening symptoms are warranted for these children. In some cases, medical intervention such as bronchodilators or corticosteroids may be considered (Malone et al., 2022).

Children with long COVID may also experience exertional dyspnea and exercise intolerance which can significantly limit mobility and participation in physical activities. Cardiopulmonary exercise testing may be beneficial for patients with these symptoms (Kersten et al., 2022; Sansone et al., 2023). Recommendations include encouraging pacing during physical activities and routine monitoring of oxygen saturation levels to determine the need for further intervention, if necessary (Malone et al., 2022).

Functional respiratory disorders such as hyperventilation and sighing dyspnea should be considered, particularly when anxiety is present (Hurvitz & Weinberger, 2021; Malone et al., 2022). Vocal cord dysfunction should also be considered when the patient endorses intermittent dyspnea that does not respond to bronchodilators combined with tightness in the throat, and inability to get air in. Referral to a speech-language pathologist with expertise in functional respiratory disorders may be helpful.

Uncommon presentations may include bronchiectasis, pulmonary fibrosis, or postinfectious bronchiolitis obliterans. These may be more common in those with more severe illness initially. Immunosuppressed children may be at higher risk for lung damage due to long COVID (Malone et al., 2022). Generally, symptoms gradually resolve in children with normal imaging.

Cardiac

Children with long COVID have reported a range of cardiac symptoms including, but not limited to, chest pain, palpitations, dizziness, and exercise intolerance (Erol et al., 2022). Chest pain is uncommon in children and adolescents with long COVID and should be differentiated from respiratory or musculoskeletal chest pain. Healthcare providers also need to be sure that chest pain is not due to MIS-C where there may be a true cardiac pathology. Red flags include chest pain with exercise, radiation of the pain to the neck, jaw, or down the arms, and/or chest pain associated with dizziness and/or loss of consciousness (Malone et al., 2022).

Cardiovascular disease including myocarditis, pericarditis, heart failure, and arrhythmias are uncommon in children with long COVID (Erol et al., 2022; Jone et al., 2022). However, it is important that these diagnoses are excluded given the potential consequences of a missed diagnosis. Prompt referral to a pediatric cardiologist is warranted if there is concern for an underlying cardiac cause (Malone et al., 2022).

Otolaryngology

Children affected by long COVID may present with a range of otolaryngology symptoms, which can vary in severity and duration. Anosmia and ageusia, the loss of smell and taste, respectively, have been reported in children and adolescents with long COVID (American Academy of Pediatrics, n.d.-a; Buonsenso et al., 2022; Funk et al., 2022; Lopez-Leon et al., 2022). The exact mechanism for anosmia and ageusia in COVID-19 is unclear; however, it is postulated to be a sensorineural deficit caused by an inflammatory response to the virus that causes damage to the olfactory bulb and taste buds (Krishnakumar et al., 2023). The presence of concurrent nasal symptoms warrants further evaluation for additional causes of altered smell (Malone et al., 2022).

The implications of loss of smell and taste in children with long COVID extend beyond the immediate impairment. Anosmia and ageusia can affect a child's ability to detect potentially dangerous odors, such as gas leaks or spoiled food. In addition, these sensory deficits can affect nutritional status and mood and impact social interactions, particularly around mealtime (American Academy of Pediatrics, n.d.-a).

Most cases of COVID-related anosmia will resolve over time without any intervention, therefore watchful waiting is an appropriate initial strategy (Rusetsky et al., 2021). Smell training should begin 2 weeks after the acute illness as resolved. Smell training involves exposing the child to pleasant and distinct smells to help stimulate the olfactory system and consists of smelling specific scents like essential oils or fragrant items multiple times per day (Hopkins et al., 2021).

Imaging is not recommended for loss of smell in the absence of other sinonasal symptoms (Hopkins et al., 2021). For patients with anosmia for more than 6 weeks combined with nasal symptoms, magnetic resonance imaging (MRI) with contrast or computed tomography without contrast is recommended. A brain MRI is warranted for all patients with loss of smell and neurological symptoms or deficits (Hopkins et al., 2021).

Consensus regarding medical treatments for COVID-related loss of smell is limited (Malone et al., 2022). Intranasal steroids are recommended only if additional nasal symptoms are present. Oral steroids may be used for isolated loss of smell lasting greater than 2 weeks. Omega 3 supplements are optional. There is insufficient evidence to recommend therapeutic use of alpha-lipoic acid or vitamin A drops (Hopkins et al., 2021). Treatment of COVID-related dysgeusia is in line with recommendations for treatment of anosmia (Malone et al., 2022).

Musculoskeletal

Myalgias, arthralgias, and weakness are common in adults with long COVID (Sapkota & Nune, 2022). These symptoms have been reported in children and adolescents as well (Buonsenso et al., 2021; Funk et al., 2022; Lopez-Leon et al., 2022; Zimmermann et al., 2022). The causes behind myalgia and arthralgia in children with long COVID are still being investigated. It is believed that the inflammatory response triggered by the virus may result in persistent muscle and joint inflammation, leading to these symptoms (Sapkota & Nune, 2022). Patients experiencing myalgia and arthralgia may report muscle soreness, weakness, stiffness, and joint pain. These symptoms may fluctuate in intensity and can significantly impact daily activities, quality of life, and overall well-being. In addition, myalgia and arthralgia can cause disruptions in sleep patterns and hinder cognitive and physical functioning (Lewandowski et al., 2011). Rheumatological diagnoses should be considered for children presenting with pain and weakness of the joints and muscles as there are several rheumatic diseases that may mimic long COVID including fibromyalgia and ME/CFS (Sapkota & Nune, 2022).

Treatment strategies for myalgia and arthralgia in children with long COVID aim to alleviate pain, improve function, and improve quality of life. The treatment plan should be individualized and may involve a combination of interventions including the use of non-steroidal anti-inflammatory drugs (NSAIDs), physical therapy, and cognitive behavioral therapy (Malone et al., 2022).

Gastrointestinal Symptoms

Commonly reported gastrointestinal symptoms in patients with long COVID include nausea, vomiting, abdominal pain, diarrhea, and decreased appetite. It is important to note that these symptoms can be associated with both acute SARS-CoV2 infection and long COVID, highlighting the importance of obtaining a detailed history that included onset and duration of symptoms. Management of GI symptoms is based on symptoms present (Malone et al., 2022).

Return to Play or Activity

The American Academy of Pediatrics recommends that a stepwise approach be implemented for the return-to-play or activity post-COVID infection. This phased progression allows for gradual increases in intensity and duration, preventing potential re-infection or exacerbation of symptoms. All children and adolescents should receive medical clearance from a HCP prior to returning to the activity. Patients and caregivers should be encouraged to promptly report any new or recurrent symptoms that occur during physical activity to their healthcare provider. This allows for ongoing assessment and ensures the appropriate adjustment of the return-to-play plan, if necessary (American Academy of Pediatrics, n.d.-c).

Accommodations for School and Other Activities

Ensuring the well-being and academic success of children with long COVID is essential. Due to its chronic, often unpredictable nature, long COVID poses a significant challenge to the physical, cognitive, and emotional health of children and adolescents. It is important for their development and overall well-being that children have regular interaction with friends and peers (American Academy of Pediatrics, n.d.-a). Some children may require accommodations related to school, sports, and other activities. This includes making necessary adjustments for children with long COVID, including academic accommodations such as a 504 plan, flexible scheduling, and additional support services. Schools are encouraged to collaborate with HCPs to implement these measures, facilitating a seamless transition back to the learning environment. Collaborative efforts between HCPs and school personnel are important to promote the development of holistic care plans, taking into consideration the academic, physical, and emotional needs of the children (American Academy of Pediatrics, n.d.-d).

Vaccinations

Vaccination against COVID-19 continues to be recommended for all children who do not have contraindications including children and adolescents with a history of SARS-CoV2 infection. In addition, children should continue to receive all routine immunizations as scheduled. Primary prevention of COVID-19 infection in children eliminates the risk of long COVID.

Barriers and Breakthroughs

Barriers in Recognizing Long COVID in Children

Diagnostic challenges: Identifying long COVID in children and adolescents can be complicated due to the varied presentation of symptoms. Some symptoms of long COVID mimic other childhood ailments making diagnosis challenging (Morello et al., 2023).

Lack of research: Given the novelty of COVID-19, research on long COVID in children is scarce limiting our understanding of this condition. The scarcity of robust scientific studies involving children hinders accurate prevalence estimates, knowledge of risk factors, and development of effective treatment strategies specific to pediatric population.

Breakthroughs and Advances

1. International collaborative efforts: Recognizing the urgency and significance of studying long COVID in children, researchers and medical professionals worldwide have come together to pool resources and establish collaborative networks. This unified approach has accelerated the exchange of knowledge and data, paving the way for a comprehensive understanding of long COVID in children (Funk et al., 2022; Malone et al., 2022; Munblit et al., 2022).
2. Symptom profiling and management guidelines: Dedicated research efforts have aided in developing symptom profiles specific to long COVID in children. This will help clinicians discern distinctive patterns and establish reliable diagnostic criteria, leading to more accurate identification and management of long COVID in pediatric patients (Malone et al., 2022; Morello et al., 2023; WHO, 2023).
3. Multidisciplinary care: The complex and multifaceted nature of long COVID necessitates a multidisciplinary approach involving healthcare professionals from various disciplines. By leveraging the expertise of respiratory specialists, neurologists, psychologists, physicians, and allied healthcare practitioners, holistic care and support systems have been established for children with long COVID (Morrow et al., 2021).

4. Longitudinal studies: Longitudinal studies following children with long COVID over extended periods have played a crucial role in capturing the natural course of the condition, understanding its long-term implications, and evaluating response to treatments and interventions. These studies contribute significantly to the evolving body of evidence and inform evidence-based care strategies (Gonzalez-Aumatell et al., 2022).

While barriers persist in recognizing and managing long COVID in children, researchers and healthcare professionals have made breakthroughs in advancing our understanding of this condition. International collaborations, well-defined diagnostic criteria, and multidisciplinary care approaches have paved the way for better recognition, management, and support for children with long COVID. Continued research and collaborative efforts will enhance our understanding of this condition, ultimately improving the outcomes and quality of life for children and adolescents long COVID.

Lessons Learned

As communities worldwide continue to face challenges brought on by the pandemic, emerging evidence has provided much needed insight on the occurrence and consequences of long COVID in children. We know that despite having mild symptoms initially, children can develop long COVID symptoms that significantly impact their quality of life. In addition, long COVID symptoms in children may be different from those in adults (Rao et al., 2022). The COVID-19 pandemic also highlighted mental and behavioral health challenges that children and adolescents face. Evidence suggests that long COVID may have a significant impact on neurodevelopment and mental health of children (Maresca et al., 2022). Cognitive impairments, attention deficits, and mood disorders have been observed, warranting long-term follow-up and support.

Calls to Action
- Create widespread awareness regarding long COVID in children. All clinicians across the care continuum and caregivers need to be equipped with the knowledge to recognize the signs and symptoms of long COVID in children, ensuring early detection, intervention, and appropriate medical care.
- Large scale research studies need to be conducted to better understand prevalence, risk factors, symptoms, and long-term effects of COVID-19 in pediatric patients, including associated health conditions and psychological distress. This will not only contribute to our understanding of long COVID in children but also inform policymakers and HCPs in designing evidence-based strategies for prevention, treatment, and long-term management.
- Professional organizations and credible health governance entities need to prioritize development of treatment guidelines to assist clinicians with appropriate management and treatment of children and adolescents with long COVID.

References

American Academy of Pediatrics. (n.d.-a). *Post-COVID-19 conditions in children and adolescents.* https://www.aap.org/en/pages/2019-novel-coronavirus-covid-19-infections/clinical-guidance/post-covid-19-conditions-in-children-and-adolescents (Accessed 22 May 2023)

American Academy of Pediatrics. (n.d.-b). *Interim guidance on supporting the emotional and behavioral health needs of children, adolescents, and families during the COVID-19 pandemic.* https://www.aap.org/en/pages/2019-novel-coronavirus-covid-19-infections/clinical-guidance/interim-guidance-on-supporting-the-emotional-and-behavioral-health-needs-of-children-adolescents-and-families-during-the-covid-19-pandemic/

American Academy of Pediatrics. (n.d.-c). *COVID-19 interim guidance: Return to spots and physical activity.* https://www.aap.org/en/pages/2019-novel-coronavirus-covid-19-infections/clinical-guidance/covid-19-interim-guidance-return-to-sports/ (Accessed 22 May 2023)

American Academy of Pediatrics. (n.d.-d). *COVID-19 interim guidance: COVID-19 guidance for safe schools and promotion of in person learning.* https://www.aap.org/en/pages/2019-novel-coronavirus-covid-19-infections/clinical-guidance/covid-19-planning-considerations-return-to-in-person-education-in-schools/ (Accessed 22 May 2023)

American Academy of Sleep Medicine. (n.d.). *Sleep deprivation.* https://aasm.org/resources/factsheets/sleepdeprivation.pdf

Asadi-Pooya, A. A., Nemati, H., Shahisavandi, M., Akbari, A., Emami, A., Lotfi, M., Rostamihosseinkhani, M., Barzegar, Z., Kabiri, M., Zeraatpisheh, Z., Farjoud-Kouhanjani, M., Jafari, A., Sasannia, F., Ashrafi, S., Nazeri, M., & Nasiri, S. (2021). Long COVID in children and adolescents. *World Journal of Pediatrics, 17*(5), 495–499. https://doi.org/10.1007/s12519-021-00457-6

Avittan, H., & Kustovs, D. (2023). Cognition and mental health in pediatric patients following COVID-19. *International Journal of Environmental Research and Public Health, 20*(6), 5061. https://doi.org/10.3390/ijerph20065061

Baptista de Lima, J., Salazar, L., Fernandes, A., Teixeira, C., Marques, L., & Afonso, C. (2023). Long COVID in children and adolescents: A retrospective study in a pediatric cohort. *The Pediatric Infectious Disease Journal, 42*(4), e109–e111. https://doi.org/10.1097/INF.0000000000003829

Breuer, A., Raphael, A., Stern, H., et al. (2021). SARS-CoV-2 antibodies started to decline just four months after COVID-19 infection in a paediatric population. *Acta Paediatrica, 110*, 3054–3062. https://doi.org/10.1111/apa.16031

Buonsenso, D., Cusenza, F., Passadore, L., Bonanno, F., De Guido, C., & Esposito, S. (2023). Duration of immunity to SARS-CoV-2 in children after natural infection or vaccination in the omicron and pre-omicron era: A systematic review of clinical and immunological studies. *Frontiers in Immunology, 13*, 1024924. https://doi.org/10.3389/fimmu.2022.1024924

Buonsenso, D., Di Gennaro, L., De Rose, C., Morello, R., D'Ilario, F., Zampino, G., Piazza, M., Boner, A. L., Iraci, C., O'Connell, S., Cohen, V. B., Esposito, S., Munblit, D., Reena, J., Sigfrid, L., & Valentini, P. (2022). Long-term outcomes of pediatric infections: From traditional infectious diseases to long COVID. *Future Microbiology, 17*, 551–571. https://doi.org/10.2217/fmb-2022-0031

Buonsenso, D., Munblit, D., De Rose, C., Sinatti, D., Ricchiuto, A., Carfi, A., & Valentini, P. (2021). Preliminary evidence on long COVID in children. *Acta Paediatrica, 110*(7), 2208–2211. https://doi.org/10.1111/apa.15870

Callard, F., & Perego, E. (2021). How and why patients made long Covid. *Social Science & Medicine, 268*, 113426. https://doi.org/10.1016/j.socscimed.2020.113426

Carter, M. J., Shankar-Hari, M., & Tibby, S. M. (2021). Paediatric inflammatory multisystem syndrome temporally-associated with SARS-CoV-2 infection: An overview. *Intensive Care Medicine, 47*(1), 90–93.

Centers for Disease Control and Prevention. (n.d.-a). *Post-COVID conditions.* https://www.cdc.gov/coronavirus/2019-ncov/long-term-effects/index.html

Centers for Disease Control and Prevention. (n.d.-b). *COVID-19. Post—COVID conditions: Information for healthcare providers: COVID overview.* https://www.cdc.gov/coronavirus/2019-ncov/hcp/clinical-care/post-covid-conditions.html#overview

Cheshire, W. P., Jr., & Goldstein, D. S. (2019). Autonomic uprising: The tilt table test in autonomic medicine. *Clinical Autonomic Research, 29*(2), 215–230. https://doi.org/10.1007/s10286-019-00598-9

Cirruzzo, C. (n.d.). *For kids with long COVID, collective help can be hard to find 2021.* https://www.usnews.com/news/health-news/articles/2021-07-13/for-kids-with-long-covidclinic-help-can-be-hard-to-find

Davis, H. E., McCorkell, L., Vogel, J. M., & Topol, E. J. (2023). Long COVID: Major findings, mechanisms, and recommendations. *Nature Reviews. Microbiology, 21*(3), 133–146. https://doi.org/10.1038/s41579-022-00846-2

Department of Health and Human Services, Office of the Assistant Secretary for Health. (2022). *National Research Action Plan on Long COVID.* Author.

Erol, N., Alpinar, A., Erol, C., Sari, E., & Alkan, K. (2022). Intriguing new faces of Covid-19: Persisting clinical symptoms and cardiac effects in children. *Cardiology in the Young, 32*(7), 1085–1091. https://doi.org/10.1017/S1047951121003693

Feldstein, L. R., et al. (2020). Multisystem inflammatory syndrome in U.S. children and adolescents. *The New England Journal of Medicine, 383*(4), 334–346. https://doi.org/10.1056/NEJMoa2021680

Funk, A. L., Kuppermann, N., Florin, T. A., Tancredi, D. J., Xie, J., Kim, K., Finkelstein, Y., Neuman, M. I., Salvadori, M. I., Yock-Corrales, A., Breslin, K. A., Ambroggio, L., Chaudhari, P. P., Bergmann, K. R., Gardiner, M. A., Nebhrajani, J. R., Campos, C., Ahmad, F. A., Sartori, L. F., Navanandan, N., et al. (2022). Post-COVID-19 conditions among children 90 days after SARS-CoV-2 infection. *JAMA Network Open, 5*(7), e2223253. https://doi.org/10.1001/jamanetworkopen.2022.23253

Gleason, M. M., & Thompson, L. A. (2022). Depression and anxiety disorder in children and adolescents. *JAMA Pediatrics, 176*(5), 532. https://doi.org/10.1001/jamapediatrics.2022.0052

Gonzalez-Aumatell, A., Bovo, M. V., Carreras-Abad, C., Cuso-Perez, S., Domènech Marsal, È., Coll-Fernández, R., Goicoechea Calvo, A., Giralt-López, M., Enseñat Cantallops, A., Moron-Lopez, S., Martinez-Picado, J., Sol Ventura, P., Rodrigo, C., & Méndez Hernández, M. (2022). Social, academic, and health status impact of long COVID on children and young people: An observational, descriptive, and longitudinal cohort study. *Children (Basel, Switzerland), 9*(11), 1677. https://doi.org/10.3390/children9111677

Gupta, M., Gupta, N., & Esang, M. (2022). Long COVID in children and adolescents. *Primary Care Companion for CNS Disorders, 24*(2), 21r03218. https://doi.org/10.4088/PCC.21r03218

Hopkins, C., Alanin, M., Philpott, C., Harries, P., Whitcroft, K., Qureishi, A., Anari, S., Ramakrishnan, Y., Sama, A., Davies, E., Stew, B., Gane, S., Carrie, S., Hathorn, I., Bhalla, R., Kelly, C., Hill, N., Boak, D., & Nirmal Kumar, B. (2021). Management of new onset loss of sense of smell during the COVID-19 pandemic—BRS consensus guidelines. *Clinical Otolaryngology, 46*(1), 16–22. https://doi.org/10.1111/coa.13636

Hurvitz, M., & Weinberger, M. (2021). Functional respiratory disorders in children. *Pediatric Clinics of North America, 68*(1), 223–237. https://doi.org/10.1016/j.pcl.2020.09.013

Jone, P.-N., John, A., Oster, M. E., Allen, K., Tremoulet, A. H., Saarel, E. V., Lambert, L. M., Miyamoto, S. D., de Ferranti, S. D., & on behalf of the American Heart Association Leadership Committee and Congenital Cardiac Defects Committee of the Council on Lifelong Congenital Heart Disease and Heart Health in the Young; Council on Hypertension, and Council on Peripheral Vascular Disease. (2022). SARS-CoV-2 infection and associated cardiovascular manifestations and complications in children and young adults: A scientific statement from the American Heart Association. *Circulation, 145*, e1037–e1052. https://doi.org/10.1161/CIR.0000000000001064

Kersten, J., Hoyo, L., Wolf, A., Hüll, E., Nunn, S., Tadic, M., Scharnbeck, D., Rottbauer, W., & Buckert, D. (2022). Cardiopulmonary exercise testing distinguishes between post-COVID-19 as a dysfunctional syndrome and organ pathologies. *International Journal of Environmental Research and Public Health, 19*(18), 11421. https://doi.org/10.3390/ijerph191811421

Komaroff, A. L., & Lipkin, W. I. (2023). ME/CFS and long COVID share similar symptoms and biological abnormalities: Road map to the literature. *Frontiers in Medicine, 10*, 1187163. https://doi.org/10.3389/fmed.2023.1187163

Krishnakumar, H. N., Momtaz, D. A., Sherwani, A., Mhapankar, A., Gonuguntla, R. K., Maleki, A., Abbas, A., Ghali, A. N., & Al Afif, A. (2023). Pathogenesis and progression of anosmia and dysgeusia during the COVID-19 pandemic. *European Archives of Oto-Rhino-Laryngology, 280*(2), 505–509. https://doi.org/10.1007/s00405-022-07689-w

Kumar, P., & Jat, K. R. (2023). Post-COVID-19 sequelae in children. *Indian Journal of Pediatrics, 90*(6), 605–611. https://doi.org/10.1007/s12098-023-04473-4

Leftin Dobkin, S. C., Collaco, J. M., & McGrath-Morrow, S. A. (2021). Protracted respiratory findings in children post-SARS-CoV-2 infection. *Pediatric Pulmonology, 56*(12), 3682–3687. https://doi.org/10.1002/ppul.25671

Lewandowski, A. S., Ward, T. M., & Palermo, T. M. (2011). Sleep problems in children and adolescents with common medical conditions. *Pediatric Clinics of North America, 58*(3), 699–713. https://doi.org/10.1016/j.pcl.2011.03.012

Lopez-Leon, S., Wegman-Ostrosky, T., Ayuzo del Valle, N. C., et al. (2022). Long-COVID in children and adolescents: A systematic review and meta-analyses. *Scientific Reports, 12*, 9950. https://doi.org/10.1038/s41598-022-13495-5

Malone, L. A., Morrow, A., Chen, Y., et al. (2022). Multidisciplinary collaborative consensus guidance statement on the assessment and treatment of postacute sequelae of SARS-CoV-2 infection (PASC) in children and adolescents. *PM & R, 14*, 1241–1269.

Maresca, G., Latella, D., Carnazza, L., Corallo, F., & Formica, C. (2022). Neuropsychological effects of COVID-19: A review. *Brain and Behavior: A Cognitive Neuroscience Perspective, 12*(9), e2602. https://doi.org/10.1002/brb3.2602

Mat Hassan, N., Salim, H. S., Amaran, S., Yunus, N. I., Yusof, N. A., Daud, N., & Fry, D. (2023). Prevalence of mental health problems among children with long COVID: A systematic review and meta-analysis. *PLoS One, 18*(5), e0282538. https://doi.org/10.1371/journal.pone.0282538

Morello, R., Martino, L., & Buonsenso, D. B. (2023). Diagnosis and management of post-COVID (Long COVID) in children: A moving target. *Current Opinion in Pediatrics, 35*(2), 184–192. https://doi.org/10.1097/MOP.0000000000001221

Morrow, A. K., Malone, L. A., Kokorelis, C., Petracek, L. S., Eastin, E. F., Lobner, K. L., Neuendorff, L., & Rowe, P. C. (2022). Long-term COVID 19 sequelae in adolescents: The overlap with orthostatic intolerance and ME/CFS. *Current Pediatrics Reports, 10*(2), 31–44. https://doi.org/10.1007/s40124-022-00261-4

Morrow, A. K., Ng, R., Vargas, G., Jashar, D. T., Henning, E., Stinson, N., & Malone, L. A. (2021). Postacute/long COVID in pediatrics: Development of a multidisciplinary rehabilitation clinic and preliminary case series. *American Journal of Physical Medicine & Rehabilitation, 100*(12), 1140–1147. https://doi.org/10.1097/PHM.0000000000001896

Munblit, D., Buonsenso, D., Sigfrid, L., Vijverberg, S. J. H., & Brackel, C. L. H. (2022). Post-COVID-19 condition in children: A COS is urgently needed. *The Lancet Respiratory Medicine, 10*(7), 628–629. https://doi.org/10.1016/S2213-2600(22)00211-9

Ormiston, C. K., Świątkiewicz, I., & Taub, P. R. (2022). Postural orthostatic tachycardia syndrome as a sequela of COVID-19. *Heart Rhythm, 19*(11), 1880–1889. https://doi.org/10.1016/j.hrthm.2022.07.014

Osmanov, I. M., Spiridonova, E., Bobkova, P., Gamirova, A., Shikhaleva, A., Andreeva, M., Blyuss, O., El-Taravi, Y., DunnGalvin, A., Comberiati, P., Peroni, D. G., Apfelbacher, C., Genuneit, J., Mazankova, L., Miroshina, A., Chistyakova, E., Samitova, E., Borzakova, S., Bondarenko, E., Korsunskiy, A. A., Konova, I., Hanson, S. W., Carson, G., Sigfrid, L., Scott, J. T., Greenhawt, M., Whittaker, E. A., Garralda, E., Swann, O. V., Buonsenso, D., Nicholls, D. E., Simpson, F., Jones, C., Semple, M. G., Warner, J. O., Vos, T., Olliaro, P., Munblit, D., & the Sechenov StopCOVID Research Team. (2022). Risk factors for post-COVID-19 condition in previously hospitalised children using the ISARIC global follow-up protocol: A prospective cohort study. *The European Respiratory Journal, 59*(2), 2101341. https://doi.org/10.118 3/13993003.01341-2021

Patient Led Research Collaborative. (2020). *Report: What does COVID-19 recovery actually look like?* https://patientresearchcovid19.com/research/report-1/

Pellegrino, R., Chiappini, E., Licari, A., Galli, L., & Marseglia, G. L. (2022). Prevalence and clinical presentation of long COVID in children: A systematic review. *European Journal of Pediatrics, 181*(12), 3995–4009. https://doi.org/10.1007/s00431-022-04600-x

Raj, S. R., Arnold, A. C., Barboi, A., Claydon, V. E., Limberg, J. K., Lucci, V. M., Numan, M., Peltier, A., Snapper, H., Vernino, S., & American Autonomic Society. (2021). Long-COVID postural tachycardia syndrome: An American Autonomic Society statement. *Clinical Autonomic Research, 31*(3), 365–368. https://doi.org/10.1007/s10286-021-00798-2

Rao, S., Lee, G. M., Razzaghi, H., Lorman, V., Mejias, A., Pajor, N. M., Thacker, D., Webb, R., Dickinson, K., Bailey, L. C., Jhaveri, R., Christakis, D. A., Bennett, T. D., Chen, Y., & Forrest, C. B. (2022). Clinical features and burden of Postacute sequelae of SARS-CoV-2 infection in children and adolescents. *JAMA Pediatrics, 176*(10), 1000–1009. https://doi.org/10.1001/jamapediatrics.2022.2800

Rusetsky, Y., Meytel, I., Mokoyan, Z., Fisenko, A., Babayan, A., & Malyavina, U. (2021). Smell status in children infected with SARS-CoV-2. *Laryngoscope, 131*(8), E2475–E2480. https://doi.org/10.1002/lary.29403

Sansone, F., Pellegrino, G. M., Caronni, A., Bonazza, F., Vegni, E., Lué, A., Bocci, T., Pipolo, C., Giusti, G., Di Filippo, P., Di Pillo, S., Chiarelli, F., Sferrazza Papa, G. F., & Attanasi, M. (2023). Long COVID in children: A multidisciplinary review. *Diagnostics (Basel, Switzerland), 13*(12), 1990. https://doi.org/10.3390/diagnostics13121990

Sapkota, H. R., & Nune, A. (2022). Long COVID from rheumatology perspective—A narrative review. *Clinical Rheumatology, 41*(2), 337–348. https://doi.org/10.1007/s10067-021-06001-1

Song, W. J., Hui, C. K. M., Hull, J. H., Birring, S. S., McGarvey, L., Mazzone, S. B., & Chung, K. F. (2021). Confronting COVID-19-associated cough and the post-COVID syndrome: Role of viral neurotropism, neuroinflammation, and neuroimmune responses. *The Lancet Respiratory Medicine, 9*(5), 533–544. https://doi.org/10.1016/S2213-2600(21)00125-9

Szperka, C. (2021). Headache in children and adolescents. *Continuum, 27*(3), 703–731. https://doi.org/10.1212/CON.0000000000000993

Tyack, C., Unadkat, S., & Voisnyte, J. (2022). Adolescent sleep—Lessons from COVID-19. *Clinical Child Psychology and Psychiatry, 27*(1), 6–17. https://doi.org/10.1177/13591045211065937

Vance, H., Maslach, A., Stoneman, E., Harmes, K., Ransom, A., Seagly, K., & Furst, W. (2021). Addressing post-COVID symptoms: A guide for primary care physicians. *Journal of American Board of Family Medicine, 34*(6), 1229–1242. https://doi.org/10.3122/jabfm.2021.06.210254

Vernino, S., Bourne, K. M., Stiles, L. E., Grubb, B. P., Fedorowski, A., Stewart, J. M., Arnold, A. C., Pace, L. A., Axelsson, J., Boris, J. R., Moak, J. P., Goodman, B. P., Chémali, K. R., Chung, T. H., Goldstein, D. S., Diedrich, A., Miglis, M. G., Cortez, M. M., Miller, A. J., Freeman, R., Biaggioni, I., Rowe, P. C., Sheldon, R. S., Shibao, C. A., Systrom, D. M., Cook, G. A., Doherty, T. A., Abdallah, H. I., Darbari, A., & Raj, S. R. (2021). Postural orthostatic tachycardia syndrome (POTS): State of the science and clinical care from a 2019 National Institutes of Health expert consensus meeting—Part 1. *Autonomic Neuroscience, 235*, 102828. https://doi.org/10.1016/j.autneu.2021.102828

Waghmare, A., & Hijano, D. R. (2023). SARS-CoV-2 infection and COVID-19 in children. *Clinics in Chest Medicine, 44*(2), 359–371. https://doi.org/10.1016/j.ccm.2022.11.014

WHO. (2021). *A clinical case definition of post—COVID-19 condition by a Delphi expert consensus.* World Health Organization. https://www.who.int/publications/i/item/WHO-2019-nCoV-Post_COVID-19_condition-Clinical_case_definition-2021.1

WHO. (2023). *A clinical case definition of post COVID-19 condition in children and adolescents by expert consensus.* World Health Organization. https://www.who.int/publications/i/item/WHO-2019-nCoV-Post-COVID-19-condition-CA-Clinical-case-definition-2023-1

Zhang, Q., Xu, B., & Du, J. (2020). Update of individualized treatment strategies for postural orthostatic tachycardia syndrome in children. *Frontiers in Neurology, 11*, 525. https://doi.org/10.3389/fneur.2020.00525

Zheng, Y. B., Zeng, N., Yuan, K., Tian, S. S., Yang, Y. B., Gao, N., Chen, X., Zhang, A. Y., Kondratiuk, A. L., Shi, P. P., Zhang, F., Sun, J., Yue, J. L., Lin, X., Shi, L., Lalvani, A., Shi, J., Bao, Y. P., & Lu, L. (2023). Prevalence and risk factor for long COVID in children and adolescents: A meta-analysis and systematic review. *Journal of Infection and Public Health, 16*(5), 660–672. https://doi.org/10.1016/j.jiph.2023.03.005

Zimmermann, P., Pittet, L. F., & Curtis, N. (2022). Long COVID in children and adolescents. *BMJ, 376*, o143. https://doi.org/10.1136/bmj.o143

Abuse and Neglect: Risk Management, Early Identification, and Evaluation

Renee Flippo, Jessica L. Peck, Katherine Hettenhaus, Kelcey King, and Kelley Rigby

It is easier to build strong children than to repair broken men.

—Frederick Douglass

Introduction and Background

On March 11, 2020, the World Health Organization (WHO) declared the COVID-19 outbreak a global pandemic (Centers for Disease Control and Prevention, 2023a). Shortly thereafter, on March 15, 2020, American states began to impose lockdowns locally and regionally to mitigate the spread of COVID-19 (Centers for Disease Control and Prevention, 2023b). This created increased stressors for families resulting in isolation, depression, anxiety, and job losses, all of which can lead to increased incidence of child maltreatment and neglect (Amick et al., 2022; Blumenthal, 2023; Whaling et al., 2023). According to Falk et al. (Falk et al., 2021), the unemployment rate topped 14.8% in 2020, which was the highest observed since 1948. Although federal funding was available to assist in covering expenses through the Coronavirus Aid, Relief, and Economic Security (CARES) Act while unemployed, only 58.6% of families categorized as at or below the federal poverty level received their allotted payments (Holtzblatt & Karpman, 2020). In their large-scale US study, Daly and Robinson (Daly & Robinson, 2021) discovered that anxiety levels for participants surveyed using the Generalized Anxiety Disorder (GAD)-2 screening tool increased significantly with the institution of local and regional lockdowns, but then declined and leveled when lockdown restrictions began to lift. Despite this plateau, levels of anxiety never returned to pre-pandemic measurements and stayed 3% above what was measured in 2019 (Daly & Robinson, 2021). For parents who were required to

R. Flippo (✉) · J. L. Peck · K. Hettenhaus · K. King · K. Rigby
Louise Herrington School of Nursing, Baylor University, Waco, TX, USA
e-mail: renee_flippo@baylor.edu; jessica_peck@baylor.edu

© The Author(s), under exclusive license to Springer Nature
Switzerland AG 2025
J. L. Peck (ed.), *COVID-19 Impacts on Child Health*,
https://doi.org/10.1007/978-3-031-80369-7_11

educate their children at home or provide childcare during the COVID-19 pandemic due to school and daycare closures, 40% met Patient Health Questionnaire (PHQ)-9 criteria for probable or severe major depression, whereas 39.9% met GAD-7 criteria for moderate or severe anxiety (Lee et al., 2021).

Child protection agencies receive more than four million reports each year (Childhelp, 2023), with the total number of referrals in 2021 alleging maltreatment for over seven million children U.S. Department of Health & Human Services [USDHHS] 2021. A report of child abuse is made every 10 s and the United States "has one of the worst records among industrialized nations" (Childhelp, 2023, "Child Abuse Statistics" section). In 2021, following the screening and investigative processes by child protection services, there were an estimated 600,000 victims of child maltreatment and neglect with children under the age of 1 year having the highest victimization rate (U.S. Department of HHS [USDHHS] 2021). According to Childhelp (Childhelp, 2023), this would fill ten modern football stadiums ("Child Abuse Statistics" section).

Adverse childhood experiences (ACEs) are traumatic events that occur to children and adolescents ages 0–17 years and have long-lasting holistic health effects into adulthood (Centers for Disease Control and Prevention, 2022, "Fast Facts: Preventing Adverse Childhood Experiences" section). "ACEs include physical, emotional, and sexual abuse and household dysfunction, such as parental mental illness, intimate partner violence (IPV), parental drug abuse, and parental separation" (Loveday et al., 2022, p. 2). Long-lasting effects of ACEs encompass chronic disease, substance abuse, and mental health disorders (Centers for Disease Control and Prevention, 2022). By preventing ACEs, as many as 1.9 million heart disease and 21 million depression diagnoses could be potentially averted. Approximately one in six adults report they've experienced four or more ACEs before 18 years of age, a factor which significantly increases the risk for experiencing seven of the leading ten causes of death in American adults (Centers for Disease Control and Prevention, 2022, "Fast Facts: Preventing Adverse Childhood Experiences" section).

The Child Abuse Prevention and Treatment Act (2010) (P.L. 111–320), and as cited by the USDHHS's Child Maltreatment Report (U.S. Department of Health, & Human Services, Children's Bureau, 2021, Summary, p. ix), defines child maltreatment and neglect as:

> Any recent act or failure to act on the part of a parent or caretaker which results in death, serious physical or emotional harm, sexual abuse, or exploitation []; or an act or failure to act, which presents an imminent risk of serious harm.

Sex trafficking was included in this definition with the passing of the Justice for Victims of Trafficking Act on May 29, 2015 (P.L. 114-22) (U.S. Department of Health, & Human Services, Children's Bureau, 2021). Child maltreatment and neglect are multi-factorial issues that include individual victim and perpetrator risk factors, as well as risk factors for the family and community (Centers for Disease Control and Prevention, 2022). Protective factors, such as positive relationships, a network of individuals or support system, and stable housing, decrease the chance of a child or adolescent being abused and incorporate individual, family, and community components (Centers for Disease Control and Prevention, 2022). Individual risk factors for victimization are children younger than the age of 4 years and those with special needs (Centers for Disease Control and Prevention, 2022, "Risk and Protective Factors" section). Risk factors for perpetrators encompass substance abuse, mental health issues, abused or neglected as children, low income, high levels of parenting stress, and use of spanking for discipline (Centers for Disease Control and Prevention, 2022, "Risk and Protective Factors" section). According to the USDHHS (U.S. Department of Health, & Human Services, Children's Bureau, 2021) for the reporting year 2021, 76.8% of perpetrators were a parent of the victim and 6.8% of perpetrators were a relative other than a parent. This supports the conclusion that most child maltreatment and neglect are occurring within the home and almost 90% of perpetrators are related to the victims.

Human Trafficking

Contrary to widely touted public attitudes exuding fear of being kidnapped by a stranger into a trafficking situation, the truth is actually far more sinister. In 2017, the International Organization of Migration estimated that in approximately 41% of child trafficking cases, a family member was the perpetrator (International Organization of Migration, n.d.). A 2023 study by the Polaris Project, an entity which runs the National Human Trafficking Hotline found 37% of 457 respondents reported experiencing familial sex trafficking (Polaris, 2023). Most persons victimized by trafficking have some sort of complicated connection to their trafficker, whether they perceive it to be a friend, a romantic partner, a caregiver, a mentor, an employer, or many other roles which leverage grooming in the presence of pre-existing vulnerabilities and risk factors to lure, force, defraud, or coerce children into trafficking. Complex trauma bonding in the presence of developmental immaturity precluding complex reasoning impedes a child's ability to recognize their own victimization or to make an outcry even when they do.

There are many other misconceptions about human trafficking that impede adequate prevention and response efforts. While the public often perceives trafficking as solely sex trafficking, the reality is that 69% of trafficking likely stems from labor trafficking. Another common misperception is that victims are primarily female, when in reality an estimated 18% of sex trafficking victims are male, and gender and sexual minority youth are particularly vulnerable to exploitation (Administration for Children and Families, n.d.; Office of Trafficking in Persons, 2019). Economic hardship and demand for frontline workers likely escalated exploitation and abuse through labor trafficking although reports for such went down in every industry except agriculture (Polaris, 2021b). It is sobering to consider, but the incredible global demand for personal protective equipment likely exacerbated supply chains leveraging labor trafficking for rapid production and distribution, including exploitation of children (Barnett et al., 2021).

Many conditions of hardship stemming from or worsened by the pandemic increase the risk of children's involvement in sex or labor trafficking, including poverty, cutbacks or closures of outreach and shelter services, unsupervised and risky social media use, family and interpersonal violence, child abuse, trauma, substance abuse in youth or caregivers, and overburdened systems (National Child Traumatic Stress Network, 2020). Economic instability and social disruption led many children to become increasingly vulnerable to the dangerous and manipulative tactics traffickers use to exploit them (Polaris, 2020). Research shows that the incidence of crisis trafficking situations increased by more than 40% during the pandemic in the United States (Polaris, 2020). Although shelter-in-place orders led to a 30% decrease in street-based trafficking, online operations rose by more than 45% (Polaris, 2021a). This stark change shows that trafficking is a dynamic crime and a severe form of child maltreatment that requires a unique approach by healthcare providers (HCPs) to recognize and respond to children presenting across the care continuum with urgent or emergent health needs resulting from trafficking abuses.

Points of Care

Incidence and Prevalence of Abuse

There is dispute among experts concerning whether child maltreatment and neglect declined or increased during the COVID-19 pandemic. Child welfare surveillance data and data from emergency room departments technically demonstrated decreases in victimization during the pandemic but this reduction aligns with school closures and a subsequent decline in child abuse reporting from educational personnel (Klika et al., 2023). Students ages 6–12 years had the steepest rate of decline in child maltreatment and neglect reporting during the pandemic, whereas, for children under the age of 1 year, the rates stayed the same (Klika et al., 2023). In contrast, data from the Adolescent Behaviors and Experiences Survey (ABES) showed that 55% of adolescents self-reported experiencing emotional abuse during the pandemic, and 10% indicated they faced physical abuse (Klika et al., 2023, p. 4). Calls and text messages to the National Child Abuse Hotline during 2020 also exceeded that of the previous year (Klika et al., 2023). Conversely, a study done by Kovski et al. (Kovski et al., 2022) discovered a decrease in child maltreatment and neglect reports following distribution of child tax credit payments.

Instead of relying on child protection services data, Amick et al. (Amick et al., 2022) used a manual chart review to investigate the incidence of emergency department (ED) visits due to child maltreatment and neglect in the state of Connecticut before and during the COVID-19 pandemic. Patient chief complaints, ICD-10-CM codes, and HCP notes were analyzed to determine whether there was an increase or decrease of child maltreatment and neglect during this time. The authors identified 1248 child maltreatment- and neglect-related visits, with 925 of those occurring pre-pandemic (Amick et al., 2022). Of the ED visits identified during the pandemic, age was the most significant difference with children 4 years of age or younger having most maltreatment-related incidents while neglect was the most frequent type of child maltreatment seen. Emergency department visits for neglect increased from a 9% pre-pandemic level to 13.9% during COVID-19 (March 16, 2020—August 31, 2020) (Amick et al., 2022). The findings of neglect as the most common form of child abuse identified during the pandemic paralleled what was discovered by Vermeulen et al. (Vermeulen et al., 2023) in the Netherlands.

Using cell phone data to track movement, Bullinger et al. (Bullinger et al., 2023) discovered that after an initial decline in reporting of child maltreatment and neglect with stay-at-home orders in the state of Georgia, each 15 min spent at home equated to an increase in material neglect referrals of 3.5% and a 1% increase for supervisory neglect (p. 339). This would seem to indicate that as the length of time that families stayed at home increased, possibly experiencing financial stressors due to job losses or the challenges of working remotely from home, material needs were not being met due to lack of funds and children were being supervised less. After the initial federal emergency declaration, reports to child protection services fell by 58%, mainly decreasing among those who are mandated reporters such as individuals in education or childcare (Bullinger et al., 2023). By child abuse type, emotional neglect and physical abuse reports saw the steepest decline, most likely due to lack of referrals from mandated reporters (p. 353).

International Studies

Although rates of child maltreatment and neglect in the United States seemed to decline during the pandemic for school-aged children according to published data, a study in the Netherlands had opposing findings. On March 15, 2020, an "intelligent lockdown" was enacted by the Dutch government to lessen the spread of COVID-19 (Vermeulen et al., 2023). Individuals were asked to work from home, social gatherings were banned, and restaurants and schools and daycares were closed. High levels of parenting stress are a risk factor for increasing child abuse, so researchers hypothesized higher stress levels experienced by individuals during the pandemic lockdown would cause an increase in child maltreatment and neglect (Vermeulen et al., 2023). Participants in their study included daycare workers and teachers from primary and secondary schools. In total, there were 444 individuals who participated in the study; 273 in the first phase and 171 in the second, reporting on children in home-based and out of home daycare settings, and children and adolescents in both primary and secondary schools (Vermeulen et al., 2023). Study participants were asked to indicate for how many of these children and adolescents they suspected child maltreatment and neglect had occurred during the 3-month period of March 16, 2020, to June 16, 2020. During the study, child maltreatment and neglect cases were identified as being in one of six categories: (1) sexual abuse,

(2) physical abuse, (3) emotional abuse, (4) physical neglect, (5) emotional/educational neglect, and (6) other abuse or neglect (Vermeulen et al., 2023).

Based on their research data, it was estimated that the prevalence rate for victims of child maltreatment and neglect in the Netherlands during the lockdown was 14 per 1000 children. The most prevalent type of child maltreatment discovered was emotional neglect with subtypes of educational neglect and witnessing domestic violence encompassing the majority. These rates are three times higher than those collected during time periods without a lockdown (Vermeulen et al., 2023). The second most prevalent reported type of abuse was physical neglect. In over 50% of the child abuse cases identified during the lockdown period of March 16, 2020, through June 16, 2020, concerns were already present for these families for child maltreatment and neglect prior to lockdown, and the circumstances within those homes worsened as lockdowns were imposed (Vermeulen et al., 2023). Results of this study indicate that vulnerable families may be more at risk for increased incidence of child maltreatment and neglect under high stress conditions, and the authors of the study emphasize that these at-risk families may need additional support and care during such times to ensure a safe home environment for all (Vermeulen et al., 2023).

Parenting Risk Factors

Abuse by parent is not based solely on individual risk factors but, rather, is multifactorial in nature and can be sensitive to environmental changes, economic and financial hardships, and stress (Blumenthal, 2023). According to the USDHHS's Child Maltreatment Report (U.S. Department of Health, & Human Services, Children's Bureau, 2021), of the more than 90% of victims abused by one or both parents, mothers of those victims have the highest percentage of acting alone as the perpetrator. Mothers are more likely to stay home while caring for their children, especially young children, and they may have minimal support and may be victims of domestic violence themselves. This held true during the pandemic as mothers continued to be the primary caregiver. According to Zamarro and Prados (Zamarro & Prados, 2021), in data collected by the Understanding Coronavirus in America Tracking Survey, 45% of women reported being the sole caretaker for their children during the pandemic compared with only 14% of men, irrespective of employment status (p. 17). Self-reported factors which amplify parenting stress for mothers are those who are the heads of their households, have low-socioeconomic means, and report being depressed (Blumenthal, 2023). Although parenting stress can be a risk factor for child maltreatment and neglect, it is not necessarily the cause of it (Blumenthal, 2023, p. 3). In unprecedented times such as a pandemic, where there are significant changes to one's environment, how parents feel about their ability to meet their family's needs during that time affects their behavior toward their children.

Using Socio-Emotional Information Processing Theory (SEIP), Rodriguez et al. (Rodriguez et al., 2023) reviewed reasons why child abuse risk may have been elevated during the pandemic, specifically for mothers who stayed home with their children. Outcome measures included parent-child aggression (PCA) approval, knowledge of discipline options, anger regulation capability, negative child attributions or a child's intention to misbehave, and PCA justification (Rodriguez et al., 2023). The results of their study indicate that a greater level of approval for PCA was associated with increased negative attributions, or a child's intention to misbehave, and a higher maternal state of anger. In addition, less knowledge of discipline options other than corporal punishment was also associated with negative attributions and a higher maternal state of anger (Rodriguez et al., 2023, p. 6). For mothers who had more effective anger management, there were fewer negative attributions, or a decreased perception that their child was intending to misbehave, and a lower maternal state of anger noted (Rodriguez et al., 2023). These results would seem to indicate a need for education related to discipline options, other than physical punishment, as well as generalized parenting techniques and anger management, may be helpful in decreasing risk for child maltreatment and neglect for mothers who are home with their children. Research supports that preventive educational training for parents can decrease the incidence of child abuse (Grzejszczak et al., 2022).

When investigating parental history of ACEs and risk of child maltreatment and neglect, Hails et al. (Hails et al., 2022) found that parental history of ACEs significantly affected the association between distress and negative parenting during the pandemic, as well as the association between pandemic distress and a child's manifestation of emotional or behavioral problems. Their study discovered that the higher level of ACEs historically for a parent, the stronger the association between these elements during the COVID-19 pandemic. This supports findings by Guyon-Harris et al. (Guyon-Harris et al., 2017) that history of exposure to child maltreatment and neglect and/or intimate partner violence may make that individual more susceptible to displaying parenting stress as adults.

As with individuals who have a history of ACEs and a higher risk for child maltreatment and neglect, the effects of lockdown during the pandemic were magnified for families who had pre-existing involvement with child protection services. In North Carolina, for families with a history of prior family violence, high levels of violence were seen in the first week following stay-at-home orders (Machlin et al., 2022). Families surveyed were categorized as having a low-socioeconomic status and a high risk for child maltreatment, and self-reported child protective services involvement, experiencing homelessness, a history of trauma in childhood, and verbal or physical conflict within the home (Machlin et al., 2022). Baseline violence for the surveyed families included children with an average of eight physical assaults in the year before the pandemic, with 76.6% of the children surveyed experiencing a pre-pandemic violent event. Violent events were classified as spanking, shoving, slapping, and beating (Machlin et al., 2022).

Despite an already pre-pandemic high level of baseline violence in the home for those surveyed, family violence peaked to its highest level 1 week after lockdown was imposed and then decreased across the months of April and May of 2020 (Machlin et al., 2022). With these results, Machlin et al. (Machlin et al., 2022) stress the importance of having policies and processes already in place during times of crisis to provide support for families identified as high risk for child maltreatment and neglect and propose that given time and the ability to adjust to environmental stressors, family violence can decrease.

Stressors for Nurses as Parents

According to the American Nurses Association (American Nurses Association, n.d.), "nurses are key to the health of the nation" (para. 12). Unfortunately, nurses are not immune to a higher risk for child maltreatment and neglect associated with pandemic stress. A study performed by Stevenson et al. (Stevenson et al., 2022) found that nurses who are also parents were at risk of not only compassion fatigue but also parental burnout during the COVID-19 pandemic. In addition to caring for very sick patients, along with dealing with a high death rate for those patients, many of these nurses were now required to tackle daycare and educational duties for their own children as facilities and schools closed, further increasing stress levels. Stevenson et al. (Stevenson et al., 2022) proposed that increased acuity of patient care, along with financial stressors and additional care of their own children due to daycare and school closures, would magnify compassion fatigue. The authors also hypothesized that the elevation of compassion fatigue would be closely associated with an increased risk of parental burnout and child maltreatment and neglect (Stevenson et al., 2022). In this study, those surveyed in May of 2020 were nurses who were also parents to children 12 years of age and younger.

Using a cross-sectional methodology, work environment and exposure to patient death and suffering were assessed, along with compassion fatigue and satisfaction, substance abuse, spousal conflict, parental burnout, and child maltreatment and neglect were measured (Stevenson et al., 2022). Participants numbered 244, with the majority being women, White, and having obtained a bachelor's degree. Most worked in an acute care hospital setting and had one child (83.2%) (Stevenson et al., 2022). Child maltreatment and neglect for study participants was measured via the Dating Violence Questionnaire, the Harsh Parenting and Ignoring scales, the Child Abuse Potential Inventory, and the Parent-Child Conflict Tactics Scale (p. 5).

Interestingly, study authors found that as the number of years of nursing experience increased, along with study participant age, the likelihood of directly caring for COVID-19 patients decreased, as did the level of spousal conflict, parental burnout, and child maltreatment and neglect (Stevenson et al., 2022). In contrast, as direct care of COVID-19 patients increased, so did levels of substance abuse, spousal conflict, parental burnout, compassion fatigue, and child maltreatment and neglect, supporting the study hypothesis (Stevenson et al., 2022). As direct care of COVID-19 patients increased, compassion fatigue also increased, as did the association with child maltreatment and neglect ($p = 0.283$) (p. 9). The authors suggest that future research be conducted to identify interventions which may decrease compassion fatigue and parental burnout for nurses [and other healthcare providers] working the front lines (Stevenson et al., 2022). Although mechanisms of decreasing compassion fatigue such as self-care and mindfulness are effective, during times of crisis nurses often prioritize others before themselves and do not take the time needed to invest in these interventions (Stevenson et al., 2022).

Human Trafficking

The coronavirus disease COVID-19 pandemic has not only unearthed inequities contributing to child abuse and neglect, it has also intensified them. The amplified impact of COVID-19 on the pediatric population has significant repercussions for children at risk of or exploited in human trafficking. Human trafficking involves substantial physical, emotional, and psychological trauma (Armitage & Nellums, 2020; Greenbaum et al., 2020). The COVID-19 pandemic crafted a harrowing landscape that increased the risk of trafficking of minors with exposure to grooming through increased child interactions with online platforms and simultaneously inhibited identification by HCPs of those who were being trafficked and those who survived trafficking because of laser-focused attention of the health system on COVID-19. These factors made it exceedingly difficult to deliver coordinated, trauma-informed, comprehensive services to support minors who had been affected by human trafficking (Armitage & Nellums, 2020; Greenbaum et al., 2020; Todres & Díaz, 2021).

Exacerbation of Risk Factors

The COVID-19 pandemic exacerbated numerous risk factors for human trafficking among pediatric populations, with experiences of homelessness and a history of child abuse emerging as particularly significant contributors to exploitation of minors during the pandemic, disproportionately impacting children representing ethnic and racial minorities as well as sexual and gender minority youth (Fedina et al., 2019; Todres & Díaz, 2021). In a 2023 study of survivors, more than half of 457 respondents responded affirmatively to experiencing ACE inquiries spanning 17 categories. Almost one-quarter reported prior encounters with the juvenile justice system while approximately one-third reported encounters with CPS (and another 20% who said CPS was not involved but should have been) (Polaris, 2023). Most tellingly, the number one reported need by 75% of survivors at the time of their trafficking exit was "accessing behavioral and mental health services with providers that understand my trauma," followed by a close second of "finding people I trust that care about me and could help me" with 73% (Polaris, 2023, p. 31). Almost one-quarter of survivors reported their own families as being a harmful or negative influence on their recovery. About 44% of survivors reported having a child during the exploitation, another complicated layer for pediatric HCPs caring for two generations who may both still be considered children. Almost one-third reported losing or almost losing custody of their child (Polaris, 2023).

The pandemic's devastating economic fallout resulted in soaring unemployment rates, leaving many individuals struggling to maintain stable housing (Agrawal & Kelley, 2020). Moreover, the closure of schools compelled children to spend more time online and in isolation, thereby heightening their vulnerability and susceptibility to traffickers employing new methods of online exploitation (Agrawal & Kelley, 2020; Todres & Díaz, 2021). Additionally, these school closures eliminated crucial opportunities for teachers and other school personnel to identify and assist at-risk or exploited youth (Agrawal & Kelley, 2020; Todres & Díaz, 2021).

However, the pandemic did not only escalate risks of entering trafficking but also worsened the already dire conditions for children experiencing trafficking (Todres & Díaz, 2021). Those who were subjected to trafficking during the pandemic's peak faced severe challenges, including limited access to essential personal protective equipment, barriers in adhering to social distancing guidelines, and restricted access to healthcare due to the overwhelming strain on healthcare institutions (Agrawal & Kelley, 2020; Todres & Díaz, 2021). The guidance to stay home from hospitals inadvertently hindered the identification of trafficked youth and their access to vital services including care coordination, accessibility to appropriate referrals, and comprehensiveness of support services for those impacted by trafficking (Agrawal & Kelley, 2020; Todres & Díaz, 2021).

Emerging Best Practices

The heightened vulnerability of minors during COVID-19 called for HCPs to adapt their practices, especially with telehealth services, when addressing minors experiencing or at risk of human trafficking. Many organizations and leading experts specializing in human trafficking emerged with new resources, education opportunities, and best practices for HCPs to reference when supporting those experiencing or at risk of human trafficking during the pandemic. The National Health Resource Center on Domestic Violence (National Health Resource Center on Domestic Violence, 2020) and Martinez-Sosa et al. (Martinez-Sosa et al., 2022) were able to accentuate strategies for healthcare professionals to utilize in overcoming the barriers created by the pandemic to ensure best practices when interacting with those affected or at risk of trafficking including:

1. Integrating information and resources specifically tailored for patient connection to human trafficking support resources.
2. Incorporating trauma-informed care communication and physical exam strategies.
3. Communicating messages of safety, including creating a safety plan.
4. Including care coordination and appropriate referrals to promote an integrated comprehensive care support model.
5. Prioritizing confidentiality best practices.
6. Providing universal information about how stress affects relationships and health status.

7. Ensuring communication pathways in which to follow up with the HCP.
8. Encouraging ways to remain connected to the health system or environment.

Barriers and Breakthroughs

Stressors

Evidence related to child maltreatment and neglect incidence and its association with the COVID-19 pandemic crisis points to a need for more efficacious policies and resources to protect children and adolescents within their home, specifically around material neglect. Many families at risk for child maltreatment and neglect experienced job loss during the pandemic, increasing financial stress, and did not receive their CARES funding because of a lack of internet access to apply for the funds, an unstable home address, and/or the requirement to have filed an IRS tax return in the previous year (Holtzblatt & Karpman, 2020). These barriers made it challenging for those in need to obtain necessary resources to provide for their families. Bullinger et al. (Bullinger et al., 2023) suggest that there should be a "robust and differentiated social policy response to reduce the economic, social, and mental health stressors that are the sources of maltreatment" (p. 354). Huang et al. (Huang et al., 2023) highlight that during times of crisis "monitoring and detection" of high-risk families need to be strengthened and emphasized and establishment of micro and macro level policies to further protect children from abuse should occur (pp. 15–16). These policies should positively affect the child and adolescent as an individual, the family unit, and society (Huang et al., 2023, p. 14). When parents were required to work remotely due to mandated lockdowns, despite being at home with their children, supervisory neglect referrals increased. Bullinger et al. (Bullinger et al., 2023) suggest that avenues to combat this issue are for employers to offer paid family leave, as well as access to "safe and affordable" childcare (p. 355). Because research supports that families who were already at risk for child maltreatment and neglect had higher initial rates of violence with stay-at-home orders, Machlin et al. (Machlin et al., 2022) stress that necessary resources be in place for such families whenever a major life transition or crisis happens. During the COVID-19 pandemic, countries such as Canada and South Africa increased resources for at-risk families and updated policies to assure protection for children and adolescents but the United States and Israel, for example, did not do the same (Marmor et al., 2023).

Telehealth

Fogarty et al. (Fogarty et al., 2022) looked at the impact of switching to a telehealth format during the COVID-19 pandemic for interventional services aimed at women and children who had experienced intimate partner violence (IPV) in Australia. Due to the pandemic and government-imposed lockdowns, the Restoring Childhood program, which typically is conducted face-to-face, transitioned to a telehealth model. Parents found that despite the telehealth format of the program, they were able to improve their parenting skills, increase their parenting confidence, understand the impact of IPV and family violence on their children, and increase their overall mental health and well-being (Fogarty et al., 2022). Overall, the telehealth experience provided the ability to (1) continue services for enrolled families despite limitations of stay-at-home orders or lockdowns, (2) increase comfort and accessibility of services for some families, and (3) provide a positive experience for children involved. Clinicians conducting telehealth visits appreciated flexibility in provision of services and the ability to see families in their home environment (Fogarty et al., 2022). Barriers to the use of telehealth were (1) work-life balance for some clinicians, (2) developing rapport with the family was more challenging, and (3) not being able to step away and process the day, because clinicians were working from home while patients were sharing their stories of family violence (Fogarty et al., 2022).

Human Trafficking

Amidst the peak of the pandemic, the implementation of social distancing, stay-at-home orders, and shelter-in-place directives imposed a new, substantial obstacle for individuals vulnerable to or experiencing human trafficking (United Nations Office on Drugs and Crime, 2021). These restrictions gave rise to heightened social isolation among youth and significantly decreased the prospects for human trafficking identification in this vulnerable population (Todres & Díaz, 2021). Throughout the pandemic, closure of clinics, prolonged appointment times, and disruptions in routine medical care resulted in a diminished number of individuals seeking assistance from HCPs (Todres & Díaz, 2021; United Nations Office on Drugs and Crime, 2021). Additionally, to adhere to the public health directives, the adoption of telehealth medicine became imperative (Junewicz et al., 2022). However, the deployment of telehealth services introduces new hindrances for youth at-risk or experiencing trafficking, including the absence of necessary devices for consultations, internet access, technological proficiency, and a confidential and safe setting for the virtual health appointment (Junewicz et al., 2022). Lastly, telehealth creates the potential barrier for HCPs to establish sound rapport and effectively assess the safety of their patients if their trafficker is present in the room or monitoring the visit, a fact perhaps unknown to the clinician conducting the visit (Wells et al. 2021).

While it's important to acknowledge the limitations of telehealth medicine, it's equally critical to recognize the advantages that contemporary technological advancements can provide to vulnerable youth at risk of trafficking. The internet, when utilized securely, can serve as a valuable means of extending support to at-risk or trafficked youth, irrespective of their geographical proximity to HCPs (UNODC 2021). Furthermore, the expansive reach of the internet enables heightened awareness initiatives via various social media platforms to occur (UNODC 2021). These benefits allow more opportunities for HCPs to receive training opportunities, provide more availability for health consults, and spread much needed awareness of the subject matter.

Other significant breakthroughs occurred through increasing awareness of human trafficking and more health entities getting engaged to help clinicians recognize and respond to risk of trafficking or experiences of trafficking. In 2021, OTIP released the landmark report *Core Competencies for Anti-Trafficking Response in Healthcare Systems*, an interprofessional report primarily authored by multidisciplinary clinicians with specific recommendations at the levels of individual practitioners, organized health systems or institutions, academic researchers, and educators (Fig. 1). There is a self-assessment tool available for free download with resources spanning six core competencies in addition to a universal competency of implementing a trauma- and survivor-informed, culturally responsive approach (National Human Trafficking Training and Technical Assistance Center, 2021). This was a tremendous breakthrough in providing evidence-based response to trafficking. Another significant step forward was NHTTAC's subsequent release of the *Toolkit for Building a Human Trafficking School Protocol* in December of 2022, the first federal resource directed to school preparedness (National Human Trafficking Training and Technical Assistance Center, 2022).

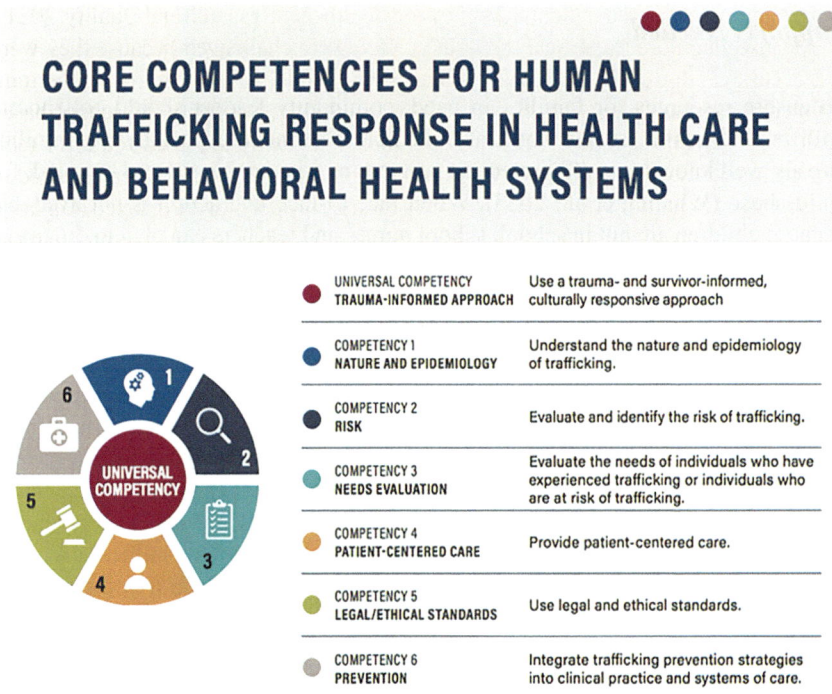

Fig. 1 Core competencies

Lessons Learned

Loss of Safety Nets

Although evidence is conflicting, there seems to be indication that child maltreatment and neglect occurred, and may have even increased, specifically during city and state-imposed lockdowns or stay-at-home orders. Children 4 years of age or younger continued to be most at risk but, with school closures, the lines are blurred as to whether school-aged children suffered more abuse during this time without the eyes of mandated reporters, such as teachers and school nurses observing them daily. During the pandemic, child protection services workers were also unable to make face-to-face visits, again removing the safety net of mandated reporters from the home. In addition, children whose exposure time to domestic violence is reduced when attending school or after school activities, were now quarantined at home, 24 h a day, without relief or access to other caring adults who are often mandated reporters (Whaling et al., 2023). It is well known that financial stressors, job loss, parental stress and burnout, anxiety, and depression increase risk for child maltreatment and neglect. In times of crisis, such as during a global pandemic, these elements are all in place, setting the stage for higher levels of abuse.

Supports Needed

To ensure resources for families in need, community leaders should collaborate with mental health, social work, and medical personnel, especially for families already well known to child protection services or who are considered high risk for child abuse (Whaling et al., 2023). When face-to-face interaction is not available because children are not in school, school nurses and teachers can plan to do virtual check-ins with families to identify any gaps in social determinants of health. According to Whaling et al. (Whaling et al., 2023), the state of Missouri instituted social media campaigns and hotlines during COVID-19, encouraging at-risk families to ask for and accept help. Educational personnel, HCPs, and social workers should also be taught how to recognize signs and symptoms of child maltreatment and neglect when doing virtual learning, telehealth visits, or with face-to-face interaction (Grzejszczak et al., 2022; Huang et al., 2023; Whaling et al., 2023). Communities as a whole need to receive education on how to recognize child abuse. Neighbors, store clerks, package and mail delivery workers, and community leaders who may have contact with the child or adolescent and their families also need training in recognizing child maltreatment and neglect and these training sessions can be offered virtually (Whaling et al., 2023). As Molnar et al. (Molnar et al., 2021) state, "Connection and intentional outreach, even if virtual, may help to support parents' health and wellbeing, as well as to promote healthy coping strategies that may reduce the risk of maltreatment" (p. 474).

Human Trafficking

The COVID-19 pandemic underscored several precarious lessons in preventing and addressing human trafficking in the pediatric population. First and foremost, the pandemic highlighted the amplified vulnerability of at-risk youth compounded by the pandemic's widespread negative socioeconomic impacts and social isolation requirements (Armitage & Nellums, 2020; Greenbaum et al., 2020). Economic hardships, social isolation, and disruption to support services and resources left many minors more susceptible to exploitation through digital media platforms (Greenbaum et al., 2020; Todres & Díaz, 2021). This susceptibility accentuates the importance of preemptive community-based outreach and coordinated early intervention efforts to identify and protect vulnerable children, especially those at risk, despite challenging circumstances (Foot et al., 2023; Greenbaum et al., 2020; Jaffe et al., 2022). Unfortunately, this increased vulnerability among youth allowed traffickers to demonstrate remarkable adaptability during the pandemic as they shifted their tactics to more online-based modalities (Jaffe et al., 2022). The digital shift encompassed grooming and exploiting minors through prevalent social media platforms, illuminating the necessity of amplifying digital literacy and online safety education for youth and their guardians (Finkelhor et al., 2021; Greenbaum et al., 2020).

Of note, a prominent children's hospital was in the news with reports of possible legal action arising from the case of a woman who was a victim of labor trafficking through services provided to a couple as a maid and a nanny. The trafficking survivor reported that she frequently encountered the health care system when bringing in her charge to access care, but she recounts she was never asked about her situation. After she was able to exit her situation, she retained legal counsel with the goal of holding the health system accountable for their alleged lack of recognition. While other industries such as hospitality and transportation have faced similar legal challenges, it has not been a common strategy in healthcare but that may change (McKim & Betancourt, 2022). These are important lessons learned: first, that not all trafficking presenting is sex trafficking of children and second, that preparedness for organizational anti-trafficking response is safest and most effective when implemented proactively, not reactively.

Another important lesson came in the polarization of the public over COVID-19 and adoption of bitter political hyperpartisanship. Politicians and legislators eager to serve their constituents were quick to support anti-trafficking legislation. However, many of these policies are not evidence-informed and could cause unintended harm. For example, several states adopted mandates for continuing education regarding trafficking response for HCPs, but without standards, there was no assurance the education would be evidence-based or effective. Texas became the first state to mandate continuing education *with clearly prescribed standards* on trafficking for HCPs (Peck et al., 2024). It is critical that policy solutions are evidence informed with careful consideration by health professionals with subject matter expertise to support the best pathway forward.

Collaborative Efforts

However, combating human trafficking during the pandemic in the pediatric population necessitates a multifaceted collaborative approach (Foot et al., 2023; Washburn et al., 2022). The increased vulnerability of youth during the pandemic demonstrated the need for cross-sector adaptive collaboration at a community, national, and global level. Human trafficking knows no borders, and the pandemic further emphasized the importance of information sharing and collaborative efforts across the United States and globally to respond to the human trafficking of minors effectively (Foot et al., 2023; United Nations Office on Drugs and Crime, 2021; Washburn et al., 2022). Effective responses to trafficking also require the coordinated efforts of particular sectors, including law enforcement, social services, education, technology companies, and healthcare to ensure integrated collaborative efforts to respond and support pediatric victims of human trafficking especially when traditional reporting channels, such as schools, are disrupted (Agrawal & Kelley, 2020; Foot et al., 2023; United Nations Office on Drugs and Crime, 2021; Washburn et al., 2022). However, to ensure resiliency of collaborative efforts across sectors, the pandemic also emphasized importance of adaptation as threats continuously evolve (Agrawal & Kelley, 2020; Todres & Díaz, 2021; United Nations Office on Drugs and Crime, 2021). Data collection and sharing by these sectors are crucial in grasping the evolving dynamics of child trafficking to guide research efforts to further develop shared nomenclature and obtain data from reliable shared sources, and effectively tailor and adapt response efforts and resources resilient to pandemic challenges (Todres & Díaz, 2021; United Nations Office on Drugs and Crime, 2021). Furthermore, we learned collaborative integrative anti-trafficking efforts for the pediatric population must be flexible, integrative, and innovative, offering remote services, telehealth, and digital support platforms to ensure minors can access critical resources and support regardless of external challenges (Finkelhor et al., 2021; Jaffe et al., 2022; United Nations Office on Drugs and Crime, 2021).

In conclusion, the COVID-19 pandemic provided profound lessons in the critical aspects of preventing and addressing human trafficking in the pediatric population. In sum, the COVID-19 pandemic has brought us face-to-face with increased vulnerabilities of at-risk youth, adaptability of traffickers, importance of digital literacy, necessity of global and national cross-sector collaboration, and the importance of flexibility to promote resiliency in our response efforts (Finkelhor et al., 2021; Foot et al., 2023; Jaffe et al., 2022; Todres & Díaz, 2021; United Nations Office on Drugs and Crime, 2021). These lessons serve as a powerful guide for our ongoing commitment as a pediatric health care community to protect minors and eradicate human trafficking in all its forms, especially in times of crisis.

Calls to Action
- Initial and continued training related to recognizing and responding to child maltreatment and neglect is needed for individuals who connect with children and families daily (e.g., social workers, teachers, school nurses, HCPs, and neighbors). This training can be face-to-face or offered virtually. Parental education programs should also be put in place for families with known child maltreatment and neglect, as well as for those at risk.
- Strengthen policies and community resources to assure protection of children from abuse, specifically during times of crisis. Frequent check-ins with at risk families should occur to assess the need for resources and assistance required, either completed via home visits or virtually.
- The increased vulnerability of youth during the pandemic, compounded by destructive socioeconomic impacts and social isolation requirements, calls for improved preventative community-based outreach, increased digital literacy among youth and their guardians, and adaptive global and sector collaboration to promote resilient integrative tailored response efforts that meet the diverse needs of youth at risk of or as victims of human trafficking.
- Clinicians, organizations, researchers, and academicians should evaluate their current practice for adoption of the Core Competencies for Anti-Trafficking Response in Health Systems.

Important Closing Notes
- It is critical for all HCPs to know and abide by the laws in the state in which you are licensed to practice, complying with all state and federal regulations governing your responsibilities as a mandated reporter. The Jones Day (Jones Day, 2022) Tool provides a listing of requirements by state that may be helpful as a starting place to explore state laws for education and reporting.
- The National Human Trafficking Hotline Number is 1-888-373-7888 and can be called 24 h 7 days a week for assistance, information, or reporting.

References

Administration for Children and Families. (n.d.). *Out of the shadows: Exposing the mths of human trafficking.* https://www.acf.hhs.gov/sites/default/files/documents/otip/trafficking_info-graphic508.pdf

Agrawal, N., & Kelley, M. (2020). Child abuse in times of crises: Lessons learned. *Clinical Pediatric Emergency Medicine, 21*(3), 100801.

American Nurses Association. (n.d.). *What is nursing?* https://www.nursingworld.org/practice-policy/workforce/what-is-nursing/

Amick, M., Bentivegna, K., Hunter, A., Leventhal, J. M., Livingston, N., Bechtel, K., & Holland, M. L. (2022). Child maltreatment-related children's emergency department visits before and during the COVID-19 pandemic in Connecticut. *Child Abuse & Neglect, 128*, 105619. https://doi.org/10.1016/j.chiabu.2022.105619

Armitage, R., & Nellums, L. B. (2020). COVID-19: Compounding the health-related harms of human trafficking. *EClinicalMedicine, 24*, 100409.

Barnett, B. S., Carlo, A. D., Mezzadri, A., & Ruwanpura, K. N. (2021). The invisible people behind our masks. *Annals of Internal Medicine, 174*, 550–551. https://doi.org/10.7326/M20-7421

Blumenthal, A. (2023). A bad time for kids in lockdown: The relationship between negative pandemic events, parenting stress, and maltreatment related parenting behaviors. *Child Abuse & Neglect, 138*, 106060. https://doi.org/10.1016/j.chiabu.2023.106060

Bullinger, L. R., Boy, A., Feely, M., Messner, S., Raissian, K., Schneider, W., & Self-Brown, S. (2023). Home but left alone: Time at home and child abuse and neglect during COVID-19. *Journal of Family Issues, 44*(2), 338–362.

Centers for Disease Control and Prevention. (2022, April 6). *Risk and protective factors.* https://www.cdc.gov/violenceprevention/childabuseandneglect/riskprotectivefactors.html

Centers for Disease Control and Prevention. (2023a, March 15). *CDC museum COVID-19 timeline.* https://www.cdc.gov/museum/timeline/covid19.html

Centers for Disease Control and Prevention. (2023b, June 29). *Fast facts: Preventing adverse childhood experiences.* https://www.cdc.gov/violenceprevention/aces/index.html

Childhelp. (2023). *Child abuse statistics.* https://www.childhelp.org/child-abuse-statistics/

Daly, M., & Robinson, E. (2021). Anxiety reported by US adults in 2019 and during the 2020 COVID-19 pandemic: Population-based evidence from two nationally representative samples. *Journal of Affective Disorders, 286*, 296–300.

Falk, G., Romero, P. D., Nicchitta, I. A., & Nyhof, E. C. (2021, August 20). *Unemployment rates during the COVID-19 pandemic.* Congressional Research Service. https://crsreports.congress.gov/product/details?prodcode=R46554

Fedina, L., Williamson, C., & Perdue, T. (2019). Risk factors for domestic child sex trafficking in the United States. *Journal of Interpersonal Violence, 34*(13), 2653–2673.

Finkelhor, D., Walsh, K., Jones, L., Mitchell, K., & Collier, A. (2021). Youth internet safety education: Aligning programs with the evidence base. *Trauma Violence Abuse, 22*(5), 1233–1247.

Fogarty, A., Savopoulos, P., Seymour, M., Cox, A., Williams, K., Petrie, S., Herman, S., Toone, E., Schroder, K., & Giallo, R. (2022). Providing therapeutic services to women and children who have experienced intimate partner violence during the COVID-19 pandemic: Challenges and learnings. *Child Abuse & Neglect, 130*, 105365. https://doi.org/10.1016/j.chiabu.2021.105365

Foot, K., Van der Watt, M., & Parks, E. S. C. (2023). Special issue "frontiers in organizing processes: Collaborating against human trafficking/modern slavery for impact and sustainability". *Societies, 13*(4), 99.

Greenbaum, J., Stoklosa, H., & Murphy, L. (2020). The public health impact of coronavirus disease on human trafficking. *Frontiers in Public Health, 8*, 561184.

Grzejszczak, J., Gabryelska, A., Gmitrowicz, A., Kotlicka-Antczak, M., & Strzelecki, D. (2022). Are children harmed by being locked up at home? The impact of isolation during the COVID-19 pandemic on the phenomenon of domestic violence. *International Journal of Environmental Research and Public Health, 19*, 13958. https://doi.org/10.3390/ijerph192113958

Guyon-Harris, K. L., Ahlfs-Dunn, S., & Huth-Bocks, A. (2017). PTSD symptom trajectories among mothers reporting interpersonal trauma: Protective factors and parenting outcomes. *Journal of Family Violence, 32*, 657–667.

Hails, K. A., Petts, R. A., Hostutler, C. A., Simoni, M., Greene, R., Snider, T. C., & Riley, A. R. (2022). COVID-19 distress, negative parenting, and child behavioral problems: The moderating role of parent adverse childhood experiences. *Child Abuse & Neglect, 130*, 105450. https://doi.org/10.1016/j.chiabu.2021.105450

Holtzblatt, J., & Karpman, M. (2020). *Who did not get the economic impact payments by mid-to-late May, and why?* Urban Institute. https://www.urban.org/

Huang, N., Yang, F., Liu, X., Bai, Y., Guo, J., & Reim, M. (2023). The prevalences, changes, and related factors of child maltreatment during the COVID-19 pandemic: A systematic review. *Child Abuse & Neglect, 135*, 105992. https://doi.org/10.1016/j.chiabu.2022.105992

International Organization of Migration. (n.d.). *Family members are involved in nearly half of child trafficking cases.* https://www.iom.int/sites/g/files/tmzbdl486/files/our_work/DMM/MAD/Counter-trafficking%20Data%20Brief%20081217.pdf

Jaffe, G., Sullivan, M. E., Angelo-Rocha, M., Cafaro, C., Crisp, J. D., & Merriweather, T. (2022). Rethinking primary prevention of child trafficking: Recommendations from the Human trafficking Task Force of the Global Alliance for Behavioral Health and Social Justice. *The American Journal of Orthopsychiatry, 92*, 616.

Jones Day. (2022). *Human trafficking and health care providers: Legal requirements for reporting and education.* https://www.jonesday.com/en/insights/2021/09/human-trafficking-and-health-care-providers

Junewicz, A., Sohn, I. E., & Walts, K. K. (2022). COVID-19 and youth who have experienced commercial sexual exploitation: A role for child mental health professionals during and in the aftermath of a pandemic. *Journal of the American Academy of Child and Adolescent Psychiatry, 61*(9), 1071–1073. https://doi.org/10.1016/j.jaac.2022.03.015

Klika, J. B., Merrick, M. T., & Jones, J. (2023). Child maltreatment during the pandemic. *Child Maltreatment, 28*(1), 3–6.

Kovski, N. L., Hill, H. D., Mooney, S. J., Rivara, F. P., & Rowhani-Rahbar, A. (2022). Short-term effects of tax credits on rates of child maltreatment reports in the United States. *Pediatrics, 150*(1), e2021054939.

Lee, S. J., Ward, K. P., Chang, O. D., & Downing, K. M. (2021). Parenting activities and the transition to home-based education during the COVID-19 pandemic. *Children and Youth Services Review, 122*, 105585. https://doi.org/10.1016/j.childyouth.2020.105585

Loveday, S., Hall, T., Constable, L., Paton, K., Sanci, L., Goldfeld, S., & Hiscock, H. (2022). Screening for adverse childhood experiences in children: A systematic review. *Pediatrics, 149*(2), e2021051884.

Machlin, L., Gruhn, M. A., Miller, A. B., Milojevich, H. M., Motton, S., Findley, A. M., Patel, K., Mitchell, A., Martinez, D. N., & Sheridan, M. A. (2022). Predictors of family violence in North Carolina following initial COVID-19 stay-at-home orders. *Child Abuse & Neglect, 130*, 105376. https://doi.org/10.1016/j.chiabu.2021.105376

Marmor, A., Cohen, N., & Katz, C. (2023). Child maltreatment during COVID-19: Key conclusions and future directions based on a systematic literature review. *Trauma Violence Abuse, 24*(2), 760–775.

Martinez-Sosa, N., Hadjikyriakou, M., Potter, J., & Alhajji, L. (2022). (PO-004) Providers' perspectives on the use of telehealth in an outpatient collaborative care clinic for human trafficking survivors during the COVID-19 pandemic. *Journal of the Academy of Consultation-Liaison Psychiatry, 63*, S2.

McKim, J. B., & Betancourt, S. (2022, October 11). *Trafficking inc: Forced labor in Massachusetts.* https://www.wgbh.org/news/local/2022-10-11/trafficking-inc-forced-labor-in-massachusetts

Molnar, B. E., Scoglio, A. A., & Beardslee, W. R. (2021). Community level prevention of childhood maltreatment: Next steps in a world with COVID-19. *International Journal on Child Maltreatment: Research, Policy and Practice, 3*, 467–481. https://doi.org/10.1007/s42448-020-00064-4

National Child Traumatic Stress Network. (2020). *The impact of COVID-19 on child sex and labor trafficking.* https://www.nctsn.org/sites/default/files/resources/fact-sheet/the_impact_of_covid-19_on_child_sex_and_labor_trafficking.pdf

National Health Resource Center on Domestic Violence. (2020). *Telehealth, COVID-19, intimate partner violence, and human trafficking: Increasing safety for people surviving abuse.*

National Human Trafficking Training and Technical Assistance Center. (2021). *Core competencies for human trafficking response in health care and behavioral health systems.* https://nhttac.

acf.hhs.gov/resource/report-core-competencies-human-trafficking-response-health-care-and-behavioral-health

National Human Trafficking Training and Technical Assistance Center. (2022). *Toolkit for building a human trafficking school safety protocol*. https://nhttac.acf.hhs.gov/system/files/2023-02/Toolkit%20for%20Building%20a%20Human%20Trafficking%20School%20Safety%20Protocol.pdf

Office of Trafficking in Persons. (2019). *Myths and facts about human trafficking*. Administration for Children and Families. https://www.acf.hhs.gov/otip/about/myths-facts-human-trafficking

Peck, J. L., Greenbaum, J., & Stoklosa, H. (2024). Mandated continuing education requirements for health care professional state licensure: The Texas model. *Journal of Human Trafficking, 10*(1), 168–173. https://doi.org/10.1080/23322705.2021.1981708

Polaris. (2020, April 1). *Crisis in human trafficking during the pandemic*. https://acrobat.adobe.com/link/review?uri=urn%3Aaaid%3Ascds%3AUS%3A7c75a904-a304-4457-8c13-73cc0918815b#pageNum=3

Polaris. (2021a, April 1). *Sexual exploitation during the pandemic*. https://polarisproject.org/wp-content/uploads/2021/07/Sexual-Exploitation-During-the-Pandemic.pdf

Polaris. (2021b). *Labor exploitation and trafficking of agricultural workers during the pandemic*. https://polarisproject.org/wp-content/uploads/2021/06/Polaris_Labor_Exploitation_and_Trafficking_of_Agricultural_Workers_During_the_Pandemic.pdf

Polaris. (2023). *In Harm's way: How systems fail human trafficking survivors*. https://polarisproject.org/wp-content/uploads/2023/07/In-Harms-Way-How-Systems-Fail-Human-Trafficking-Survivors-by-Polaris-modifed-June-2023.pdf

Rodriguez, C. M., Lee, S. J., & Ward, K. P. (2023). Applying socio-emotional information processing theory to explain child abuse risk: Emerging patterns from the COVID-19 pandemic. *Child Abuse Neglect, 135*, 105–954. https://doi.org/10.1016/j.chiabu.2022.105954

Stevenson, M. C., Schaefer, C. T., & Ravipati, V. M. (2022). COVID-19 patient care predicts nurses' parental burnout and child abuse: Mediating effects of compassion fatigue. *Child Abuse Neglect, 130*, 105–458. https://doi.org/10.1016/j.chiabu.2021.105458

Todres, J., & Díaz, Á. (2021). COVID-19 and human trafficking—The amplified impact on vulnerable populations. *JAMA Pediatrics, 175*(2), 123. https://doi.org/10.1001/jamapediatrics.2020.3610

U.S. Department of Health & Human Services, Children's Bureau. (2021). *Child maltreatment*. https://www.acf.hhs.gov/cb/report/child-maltreatment-2021

United Nations Office on Drugs and Crime. (2021). *The effects of the COVID-19 pandemic on trafficking in persons and responses to the challenges*. https://www.unodc.org/documents/human-trafficking/2021/The_effects_of_the_COVID-19_pandemic_on_trafficking_in_persons.pdf

Vermeulen, S., Alink, L. R. A., & van Berkel, S. R. (2023). Child maltreatment during school and childcare closure due to the COVID-19 pandemic. *Child Maltreatment, 28*(1), 13–23.

Washburn, T., Diener, M. L., Curtis, D. S., & Wright, C. A. (2022). Modern slavery and labor exploitation during the COVID-19 pandemic: A conceptual model. *Global Health Action, 15*(1), 2074784.

Whaling, K. M., Der Sarkissian, A., Larez, N., Sharkey, J. D., Allen, M. A., & Nylund-Gibson, K. (2023). Child maltreatment prevention service cases are significantly reduced during the COVID-19 pandemic: A longitudinal investigation into unintended consequences of quarantine. *Child Maltreatment, 28*(1), 34–41.

Zamarro, G., & Prados, M. J. (2021). Gender differences in couples' division of childcare, work and mental health during COVID-19. *Review of Economics of the Household, 19*, 11–40. https://doi.org/10.1007/s11150-020-09534-7

Children with Special Care Needs: Principles of Management for Complex Patients

Kathleen A. Kent, Julie LaMothe, Cindy Hill, and Beth Morton

We cannot direct the wind, but we can adjust the sails.

—Dolly Parton

Introduction and Background

Children and youth with special health care needs (CYSHCN) are defined by Human Resources and Services Administration (HRSA) and the Maternal and Child Health Bureau (MCHB) as "those children who are at increased risk for chronic physical, developmental, behavioral, or emotional conditions and require health and related services of a type or amount beyond that required for children generally" (Maternal and Child Health Bureau, 2020). According to the 2017–2018 National Survey of Children's Health (NSCH), there are about 13.6 million children in the United States (U.S.) under 18 years of age with special health care needs and 25% of homes had one or more children with a special health care need (Maternal and Child Health Bureau, 2020). These needs impact the child's and family's daily life with increased service use, challenges when accessing care and prescription medications, and a heavy financial burden. Children with underlying conditions, such as respiratory, cardiac, or immunocompromise, may be more susceptible to severe disease if infected by COVID-19. Many do not have medical homes for primary care and have higher rates of emergency department use than those without special health care needs (Maternal and Child Health Bureau, 2020). The NSCH reports that CYSHCN have functional limitations and increased rates of anxiety and depression leading to missed school days and needs for services at home, resulting in a higher burden of care on caregivers. In addition, many children with complex needs require medical technology and extensive care to meet their daily needs (Giambra & Spratling, 2023). Examples of technologies include tracheostomies, ventilators,

K. A. Kent · J. LaMothe (✉) · C. Hill · B. Morton
Indiana University School of Nursing, Indianapolis, IN, USA
e-mail: kaakent@iu.edu; vlamothe@iu.edu; cindhill@iu.edu; bemorton@iu.edu

J. L. Peck (ed.), *COVID-19 Impacts on Child Health*,
https://doi.org/10.1007/978-3-031-80369-7_12

219

noninvasive respiratory support, and feeding tubes. Expert caregivers are needed to be available at home to care for children and coordinate their care including visits to the emergency department (ED), healthcare provider (HCP) visits, and hospitalizations (Giambra & Spratling, 2023).

The COVID-19 pandemic significantly impacted CYSHCN (Aishworiya & Kang, 2021). These children had higher health needs and lack of access to health care specialists during the pandemic, creating major challenges in the continuity of care (Aishworiya & Kang, 2021; Ameis et al., 2020). This likely leads to delays in diagnosis and treatment and impaired access to necessary services for optimal functioning (Brandenburg, Holman, et al., 2020). In addition, COVID-19-related school closures and suspended therapies had a significant negative impact on CYSHCN (Ameis et al., 2020). These children are especially vulnerable to disruptions in their routines and therapies, which are essential for meeting their daily goals (Brandenburg, Holman, et al., 2020). The pandemic led to an increase in mental health issues such as isolation, depression, and generalized anxiety among children, including CYSHCN (Yusuf et al., 2022). These children often struggle to understand changes in their routines and the reasons behind them leading to greater anxiety and depression (Ameis et al., 2020; Yusuf et al., 2022).

Families of CYSHCN experience additional stressors when caring for their children with physical and developmental disabilities, and the COVID-19 epidemic has only exacerbated these challenges. Many families had to adapt to homeschooling or video online education and health services, which can be difficult for children who require additional support and accommodations (Vanegas et al., 2022). Access to necessary therapies and medications was reduced, which further impacted the child's health and well-being (Vanegas et al., 2022). Coordination of homecare was disrupted by limited services, lack of supplies, and limited access to HCPs. Health care transition from child to adult care for CYSHCN is disrupted during a time of crisis, which further challenges access to care. This places children at risk of not receiving community or school services and further delays the transition to an adult health care provider (Lebrun-Harris et al., 2018).

CYSHCN are more likely to live in poverty than non-CYSHCN, which can further impact the challenges faced by these families (Maternal and Child Health Bureau, 2020). CYSHCN are twice as likely to experience one or more unmet health care needs (Maternal and Child Health Bureau, 2020). This highlights the need for policies and programs that support the needs of these families, including access to health care, education, and financial assistance. These challenges can be particularly difficult for families already experiencing COVID-19's impact on their jobs, finances, lack of respite services, transportation issues, and health risks. It is important to recognize and support the needs of these families, both during the pandemic and beyond.

Points of Care

With one in four U.S. households having at least one child with special health care needs, HCPs must consider the impact that COVID-19 infection has on these children and their health status specific to their diagnoses (Maternal and Child Health Bureau, 2020). CYSHCN require more care and resources to meet the physical, behavioral, developmental, and emotional needs associated with a variety of conditions than their peers without special health care needs. While CYSHCN often have intellectual or neurodevelopmental disabilities, this group also includes typically developing children with chronic diseases such as asthma, diabetes, epilepsy, and bleeding disorders (Centers for Disease Control and Prevention, 2021). Data on the impact of COVID-19 in CYSHCN in the U.S. is very limited; however, other countries have contributed to research on the impacts of COVID-19 infection on CYSHCN and must be included for a truly global experience and perspective. In the U.S., there is significant data on risk factors leading to more severe COVID-19 infection in the adult population, including pre-existing medical conditions and disabilities that also affect the pediatric population. In addition to complex comorbidities in CYSHCN, they are more likely to experience access to care barriers or live in group facilities. It is these combined factors that place CYSHCN at a higher risk to experience severe COVID-19 infection with increased hospitalization and required mechanical ventilation (Centers for Disease Control and Prevention, 2023). Additionally, CYSHCN often have an interprofessional team of HCPs across many settings for primary care, ambulatory specialty services, inpatient acute care facilities, school-based therapies, and long-term care institutions, making communication and assuring continuity of care more challenging. Telehealth visits can pose challenges for providers and CYSHCN when certain specialties rely on hands-on examination and not just observation (Houtrow et al., 2020).

According to the National Institute of Health (NIH), severe COVID-19 infection is defined as oxygen saturation measured by pulse oximetry (SpO_2) "<94% on room air at sea level, a ratio of arterial partial pressure of oxygen to fraction of inspired oxygen (PaO_2/FiO_2) < 300 mmHg, a respiratory rate >30 breaths/min, or lung infiltrates >50%" (U.S. Department of Health and Human Services, 2023). Age differences in respiratory rate and higher prevalence of abnormal chest radiographs must be considered in determining the severity of COVID-19 infection in children (U.S. Department of Health and Human Services, 2023). The Centers for Disease Control and Prevention (CDC) compiled a list of certain medical conditions that increase these risks for severe disease in the COVID-19 epidemic (Centers for Disease Control and Prevention, 2023). These conditions are diagnosed in children of all ages, and evidence suggests that CYSHCN (including those with immunocompromise, obesity, congenital heart disease, and genetic, neurologic, hematologic, pulmonary, and metabolic disorders) are at risk for complications from severe COVID-19 infection. Preterm birth was a common risk factor for severe COVID-19 illness in children aged 1 year or younger (Kompaniyets et al., 2021). In addition to CYSHCN, there is a subset of children with medical complexity (CMC) who have significant health care needs due to multiple chronic disorders and other limitations (American Academy of Pediatrics, 2022a). Even with limited data on CYSHCN and CMC for specific disorders, it is important to look at the comorbidities associated with them. For example, Down Syndrome (DS) is often associated with obesity, along with hypothyroidism, low muscle tone, and congenital heart disease. These comorbidities make children with DS more vulnerable to severe respiratory illnesses. In a global retrospective study, Emes et al. found that children with DS and COVID-19 infections were more likely to require mechanical ventilation (24.8% DS vs. 5.8% controls) and had a higher mortality rate (5.0% DS vs. 0.5% controls) than their peers without DS (Emes et al., 2021). Children with DS also had significantly higher complication rates for pneumonia (36.9% vs. 11.1% controls), acute respiratory distress syndrome (32.8% DS vs. 1.9% controls), and acute renal failure (17.3% DS vs. 2.9% controls) (Emes et al., 2021). Table 1 summarizes the considerations associated with common disorders in CYSHCN who are impacted by complications of COVID-19 infection or the pandemic's interruptions to the health care system.

Social, Emotional, and Mental Health Implications

In addition to the information provided in Table 1 on conditions in CYSHCN and their risks and other impacts from the COVID-19 illness and pandemic, it is very important to have a comprehensive understanding of the implications of the COVID-19 pandemic on youth mental health. These striking effects were immediately observed, and long-term sequelae continue to be evident years later. Stressors and hardships during the pandemic included social disruption including lockdowns, social distancing, and home confinement (Prime et al., 2020). Caregiver stressors impacting children included financial insecurity due to caregiver job loss (and/or illness/hospitalization), personal psychological distress, and other effects that may impact parenting (Prime et al., 2020). Social and mental health effects specific to CYSHCN, related to the disruption of their health care services, schooling, and community activities, include delay in development, learning deficiencies, and mental health challenges (American Academy of Pediatrics, 2022b). Adjustment disruptions included the cancellation of in-person school and/or remote online schooling, which affected academic progress and caused strain and challenges with peer relationships (Prime et al., 2020). Quarantine and isolation often result in post-traumatic stress syndrome symptoms, confusion, and anger (Brooks et al., 2020). The CDC described that over one-third of high school students reported poor mental health and about half reported persistent sadness or hopelessness early in the pandemic (Centers for Disease Control and Prevention, 2022). In 2020, emergency department visits related to mental health crises increased by over 30% among adolescents compared to the prior year (Centers for Disease Control and Prevention, 2020). These longstanding mental health effects have proven especially dire, leading the American Academy of Pediatrics, the American Academy of Child and Adolescent Psychiatry, and the Children's Hospital Association to jointly declare a

Table 1 Considerations for CYSHCN during the COVID-19 pandemic

Comorbidities	Considerations
Pulmonary	
Asthma (Choi et al., 2022; Zhang et al., 2022)	More likely to be hospitalized but not for severe COVID-19 infection
	Not related to increased ICU admission for COVID-19 management
Chronic lung disease/ bronchopulmonary dysplasia (Choi et al., 2022)	More likely to develop severe COVID-19
Cystic fibrosis (Brackenborough et al., 2022)	Solid organ transplant is a risk factor for ICU admission and death
	Limitations of lung transplant availability
	Delayed transition to adult health care services
Tuberculosis (Mane et al., 2022)	No statistically significant differences between children with and without tuberculosis
	Potential risk reactivation of latent tuberculous with the use of immunosuppressant medication in the treatment of COVID-19 infection
Cardiovascular	
Congenital heart disease (Soleimani & Soleimani, 2022)	Complications include heart failure, arrhythmias, stroke, pulmonary hypertension, and increased mortality
	Longer hospital stays
Any cardiac disease (Choi et al., 2022)	Higher prevalence of ICU admission
Neurological	
Epilepsy (Choi et al., 2022; Thongsing et al., 2022)	The prevalence of severe COVID-19 infection is significantly higher in children with seizures
	Prolonged seizures
Traumatic brain and spinal cord injuries (Pollock et al., 2022)	No data on the severity of COVID-19 infection
	Significant interruptions of rehabilitation services leading to caregiver distress
Cerebral palsy (Bhaskar et al., 2022; Brandenburg, Fogarty, & Sieck, 2020)	Interruptions of therapies
	Lack of support for new or modifications to orthoses or splints
	Deterioration in ambulatory status and increased contractures due to lack of therapy
	Surgery delays
	Weight gain
	Alterations in behavior—Irritability, anger
	Higher risk of severe respiratory symptoms with COVID-19 infection

(continued)

Table 1 (continued)

Comorbidities	Considerations
Hematology and Oncology	
Cancer (Belsky et al., 2021)	Fewer COVID-19 symptoms than adults with cancer
	Lower mortality from COVID-19 than adults with cancer
Solid organ (SOT) or stem cell (HCT) transplant (Dulek et al., 2022; Feldman & Danziger-Isakov, 2022)	Chronic immunosuppressive therapy might be protective against severe COVID-19 infection
	Limited data but immunogenicity post-COVID-19 mRNA vaccine is modestly higher in children with SOT than in adults with SOT but less than the general population. Booster doses may be recommended
Sickle cell disease (Martin et al., 2023)	Higher rate of severe COVID-19 infection and hospitalization
	ICU admissions due to multi-lobar infiltrates, acute chest syndrome, and hypoxia
	Vaso-occlusive pain crisis was more likely
	Patients taking hydroxyurea were less likely to be hospitalized
Metabolic	
Diabetes mellitus (Choi et al., 2022; Kompaniyets et al., 2021)	Higher rate of severe COVID-19 infection and hospitalization
	ICU admissions for management of hyperglycemia diabetic ketoacidosis (DKA)
	Delayed diagnoses for new onset of diabetes type 1, leading to more cases of DKA
Chronic kidney disease (Dulek et al., 2022; Feldman & Danziger-Isakov, 2022)	Reduction of available kidneys for transplant during the early pandemic leading to kidney waitlist removal from death or deterioration of kidney disease
Liver disease (Dulek et al., 2022; Feldman & Danziger-Isakov, 2022)	Reduction of available livers for transplant during the early pandemic leading to liver waitlist removal from death or deterioration of liver disease
Behavioral and mental health	
Intellectual and developmental disabilities (Gleason et al., 2021)	More likely to require hospital admission
	Higher mortality rates
ADHD (Merzon et al., 2021)	Increased likelihood of severe symptoms, thus hospitalization
	Related to inadequate self-care and prevention
	Impulsivity increases exposure
Substance use disorder (U.S. Department of Health and Human Services, 2022)	1.5× more likely to contract CV-19 than general population
	More likely to have severe outcomes including hospitalization and death
Autism Spectrum Disorder (ASD) (Al-Beltagi et al., 2022)	One in four children with ASD has immune deficiency or dysfunction, increasing the risk of severe infection/complications
	Behavioral risk factors (oral sensory-seeking and/or pica) increase exposure to risk
	Sensory disturbances can limit infection prevention practices (mask-wearing, handwashing)

state of emergency in response to the "soaring rates of mental health challenges in children, adolescents, and their families over the course of the COVID-19 pandemic" in October of 2021 (American Academy of Pediatrics, 2021).

When in-person medical visits are not an option such as during the lockdown period of the pandemic, to maintain consistency for CYSHCN and those who may have higher mental health needs such as autism spectrum disorder, anxiety, depression, and mood disorders, it is recommended to provide telemedicine approaches to complete visits (American Academy of Pediatrics, 2022b). Providers and pediatric offices should also proactively plan and assist with connection to socialization opportunities, respite options, support groups, and parent-to-parent groups/information centers to address social isolation and increased stress and dependence on caregivers (American Academy of Pediatrics, 2022b). Immunizations need to be prioritized by HCPs and those who care for CYSHCN. Since many of these children are considered high risk by the CDC, they qualify for early rounds of immunizations. Families need to be aware of this, educated, and encouraged to get their children immunized to reduce their risk as much as possible. Pediatric HCPs, schools, and caregivers for this population can assist through educational materials such as posters and pamphlets, transportation assistance, and electronic/text reminders.

Adding to the social implications of a pandemic, CYSHCN may have unique behavioral, physical, immunological, and genetic attributes that can increase their risk of acquisition of the disease, severity of infections, and response to treatment. Approximately 25% of children with ASD have immune deficiency or dysfunction, increasing their risk of severe infection or complications from COVID-19 infection (Al-Beltagi et al., 2022). There are also behavioral risk factors, including oral sensory-seeking activities and pica, which is more common in this population and increases the risk of exposure (Al-Beltagi et al., 2022). Because of sensory disturbances, infection prevention measures such as mask-wearing, handwashing, and distance-keeping efforts are challenging (Al-Beltagi et al., 2022). Merzon et al. found that people with ADHD were more likely to experience severe symptoms of COVID-19 and had a higher likelihood of hospitalization (Merzon et al., 2021). This study hypothesized that this was related to inadequate self-care and prevention efforts. Also, there is a higher likelihood of exposure, and thus increased viral load, due to impulsivity (Merzon et al., 2021). Children with DS have also been identified by the CDC as a high-risk group for COVID-19 infection. A study out of the United Kingdom noted that they are four times more likely to be hospitalized and ten times more likely to die than the general population (Kieran Clift et al., 2021). This may be related to improper mask usage as well as specific anatomical risk factors like enlarged tongues, tonsils and adenoids, and immune system abnormalities (MacMillan, 2021). Other behavioral considerations related to the increase in morbidity during the pandemic within the population of CYSHCN included decreased treatment adherence. Nonadherence, which increases health care utilization was found to be related to emotional lability, exacerbated chronic stress, and supply chain disruptions during the pandemic (Logan, 2022; Plevinsky et al., 2020). Also affecting adherence was unstable caregiver availability, likely related to illness, job loss, financial stress, and other variables (Plevinsky et al., 2020).

Educational Implications

Children spend over half of their waking hours in school with a set routine for learning and achieving goals. Of the children in public schools in the US, 14% are students with disabilities and receive services under the Individuals with Disabilities Education Act (IDEA) (IDEA, 2023). IDEA became federal law in 1975 to ensure children with disabilities the right to an equitable public education. Before the law, only 20% of CYSHCN attended public school and were afforded an education while the remaining 80% of this population remained at home or in institutions (IDEA, 2023). Section 504 of the Rehabilitation Act protects people with disabilities from being discriminated against (IDEA, 2023). Furthermore, each child in special education must have an individual education plan (IEP) for the protection of the right to an equitable education. This legal document assists and manages the attainment of goals and is vital for the long-term principles of management for this population. For CYSHCN and their families, the IEP communicates to school staff what is needed for each child's individual education and is updated multiple times during the school year. Presently, parents are often uninformed about their child's rights under the IDEA ruling and revisions stressing the need for HCPs to continually advocate and explain these resources for critical management of this population.

The pandemic changed everything stable and consistent in a child's life (Benner & Mistry, 2020). School closures upended the daily routine and resulted in remote learning that lasted over a year with several repercussions (Colvin et al., 2022). While over 80% of children worldwide were impacted by school closures, CYSHCN were significantly impacted due to the additional interruption of vital health interventions and therapies (Brandenburg, Holman, et al., 2020). The reality was unmet health needs, causing the United States Department of Education to send reminders to schools that the required evaluations and therapies for CYSHCN were still mandated during the pandemic (IDEA, 2023). Difficulties in meeting these required evaluations resulted in a downward spiral of unmet social, cognitive, and physical health needs for these children. Management of these now unmet needs for CYSHCN during the COVID-19 pandemic became an interprofessional goal in the communities and nationally, including the government providing compensation to families who were harmed by a lack of needed health therapies (Harris et al., 2021). The pandemic highlighted the important need to advocate for a solution to these health inequities of our youth, especially those with disabilities (Masonbrink & Hurley, 2020).

Upon school closures being initiated, remote learning was quickly set up as a replacement for in-person learning. Globally, this was a new era of public education. School settings strive for equal educational opportunities, yet remote learning highlighted inequities among home learning environments (Watson et al., 2021). The impact of social determinants of health became clear as not all family units had access to reliable internet, laptops for learning, or a safe home environment conducive to learning. Food insecurity during lockdowns was a vital concern, considering before the pandemic 35 million American children relied on national school breakfast and lunch programs (Dunn et al., 2020). Adding to the challenge of home learning, parents/guardians became teachers for their multiple school-aged children without any training. Children were even more impacted as digital literacy also was a barrier (Klosky et al., 2022) and parents/guardians cited concerns over educating in the home environment with the loss of essential therapies (Neece et al., 2020). During the time of school closures, both parents and CYSHCN had increased anxiety and depressive symptoms (Asbury et al., 2021) and parents were unable to have pre-pandemic routines such as being able to secure respite care due to the pandemic mandates (Brandenburg, Holman, et al., 2020).

One of the most notable deficits in this vulnerable population due to remote learning was social isolation. CYSHCN thrive on routines and need dependability in their day (Brandenburg, Holman, et al., 2020). They went from seeing their peers daily to being sequestered in their homes. Not only did children lose their routine of school, but peer connections were also lost (Larsen et al., 2021). Children were no longer in a setting where they could learn with and from peers. Social isolation had a greater impact on the family unit as well demonstrating that children who previously depended on school social support did not participate in remote learning and meet goals as well as before the pandemic (Baten et al., 2022). This lack of student success at home via online learning compounded the stressors parents/guardians were facing.

When students returned to school, it looked vastly different, including the addition of shields and partitions around desks, social distancing, and multiple disruptions to the school day. Of greater importance was how difficult it was for CYSHCN to return to school at the same time as their peers (Brandenburg, Holman, et al., 2020). Expert opinion was unclear at first regarding the timing of allowing this vulnerable population to return to in-person learning safely due to CYSHCN's increased risk for contracting COVID-19 and the possible inability to consistently take needed precautions for safety (Kelly et al., 2022).

Parents/guardians of CYSHCN in the school setting depend on their child's education plan (IEP) to guide teachers and health personnel in achieving measurable student goals during the school day. Students with complex health issues normally would receive therapies during the school day, but with remote learning, treatments were paused due to the emergency of the pandemic and IEPs were also not maintained (Brandenburg, Holman, et al., 2020). This pause in health interventions significantly impacted the health and development of CYSHCN, and consequently, furthered this population's education gap and health inequities (Van Lancker & Parolin, 2020).

Barriers and Breakthroughs

From birth, parents of CYSHCN are faced with the necessity of navigating the complex needs of their children. CYSHCN and their families face multiple barriers that can impede their right to healthcare equity. Compared to the general pediatric population, CYSHCN experienced additional barriers to appropriate comprehensive care during the COVID-19 pandemic. At baseline, CYSHCN have increased medical needs including the use of multiple medications, the need for a steady stream of supplies, as well as equipment needs and repairs. Also, this population has more specialty HCPs, physicians, and therapists, such as speech, occupational, physical, and behavioral. Management of this complex care before the pandemic was unyielding and often near impossible for families; the immense struggle during the pandemic to meet these children's comprehensive care needs was unsubstantiated, especially without tremendous amounts of support financially, physically, and emotionally from the medical community, friends, and family.

The COVID-19 pandemic led to disruptions in routine care including regular visits to HCPs resulting in a decline in immunization administration and delays or gaps in essential health care. The lack of HCP access increased the fragmentation of health care for CYSHCN. Children with underlying conditions needed more hospitalizations during COVID-19 but could not have caregivers at the bedside, leading to widening communication and isolation gaps. A paucity of large studies on the impacts of CYSHCN continues throughout the pandemic with the available data derived from small, single-institution research or meta-analyses.

Educational barriers include school closures which lead to developmental gaps because these children rely on specialized educational support, IEPs, or therapies provided in school settings. Increased isolation and reduced opportunities for social interaction were particularly difficult for CYSHCN, and can lead to anxiety, depression, stress, or other mental health concerns due to the disruption of their routines and support systems.

Barriers during COVID-19 can promote new breakthroughs. Healthcare access became a priority during the COVID-19 epidemic and resulted in new healthcare models including telehealth. This ensured continued access to essential health care services for these children. However, telehealth does have limitations for this population such as technological access and greater need for in-person examinations related to medical complexities.

Air quality improved during the pandemic shutdown around the world due to fewer automobiles on the road and less plane travel, resulting in a positive impact on those with respiratory disorders (Venter et al., 2020). There was also less antibiotic usage for those with cystic fibrosis related to fewer infections and less influenza. Medications and medical supplies needed to become more readily available for families isolated in their homes, resulting in new models of delivery and coordination for healthcare supplies and medicines.

Collaboration between healthcare specialists, therapists, primary care providers, and families became a necessity and model for safe patient-centered care. Open and effective communication between all stakeholders is a priority for the coordination of care for patients and families. Interprofessional education is an essential competency for all health science students, which results in safer health care for all children and families.

Schools were challenged to meet the special educational needs by developing strategies to support CYSHCN during and after the pandemic. The use of clear masks by educators and staff, as recommended as best practice, improved communication in schools for children and staff who are deaf or hard of hearing (National Association of the Deaf, n.d.). The use of computer and internet technology allowed online schooling access to teachers and support staff. Speech and language therapists improved the delivery of services through telehealth therapy sessions (Telehealth.HHS.gov, 2023). Mental health became a priority which improved online access to mental health therapists for CYSHCN and their caregivers (American Academy of Pediatrics, 2021; Asbury et al., 2021). Targeted interventions such as virtual support can be incorporated into individualized learning plans to bridge educational gaps.

Lessons Learned

The COVID-19 pandemic allowed for essential lessons to be learned by the healthcare community about the effect that isolation, serious illness, and lockdowns can have on CYSHCN and their families' lives, livelihoods, and mental health. Later practices have been integrated into United States healthcare culture and can be expected in healthcare use in future pandemics. A major focus needs to be on the prevention of disruption of healthcare access in the future in the form of the implementation of safety measures and the use of telemedicine practices. Mental health challenges were critically exacerbated during the pandemic and are to be anticipated and proactively addressed in the future by decreasing isolation, providing mental healthcare resources and supports, and accommodating the continuance of therapies, medication management, education, and group activities in modified scenarios/environments or in virtual environments as a last resort.

The importance of the role school plays in children's lives proves immeasurable, from education and independent living skills development, socialization, structure, safety, and stability to school health care—including nursing care, medical and developmental screenings, and meal insecurity programs. Abruptly closing in-person school proved catastrophic for CYSHCN including mental health crises, cognitive declines, and behavioral and physical regressions along with caregiver burnout, mental health concerns, and job loss/financial strain due to diminished opportunities for respite and childcare.

The COVID-19 epidemic contributed to childhood illnesses and can have lasting health implications requiring a diverse group of HCPs. As of May of 2023, children aged 0–19 years accounted for approximately 18% of all reported COVID-19 cases since the beginning of the pandemic (American Academy of Pediatrics, 2023). With (2%) of deaths among this age-group, COVID-19 subsequently has been ranked eighth among causes of death in children (Flaxman et al., 2023). Collaborative communication and interprofessional teamwork between providers are essential for optimal health outcomes of CSHCN and the key to the delivery of effective care systems.

Calls to Action

- Prioritize access to healthcare during shutdowns for CYSHCN by optimizing telehealth visits and consultations by having HCP offices include interpreters, use live captioning programs, automatic transcription, high-contrast displays, and allow the use of landline telephone as an alternative to video (Telehealth.HHS.gov, 2023).
- Continue to emphasize the importance of vaccines in vulnerable populations and their caregivers. CYSHCN including children with physical disabilities such as cerebral palsy and those with cognitive impairment, including Down syndrome, are currently included on the CDC's "People with Certain Medical Conditions" list which places them as a higher priority group in most states for vaccination (Centers for Disease Control and Prevention, 2023). For these healthcare risks, maintaining current COVID-19 vaccinations in CYSHCN is a healthcare priority and the best preventive strategy for severe COVID-19 infection as well as practicing physical distancing, good hand hygiene, minimizing trips to public places such as stores and restaurants, and thorough cleaning of any equipment that is used outside the home (i.e., walkers and wheelchairs). Additionally, it is important to encourage COVID-19 vaccination in parents, caregivers, and other household contacts of CYSHCN.
- Increase support in the community for families of CYSHCN by ensuring state/national funding for coordination of care (primary care, medical home, tertiary programs, community, and school). This should include an emphasis on collaboration in the transition of care, highlighting the need for school support personnel (nurses, therapists, psychologists) to continually assist student transition (IEP) and address these special needs in school policy and legislation (Brandenburg, Holman, et al., 2020). Further, this includes additional services in the home, training for parents, and increased hours for respite care (Watson et al., 2021) that would provide improved health outcomes in the management of this population.

References

Aishworiya, R., & Kang, Y. Q. (2021). Including children with developmental disabilities in the equation during this COVID-19 pandemic. *Journal of Autism and Developmental Disorders, 51*(6), 2155–2158. https://doi.org/10.1007/s10803-020-04670-6

Al-Beltagi, M., Saeed, N. K., Bediwy, A. S., Alhawamdeh, R., & Qaraghuli, S. (2022). Effects of COVID-19 on children with autism. *World Journal of Virology, 11*(6), 411–425. https://doi.org/10.5501/wjv.v11.i6.411

Ameis, S. H., Lai, M.-C., Mulsant, B. H., & Szatmari, P. (2020). Coping, fostering resilience, and driving care innovation for autistic people and their families during the COVID-19 pandemic and beyond. *Molecular Autism, 11*(1), 61. https://doi.org/10.1186/s13229-020-00365-y

American Academy of Pediatrics. (2021). *AAP-AACAP-CHA Declaration of a national emergency in child and adolescent mental health.* https://www.aap.org/en/advocacy/child-and-adolescent-healthy-mental-development/aap-aacap-cha-declaration-of-a-national-emergency-in-child-and-adolescent-mental-health

American Academy of Pediatrics. (2022a). *Children with medical complexity.* https://www.aap.org/en/patient-care/children-with-medical-complexity/

American Academy of Pediatrics. (2022b). *Caring for children and youth with special health care needs during the COVID-19 pandemic.* https://www.aap.org/en/pages/2019-novel-coronavirus-covid-19-infections/clinical-guidance/caring-for-children-and-youth-with-special-health-care-needs-during-the-covid-19-pandemic/

American Academy of Pediatrics. (2023). *Children and COVID-19: State-level data report.* http://www.aap.org/en/pages/2019-novel-coronavirus-COVID-19-infections/children-and-COVID-19-state-level-data-report/

Asbury, K., Fox, L., Deniz, E., Code, A., & Toseeb, U. (2021). How is COVID-19 affecting the mental health of children with special educational needs and disabilities and their families? *Journal of Autism and Developmental Disorders, 51*(5), 1772–1780. https://doi.org/10.31234/osf.io/sevyd

Baten, E., Vlaeminck, F., Mues, M., Valcke, M., Desoete, A., & Warreyn, P. (2022). The impact of school strategies and the home environment on home learning experiences during the COVID-19 pandemic in children with and without developmental disorders. *Journal of Autism and Developmental Disorders, 53*, 1642–1672. https://doi.org/10.31219/osf.io/b2a7r

Belsky, J. A., Tullius, B. P., Lamb, M. G., Sayegh, R., Stanek, J. R., & Auletta, J. J. (2021). COVID-19 in immunocompromised patients: A systematic review of cancer, hematopoietic cell and solid organ transplant patients. *The Journal of Infection, 82*(3), 329–338. https://doi.org/10.1016/j.jinf.2021.01.022

Benner, A. D., & Mistry, R. S. (2020). Child development during the COVID-19 pandemic through a life course theory lens. *Child Development Perspectives, 14*(4), 236–243. https://doi.org/10.1111/cdep.12387

Bhaskar, A. R., Gad, M. V., & Rathod, C. M. (2022). Impact of COVID pandemic on the children with cerebral palsy. *Indian Journal of Orthopaedics, 56*(5), 927–932. https://doi.org/10.1007/s43465-021-00591-3

Brackenborough, K., Ellis, H., & Flight, W. G. (2022). Respiratory viruses and cystic fibrosis. *Seminars in Respiratory and Critical Care Medicine, 44*(2), 196–208. https://doi.org/10.1055/s-0042-1758728

Brandenburg, J. E., Fogarty, M. J., & Sieck, G. C. (2020). Why individuals with cerebral palsy are at higher risk for respiratory complications from COVID-19. *Journal of Pediatric Rehabilitation Medicine, 13*(3), 317–327. https://doi.org/10.3233/prm-200746

Brandenburg, J. E., Holman, L. K., Apkon, S. D., Houtrow, A. J., Rinaldi, R., & Sholas, M. G. (2020). School reopening during COVID-19 pandemic: Considering students with disabilities. *Journal of Pediatric Rehabilitation Medicine, 13*(3), 425–431. https://doi.org/10.3233/prm-200789

Brooks, S. K., Webster, R. K., Smith, L. E., Woodland, L., Wessely, S., Greenberg, N., et al. (2020). The psychological impact of quarantine and how to reduce it: Rapid review of the evidence. *Lancet, 395*(10227), 912–920. https://doi.org/10.1016/s0140-6736(20)30460-8

Centers for Disease Control and Prevention. (2020). *Mental health–related emergency department visits among children aged 18 years during the covid-19 pandemic—United States, January 1–October 17, 2020.* https://www.cdc.gov/mmwr/volumes/69/wr/mm6945a3.htm

Centers for Disease Control and Prevention. (2021). *Children and youth with special health care needs in emergencies.* http://www.cdc.gov/childrenindisasters/children-with-special-healthcare-needs.html

Centers for Disease Control and Prevention. (2022). *New CDC data illuminate youth mental health threats during the COVID-19 pandemic.* https://www.cdc.gov/media/releases/2022/p0331-youth-mental-health-covid-19.html

Centers for Disease Control and Prevention. (2023). *People with certain medical conditions*. http://www.cdc.gov/coronavirus/2019-ncov/need-extra-precautions/people-with-medical-conditions.html

Choi, J. H., Choi, S.-H., & Yun, K. W. (2022). Risk factors for severe COVID-19 in children: A systematic review and meta-analysis. *Journal of Korean Medical Science, 37*(5), e35. https://doi.org/10.3346/jkms.2022.37.e35

Colvin, M. K., Reesman, J., & Glen, T. (2022). The impact of covid-19 related educational disruption on children and adolescents: An interim data summary and commentary on ten considerations for neuropsychological practice. *The Clinical Neuropsychologist, 36*(1), 45–71. https://doi.org/10.1080/13854046.2021.1970230

Dulek, D. E., Ardura, M. I., Green, M., Michaels, M. G., Chaudhuri, A., Vasquez, L., et al. (2022). Update on COVID-19 vaccination in pediatric solid organ transplant recipients. *Pediatric Transplantation, 26*(5), e14235. https://doi.org/10.1111/petr.14235

Dunn, C. G., Kenney, E., Fleischhacker, S. E., & Bleich, S. N. (2020). Feeding low-income children during the COVID-19 pandemic. *The New England Journal of Medicine, 382*(18), e40. https://doi.org/10.1056/nejmp2005638

Emes, D., Hüls, A., Baumer, N., Dierssen, M., Puri, S., Russell, L., et al. (2021). COVID-19 in children with down syndrome: Data from the Trisomy 21 Research Society Survey. *Journal of Clinical Medicine, 10*(21), 5125. https://doi.org/10.3390/jcm10215125

Feldman, A. G., & Danziger-Isakov, L. A. (2022). The impact of COVID-19 on the pediatric solid organ transplant population. *Seminars in Pediatric Surgery, 31*(3), 151178. https://doi.org/10.1016/j.sempedsurg.2022.151178

Flaxman, S., Whittaker, C., Semenova, E., Rashid, T., Parks, R. M., Blenkinsop, A., et al. (2023). Assessment of covid-19 as the underlying cause of death among children and young people aged 0 to 19 years in the US. *JAMA Network Open, 6*(1), e2253590. https://doi.org/10.1001/jamanetworkopen.2022.53590

Giambra, B. K., & Spratling, R. (2023). Examining children with complex care and technology needs in the context of social determinants of health. *Journal of Pediatric Health Care, 37*(3), 262–268. https://doi.org/10.1016/j.pedhc.2022.11.004

Gleason, J., Ross, W., Fossi, A., Blonsky, H., Tobias, J., & Stephens, M. (2021). The devastating impact of COVID-19 on individuals with intellectual disabilities in the United States. *Massachusetts Medical Society*. https://doi.org/10.1056/CAT.21.0051

Harris, B., McClain, M. B., O'Leary, S., & Shahidullah, J. D. (2021). Implications of COVID-19 on school services for children with disabilities: Opportunities for interagency collaboration. *Journal of Developmental and Behavioral Pediatrics, 42*(3), 236–239. https://doi.org/10.1097/dbp.0000000000000921

Houtrow, A., Harris, D., Molinero, A., Levin-Decanini, T., & Robichaud, C. (2020). Children with disabilities in the United States and the COVID-19 pandemic. *Journal of Pediatric Rehabilitation Medicine, 13*(3), 415–424. https://doi.org/10.3233/prm-200769

IDEA. (2023). *A history of the individuals with disabilities education act*. https://sites.ed.gov/idea/IDEA-History

Kelly, M. M., GP, D. M., Barton, H. J., Nacht, C. L., Butteris, S. M., Katz, B., et al. (2022). Priorities for safer in-person school for children with medical complexity during COVID-19. *Pediatrics, 149*(3), e2021054434. https://doi.org/10.1542/peds.2021-054434

Kieran Clift, A. K., Coupland, C. A. C., Keogh, R. H., Hemingway, H., & Hippisley-Cox, J. (2021). COVID-19 mortality risk in down syndrome: Results from a cohort study of eight million adults. *Annals of Internal Medicine, 174*(4), 572–576. https://doi.org/10.7326/m20-4986

Klosky, J. V., Gazmararian, J. A., Casimir, O., & Blake, S. C. (2022). Effects of remote education during the COVID-19 pandemic on young children's learning and academic behavior in Georgia: Perceptions of parents and school administrators. *The Journal of School Health, 92*(7), 656–664. https://doi.org/10.1111/josh.13185

Kompaniyets, L., Agathis, N. T., Nelson, J. M., Preston, L. E., Ko, J. Y., Belay, B., et al. (2021). Underlying medical conditions associated with severe covid-19 illness among children. *JAMA Network Open, 4*(6), e2111182. https://doi.org/10.1001/jamanetworkopen.2021.11182

Larsen, L., Helland, M. S., & Holt, T. (2021). The impact of school closure and social isolation on children in vulnerable families during COVID-19: A focus on children's reactions. *European Child & Adolescent Psychiatry, 31*(8), 1–11. https://doi.org/10.31234/osf.io/deju9

Lebrun-Harris, L. A., McManus, M. A., Ilango, S. M., Cyr, M., McLellan, S. B., Mann, M. Y., et al. (2018). Transition planning among US youth with and without special health care needs. *Pediatrics, 142*(4), e20180194. https://doi.org/10.1542/peds.2018-0194

Logan, B. A. (2022). The impact of the COVID-19 pandemic on pediatric chronic illness groups. *The Brown University Child and Adolescent Behavior Letter, 38*(5), 1–4. https://doi.org/10.1002/cbl.30623

MacMillan, C. (2021). Those with down syndrome are at increased risk of COVID-19 severity. *Yale Medicine.* https://www.yalemedicine.org/news/down-syndrome-covid-19

Mane, S. S., Janardhanan, J., Pustake, M., Wanvat, A., Khan, G. I., & Chopade, R. (2022). Outcome of COVID-19 in children with tuberculosis: Single-center experience. *Indian Pediatrics, 59*(8), 617–619. https://doi.org/10.1007/s13312-022-2574-6

Martin, O. Y., Darbari, D. S., Margulies, S., Nickel, R. S., Leonard, A., Speller-Brown, B., et al. (2023). Clinical outcomes of children and adolescents with sickle cell disease and covid-19 infection: A year in review at a Metropolitan Tertiary Pediatric Hospital. *Frontiers in Medicine, 10*, 987194. https://doi.org/10.3389/fmed.2023.987194

Masonbrink, A. R., & Hurley, E. (2020). Advocating for children during the COVID-19 school closures. *Pediatrics, 146*(3), e20201440. https://doi.org/10.1542/peds.2020-1440

Maternal and Child Health Bureau. (2020). *Children with special health care needs NSCH data brief Health Resources and Services Administration*

Merzon, E., Weiss, M. D., Cortese, S., Rotem, A., Schneider, T., Craig, S. G., et al. (2021). The association between ADHD and the severity of COVID-19 infection. *Journal of Attention Disorders, 26*(4), 491–501. https://doi.org/10.1177/10870547211003659

National Association of the Deaf. (n.d.). *Best practices for wearing masks when communicating with deaf and hard of hearing people transcript.* https://www.nad.org/best-practices-for-wearing-masks-when-communicating-with-dhh-transcript/

Neece, C., McIntyre, L. L., & Fenning, R. (2020). Examining the impact of COVID-19 in ethnically diverse families with young children with intellectual and developmental disabilities. *Journal of Intellectual Disability Research, 64*(10), 739–749. https://doi.org/10.1111/jir.12769

Plevinsky, J. M., Young, M. A., Carmody, J. K., Durkin, L. K., Gamwell, K. L., Klages, K. L., et al. (2020). The impact of COVID-19 on pediatric adherence and self-management. *Journal of Pediatric Psychology, 45*(9), 977–982. https://doi.org/10.1093/jpepsy/jsaa079

Pollock, A., D'Cruz, K., Scheinberg, A., Botchway, E., Harms, L., Amor, D. J., et al. (2022). Family-centred care for children with traumatic brain injury and/or spinal cord injury: A qualitative study of service provider perspectives during the COVID-19 pandemic. *BMJ Open, 12*(6), e059534. https://doi.org/10.1136/bmjopen-2021-059534

Prime, H., Wade, M., & Browne, D. T. (2020). Risk and resilience in family well-being during the COVID-19 pandemic. *The American Psychologist, 75*(5), 631–643. https://doi.org/10.1037/amp0000660

Soleimani, A., & Soleimani, Z. (2022). Presentation and outcome of congenital heart disease during COVID-19 pandemic: A review. *Current Problems in Cardiology, 47*(1), 100905. https://doi.org/10.1016/j.cpcardiol.2021.100905

Telehealth.HHS.gov. (2023). *Improving access to telehealth.* https://telehealth.hhs.gov/providers/health-equity-in-telehealth/improving-access-to-telehealth

Thongsing, A., Eizadkhah, D., Fields, C., & Ballaban-Gil, K. (2022). Provoked seizures and status epilepticus in a pediatric population with COVID-19 disease. *Epilepsia, 63*(8), e86–e91. https://doi.org/10.1111/epi.17293

U.S. Department of Health and Human Services. (2022). *Covid-19 and substance use*. https://nida. nih.gov/research-topics/comorbidity/covid-19-substance-use

U.S. Department of Health and Human Services. (2023). *Clinical spectrum*. https://www. covid19treatmentguidelines.nih.gov/overview/clinical-spectrum/

Van Lancker, W., & Parolin, Z. (2020). Covid-19, school closures, and Child poverty: A social crisis in the making. *The Lancet Public Health, 5*(5), e243–e244. https://doi.org/10.1016/ s2468-2667(20)30084-0

Vanegas, S. B., Dueñas, A. D., Kunze, M., & Xu, Y. (2022). Adapting parent-focused interventions for diverse caregivers of children with intellectual and developmental disabilities: Lessons learned during global crises. *Journal of Policy and Practice in Intellectual Disabilities, 20*(1), 45–57.

Venter, Z. S., Aunan, K., Chowdhury, S., & Lelieveld, J. (2020). Covid-19 lockdowns cause global air pollution declines. *Proceedings of the National Academy of Sciences, 117*(32), 18984–18990. https://doi.org/10.1073/pnas.2006853117

Watson, K. R., Astor, R. A., Benbenishty, R., Capp, G., & Kelly, M. S. (2021). Needs of children and families during Spring 2020 COVID-19 school closures: Findings from a national survey. *Social Work, 67*(1), 17–27. https://doi.org/10.1093/sw/swab052

Yusuf, A., Wright, N., Steiman, M., Gonzalez, M., Karpur, A., Shih, A., et al. (2022). Factors associated with resilience among children and youths with disability during the COVID-19 pandemic. *PLoS One, 17*(7), e0271229. https://doi.org/10.1371/journal.pone.0271229

Zhang, J., Dong, X., Liu, G., & Gao, Y. (2022). Risk and protective factors for COVID-19 morbidity, severity, and mortality. *Clinical Reviews in Allergy and Immunology, 64*(1), 90–107. https:// doi.org/10.1007/s12016-022-08921-5

Poverty and Food Insecurity: Assessment of Impacts of Children and Families

Janine Bruce

> *"Clinicians always inherit the results of bad social policy. Sooner or later, deleterious or ineffective policies will find clinical expression in patterns of illness, hospitalization, and ultimately death. History has shown that this cascade is never more intense than for children, a group exquisitely dependent on the adequacy of societal nurturance and protection."*
>
> —Wise (2009)

Introduction

The COVID-19 pandemic shone a critical light on existing and widening inequities in the United States (Ambrose, 2020). Individuals and families faced reductions in household income, heightened levels of housing and food insecurity and increased stress and mental health (Abrams et al., 2022). At the start of the pandemic, difficulties accessing food were quickly elevated locally and nationally as shelter in place orders went into effect, work slowed, and layoffs rose.

Food insecurity in the United States was a leading public health crisis in terms of the national scope and severity of consequences prior to the onset of the pandemic (Gundersen, 2013). The systems and policies addressing food insecurity were already strained and tenuous for decades, making this issue primed for fracture when the pandemic hit. In 2019 prior to the pandemic, 10.5% of US households (13.7 million households) were food insecure at some time during the year, meaning they experienced limited or uncertain access to adequate food as a result of lack of money and other resources at times during the year (Coleman-Jensen, 2019).

J. Bruce (✉)
Stanford School of Medicine, Stanford, CA, USA
e-mail: jsbruce@stanford.edu

J. L. Peck (ed.), *COVID-19 Impacts on Child Health*,
https://doi.org/10.1007/978-3-031-80369-7_13

Impact of Food Insecurity on Children

The pre-pandemic period demonstrated decreases in food insecurity in households with children to 6.5% of households (2.4 million households) in 2019 (down from 7.1% in both 2017 and 2018). Less than one precent of these households reported "very low" food security (Coleman-Jensen, 2019), experiences where children went hungry, skipped meals, or did not eat for the whole day because the household/family could not afford enough food (Defeyter et al., 2015; Oberg, 2011). Food insecurity in children is shown to be associated with poor physical and behavioral outcomes such as inadequate intakes of important nutrients (Lozoff et al., 2000; Rose, 1999; Rose & Oliveira, 1997), cognitive developmental delays, and psychosocial dysfunction (Lozoff et al., 2000; Murphy et al., 1998; Rose-Jacobs et al., 2008). Children who are food insecure can suffer from poor overall health (Alaimo et al., 1998; Cook et al., 2004) with effects lasting into adulthood (Gitterman et al., 2015; Stuff et al., 2004). Food insecurity further strains households by increasing the risk of maternal mental health problems including depression, stress and anxiety, poor physical health, and current or past substance use (Chilton & Booth, 2007; Gundersen & Ziliak, 2014; Whitaker et al., 2006). Maternal health outcomes can subsequently have detrimental impacts on children, amplifying the consequences of food insecurity on the entire family (Petterson & Albers, 2001).

Food insecurity does not equitably impact individuals. Households at higher risk include those with incomes near or below the federal poverty level (FPL), and households headed by a single parent (Coleman-Jensen et al., 2016), individuals with low education (Coleman-Jensen et al., 2013), or immigrant mothers (Chilton et al., 2009). Studies document the disproportionate impact of food insecurity on under-represented minority populations such as Black and Hispanic households (Alaimo et al., 1998; Bowen et al., 2021; Morales et al., 2021; Willems et al., 2022).

Existing Programs to Address Food Security

The U.S. Department of Agriculture's Food and Nutrition Service (USDA-FNS) oversees numerous programs aimed at increasing food security and reducing hunger among low-income Americans by promoting access to healthy foods and nutrition education. The most notable anti-hunger program is the Supplemental Nutrition Assistance Program (SNAP). Originally established as the Food Stamp Program in 1939, the program underwent years of modifications, expansion, and changes to eligibility and benefits (Caswell & Yaktine, 2013).

The SNAP program of today was rebranded in 2008, providing support to low-paid working families, low-income older adults aged 60 years and older, and individuals with disabilities meeting income eligibility. Prior to the pandemic, children under 18 years represented nearly half (43%) of all SNAP participants, and more than two-thirds of participants were school aged children 5–17 years. During the 2019 fiscal year, (October 1, 2018 to September 30, 2019) approximately 35.7 million people (18 million households) received SNAP benefits in an average month.

Among the 7.4 million households with children receiving SNAP benefits in an average month, the approximate monthly benefit for a single-adult household with children benefit was $373 (Cronquist, 2021).

The Special Supplemental Nutrition Program for Women, Infants, and Children (WIC) program, established in 1972, is another key USDA-FNS nutrition safety net program focused on the period of early childhood where growth and development are critical. The program provides food and nutrition education to nutritionally at-risk pregnant, breastfeeding, and postpartum women, and infants and children under 5 years old (Bartholomew et al., 2017). WIC is an entry point to other health and social services to promote important nutrition linkages early in a child's life course.

Two of the most prominent and important nutrition safety net programs for children also under the purview of the USDA-FNS are the National School Lunch Program (NSLP, created in 1946) and School Breakfast Program (SBP, created in 1966). Both programs provide children living in low-income households with free (<130% of the FPL) or reduced-price meals (130–185% of the FPL) (U. S. Department of Agriculture Food and Nutrition Service, 2017; Gitterman et al., 2015; Gundersen et al., 2012; Gundersen & Ver Ploeg, 2015). Prior to the pandemic (2019 fiscal year), the NSLP served 29.6 million students (20.1 million free, 1.7 million reduced-price, and 7.7 million full price). Similarly, the SBP distributed breakfasts to 14.77 million students (11.8 million free, 0.74 million reduced-price, 2.23 million full price) (U.S. Department of Agriculture, 2023). Recognizing that these two programs do not meet the food security needs of all children living in low-income households, the USDA-FNS authorized funding for the Summer Food Service Program (SFSP) and the Child and Adult Care Food Program (CACFP) in 1975 (U.S. Department of Agriculture Food and Nutrition Service, 2019). These programs provide meals and snacks to school aged children during the summer months through SFSP and to preschool-aged children enrolled in participating child care programs eligible for CACFP (Ralston et al., 2017).

While federal food assistance programs and child nutrition programs are not enough to reverse the effects of food insecurity, they are an essential part of the food safety net for children living in low-income households (Gundersen et al., 2012). The programs supplement the economic needs of households and offer children access to a reliable source of healthy and nutritious meals (Ralston et al., 2017). These programs provide the foundation for addressing child and family food insecurity during the pandemic and are discussed below as pandemic-era programs and breakthroughs.

Points of Care

Pediatric providers have a long history of addressing the social needs of their patients (Berman et al., 2018; Chung et al., 2016; Council on Community Pediatrics et al., 2013). In 2013, American Academy of Pediatrics (AAP) released a Policy Statement that outlined the pediatrician's role in recognizing the context in which their patients and families live, specifically the social determinants of health

(Council on Community Pediatrics et al., 2013). This was followed by the 2015 AAP policy statement on promoting food security for all children. This statement not only outlined the health, behavioral, and emotional consequences of food insecurity for children, but it also affirmed the central role that pediatricians and other pediatric healthcare providers (HCPs) play in screening and identifying children at risk for food insecurity and hunger and advocating for local and federal policies in favor of increasing children's access to adequate healthy foods for optimal health and well-being (Council on Community Pediatrics; Committee on Nutrition, 2015; Hager et al., 2010).

The pandemic posed unforeseen challenges to individuals, HCPs, systems, and institutions. Despite these challenges, service providers caring for the most under-resourced and marginalized communities responded in an unprecedented manner. It is important to recognize the important role that pediatric providers played in addressing children and families access to food resources during the pandemic. They screened and provided resources for key social and financial needs, they developed critical partnerships with community and policy partners, and they advocated for stronger policies to support the children and families impacted by the pandemic.

Barriers and Breakthroughs

A review of efforts to address pandemic emergency food needs shows the extent to which programs were expanded and modified, and new programs were quickly developed—all in a herculean effort to respond to the new challenges posed by the pandemic. The synthesis of these efforts is aided by the social ecological framework (McLeroy et al., 1988), demonstrating the multi-level impact of food insecurity and the corresponding opportunities to provide emergency programming and interventions (Fig. 1). The adapted model presented here takes into account the individual level factors and the context in which patients and families live, as well as the interpersonal, community, institutional, and policy factors that are key to providing needed programs and interventions. A deeper dive into each level provides a snapshot of the response that was launched at the onset of the pandemic (Table 1). While the individual factors are not explicitly outlined, it is widely accepted that an individual's experiences with poverty, racism, housing insecurity, and mental health struggles, to name a few, impact levels of food insecurity (Alaimo et al., 1998; Chilton et al., 2009; Coleman-Jensen et al., 2013; Coleman-Jensen et al., 2018) and the ability to access needed resources. Individual level risk factors are discussed along with interpersonal level strategies below.

Finally, the model provides an opportunity to recognize the ways in which pediatric HCPs interface with individuals and partners at each of these levels, with unique contributions to addressing food insecurity for their patients and the larger communities they serve (Fig. 1). The unique role that pediatric HCPs played across multiple systems is described in detail below.

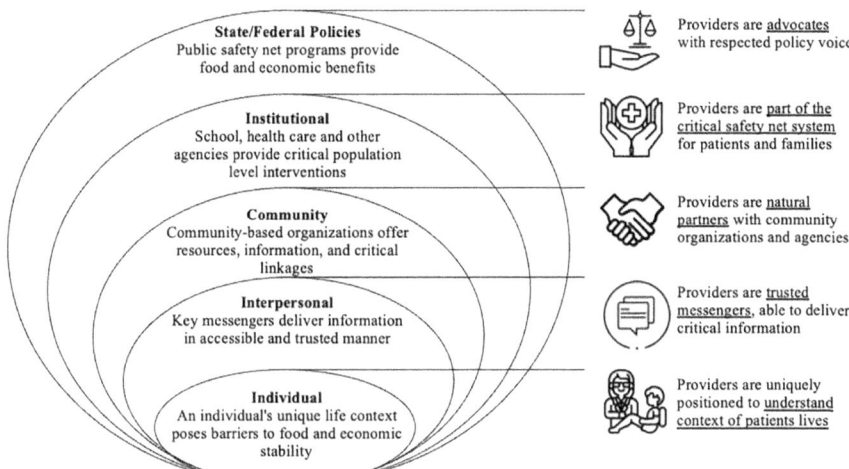

Fig. 1 Addressing food insecurity during COVID-19, application of the socioecological model and provider points of care

Table 1 Strategies to address COVID-19 social and economic needs with points of care models for providers

Framework	Targeted programs	Breakthroughs	Points of care (Models)
Individual and interpersonal levels	1. Community health workers and promotores engaged in community outreach (Akseer et al., 2020; Garba et al., 2022; Montiel et al., 2021; Parolin, 2021; Peretz et al., 2020)	1. Employment of grassroots strategies using trusted messengers and networks to distribute important information to hard-to-reach communities and high-need populations (Jablonski et al., 2020; Parolin, 2021)	1. Providers understand the unique life context of patients and families (e.g., poverty, employment, immigration status, racism, mental health) and screen for key social needs, and make community referrals to trusted organizations (Ambrose, 2020; Hetrick et al., 2020; Tester et al., 2020)
	2. Accessible and trusted social media campaigns supported through multiple communication channels (e.g., Facebook, CBO social media)	2. Recognition of the context of distrust in government systems, agencies, and public programs to craft messaging to dispel misinformation and eliminate barriers (Escobar et al., 2021)	

(continued)

Table 1 (continued)

Framework	Targeted programs	Breakthroughs	Points of care (Models)
Community level	1. Food bank sponsored pantries	1. Centralization and wide distribution of information about meal programs and food resources (Dunn et al., 2020) in multiple languages, using inclusive messaging and images (McLoughlin et al., 2020)	1. Providers partner with trusted local community organizations to learn about key social safety net programs and accessible resources
	2. Meals for pick-up or delivery from community organizations	2. Community-level assistance with online and in-person applications, dissmination of highly accurate information in multiple languages and formats, technology support, and transparent eligibility information	2. Providers leverage clinical interactions to disseminate community-level information to patients, reinforcing consistent and accurate information through multiple modes and in a language-specific and culturally relevant manner (Brochier et al., 2022; Escobar et al., 2021)
	3. Culturally tailored food boxes for pick-up or delivery (Garba et al., 2022)	3. Development of cross-sector collaboration among public and private partners to discuss emergency food provision and resource allocation (e.g., city and county, existing task forces, social services, schools, first responders, community organizations) (Ashikkali et al., 2020; Jablonski et al., 2020; Jowell et al., 2021; McLoughlin et al., 2020; Reimold et al., 2021)	3. Providers engage in advocacy efforts to promote systems and policy solutions to increase program participation
	4. Food vouchers (Sharma et al., 2022; Tester et al., 2020)		
	5. Neighborhood mutual aid food sharing (Lofton et al., 2022)		
	6. Bundling meals and resources (e.g., material goods, educational resources)		
	7. Economic stability (e.g., financial, rent and mortgage, utility) (McLoughlin et al., 2020)		

Table 1 (continued)

Framework	Targeted programs	Breakthroughs	Points of care (Models)
Institutional level	School and childcare	1. Assessment of barriers to participation in programs and apply innovative solutions (e.g., drive up or delivery options; batched meal pick-up at centralized sites and/or days of the week; culturally tailored foods) (Dunn et al., 2020; Jablonski et al., 2020; Kinsey et al., 2020b; Sharma et al., 2022)	1. Providers deliver information about available school meals, strengthen the communication channels needed to get critical information out and dispel any fears or worries regarding accessing pandemic-era meals
	1. School meals (Jowell et al., 2021; Kinsey et al., 2020a; McLoughlin et al., 2020)	2. Consideration of heightened barriers and service gaps for high-need populations (e.g., those with diabetes, chronic illnesses, disabilities) and populations disproportionately impacted by the pandemic (Jablonski et al., 2020)	
	2. School meals through summer seamless summer option (McLoughlin et al., 2020)	3. Utilization of school meal waivers to remove participation barriers, increase operational flexibility, and ensure safety of students and staff (Jowell et al., 2021; Kinsey et al., 2020a, 2020b)	
	3. After school meals and snacks	4. Observation of strains to systems and capacity (e.g., meal deliveries) (Jowell et al., 2021; Kinsey et al., 2020b)	
	4. Friday food backpacks students only or open to community (Jablonski et al., 2020)		
Federal and state policy level	Food programs	1. Emergency expansion of existing safety net programs addressed urgent economic needs (Akseer et al., 2020; Dunn et al., 2020; Kinsey et al., 2020a)	1. Providers examine unique barriers faced by immigrants (e.g., fear of public charge, documentation, eligibility) when accessing resources (Cadenas et al., 2022) and provide testament to patients' needs

(continued)

Table 1 (continued)

Framework	Targeted programs	Breakthroughs	Points of care (Models)
Public safety net programs	1. USDA nutrition waivers for school meals (Jowell et al., 2021; Kinsey et al., 2020a)	2. Creation of nutrition waivers allowed flexibility for program implementation to remove (Jowell et al., 2021; Kinsey et al., 2020a) participation barriers, as with school meals (Hetrick et al., 2020)	2. Providers advocate for systems and policy changes to enhance program participation in public safety net programs partnership with community and policy partners (Ambrose, 2020)
	2. Supplemental nutrition assistance program (SNAP)/food stamps	3. Authorization of emergency benefits beyond the COVID-19 period (Dunn et al., 2020)	
	3. Pandemic emergency benefit (P-EBT) (Kinsey et al., 2020a; Reimold et al., 2021; Wolfson & Leung, 2020)	4. Examination and amendment of policies aimed at reducing or deterring access to and utilization of public programs (Dunn et al., 2020); particularly for immigrants during times of crisis (e.g., pathway to citizenship, poverty alleviation) (Cadenas et al., 2022; Sinha et al., 2020)	
	4. Women infants and children (WIC)		
	5. Child and adult care food program (CACFP) (Dunn et al., 2020) economic stability programs		
	6. TANF and other cash support programs (Akseer et al., 2020; Sharma et al., 2022)		
	7. Housing subsidies and payment deferrals (Parolin, 2021)		
	8. Tax breaks (Parolin, 2021)		

EMR electronic medical records, *SNAP* supplemental nutrition assistance program, *WIC* women infants and children program, *CACFP* child and adult care food program

Individual and Interpersonal Level Strategies

The pandemic caught most of America off guard, with individuals unsure of the impact and how to protect themselves and their loved ones. Lack of accurate information and deliberate forms of misinformation (i.e. disinformation) were rampant, particularly with respect to vaccines (Loomba et al., 2021), posing problems for community-based organizations (CBOs) and HCPs struggling to assuage the worries of the community at large. Key to these challenges was the reliance on word of mouth and grassroots dissemination of information using trusted messengers and communication networks. As sheltering in place mandates went into effect, information was transmitted through multiple channels including television, radio, web-based, and social media platforms (Tsao et al., 2021) and via more proximal and trusted networks of family, friends, and neighbors (Merchant et al., 2021).

Engagement of community health workers and promotores was not a new strategy (Elder et al., 2009; Rosenthal et al., 2010; Scott et al., 2018), but one that was quickly recognized as critical for meeting needs of the hardest to reach individuals living in rural and marginalized communities (Akseer et al., 2020; Garba et al., 2022; Jablonski et al., 2020; Parolin, 2021), and those with inequitable access to reliable and accurate information. The ability of community health workers to reach out to their own communities, or those with which they were familiar, jump-started the transmission of necessary information (Peretz et al., 2020). These and other trusted messengers not only recognized families' distrust in government systems, agencies, and public programs but they were able to dispel mis- and disinformation and eliminate barriers to resource utilization (Escobar et al., 2021).

Varied and trusted social media channels were similarly important for disseminating information and increasing access to resources. Community organizations and CHWs were able to leverage communication networks and strategies relied on by community residents. In some cases, this included known channels such as Facebook and X (formerly Twitter), but there was also increased reliance on local community organizations to use internal platforms, texting, and email listservs to disseminate information. Communication format was also an important consideration, recognizing that individuals with limited time and literacy might prefer videos delivered by trusted messengers who represented the community. CBOs stressed the importance of any and all information delivered in a culturally sensitive manner, by individuals who looked liked and represented the community, and in the language concordant manner (Merchant et al., 2021; Peretz et al., 2020).

Disseminating information about eligibility for programs was particularly important for immigrant populations worried about the impact of documentation status on their ability to access health resources and economic assistance (Martínez et al., 2021). The evident hesitation among immigrants was driven in part by the increasing anti-immigrant policies and sentiment that plagued immigrants nationwide (Garcini et al., 2020). The experiences of immigrants and other marginalized communities highlighted the need for effective and innovative strategies necessary to address the interpersonal barriers to food access (Montiel et al., 2021).

Intersection of Clinical Care

Pediatric HCPs are uniquely positioned to understand the context in which their patients and families live. They quickly recognized how COVID-19 impacted families already experiencing poverty and its associated outcomes. Despite this, many HCPs were unprepared for unprecedented levels of unemployment, new immigration fears, heightened experiences of racism, and devastating mental health struggles that resulted. These levels of trauma reinforced the need for additional trusted messengers, individuals experienced in asking sensitive questions and ready to respond with resources and support (Table 1).

Healthcare providers had over a decade of experience screening for food insecurity (Goldman et al., 2014; Hager et al., 2010) and broader screenings for other social determinants (Berman et al., 2018; Chung et al., 2016; Council on Community Pediatrics et al., 2013). Many practices already had established clinic-based systems to screen for social determinants and make necessary community referrals (Ambrose, 2020; Hetrick et al., 2020; Tester et al., 2020), while others launched new systems to address the growing needs of patients and families. Some practices integrated social screenings with the electronic medical records (EMR), moving beyond paper-based screenings and data entry. As trusted messengers, HCPs were well positioned to make necessary referrals to public programs and community resources (Tester et al., 2020).

Clinic practices with additional resources and infrastructure were able to set up clinic-based food pantries to allow HCPs to provide food prescriptions and give families easy access to food onsite. Additionally, in states with value-based Medicaid payment models, providers were incentivized to address food insecurity and provide social supports to address the consequences of adverse social determinants of health (Brochier et al., 2022).

Community-Level Strategies

The social safety net supported by community organizations was quick to respond to food insecurity across the country. Food banks notably were at the forefront of the crisis, having the experience and knowledge to quickly address emergency food needs. They saw unprecedented numbers of individuals coming to their existing food sites. They mobilized drive-through and delivery models to address COVID-19 infection risks, and they continued to provide food to a myriad of community organizations and agencies (e.g., core social service agencies, schools, and libraries) already partnering with food banks to disseminate food throughout the community. These organizations strove to centralize and widely distribute information about meal programs and food resources (Dunn et al., 2020) in multiple languages, using inclusive messaging and images to increase utilization and remove added stress already present among individuals and families (McLoughlin et al., 2020). Community-level assistance with online and in-person applications, highly accurate program information (e.g., days, times, locations) in multiple languages and formats, technology support, and transparent eligibility information was a critical part of ensuring information dissemination and removal of access barriers.

Other existing and new strategies for food distribution were utilized. For example, culturally tailored food box programs offered food pick-up and delivery options (Garba et al., 2022), allowing more safe and accessible options for receiving food.

Delivery models were expensive and particularly hard to operationalize; however, they were critical for overcrowded households with inability to socially isolate when one family may have been living in one room in a house and/or multiple families shared food storage and cooking spaces. In some cases, this resulted in whole households being simultaneously COVID-19 positive and unable to leave the house to get food and other essential goods. Without viable food delivery options, already under-resourced families were further impacted by inequitable food access.

Neighborhood mutual aid food sharing programs were utilized in some communities. They leveraged neighbors willing to stock and share surplus foods in designated storage containers for easy access (Lofton et al., 2022). While there were barriers to this method of short-term food assistance, it demonstrated the power of community members coming together in an emergency to support one another and engage in innovative community-level solutions.

Voucher programs were also recommended as an option for addressing food insecurity, given they allow individuals to receive vouchers through clinic, county, and community service providers and utilize funds to purchase food at farmer's markets and local stores (Sharma et al., 2022; Tester et al., 2020). This gave individuals and families more choice in the foods they select to purchase, promoting dignity and access to culturally relevant foods. Despite this recommendation, vouchers may not have been highly utilized during the pandemic given temporary closures of farmer's markets and concerns for social distancing, but they are still a viable option for emergency food assistance when infrastructure, safety, and resources permit.

A key community-level breakthrough was the power of collaboration. County agencies, community-based organizations, and other service providers recognized the importance of developing cross-sector collaborations among public and private partners to discuss emergency food provision and resource allocation (e.g., city and county, existing task forces, social services, schools, first responders, and community organizations) (Ashikkali et al., 2020; Jablonski et al., 2020; Jowell et al., 2021; McLoughlin et al., 2020; Reimold et al., 2021). A wonderful case in New Haven, Connecticut, documented the development of a food assistance coalition that emerged during the pandemic that represented 63 organizations (165 individuals) and engaged in 50 initiatives to promote greater food access and health in their community (Santilli et al., 2022). These and other collaborative efforts developed in response to COVID-19 demonstrated the importance of bringing together volunteer organizations and service providers to amplify efforts, and collectively reach the hardest to reach populations in need.

Community collaborations supported the opportunity to strengthen the dissemination of important resources. For example, many organizations partnered to bundle food with material goods (e.g., diapers, masks, COVID-19 tests, and cleaning supplies), economic stability resources (e.g., financial, rent and mortgage, and utility) (McLoughlin et al., 2020), and educational materials. For example, libraries with existing pick-up meal distribution programs leveraged their food program to also distribute educational packets for kids and community resource information.

Intersection of Clinical Care

At the start of the pandemic, pediatric HCPs were sought after and relied upon, trusted messengers. As community-level strategies emerged to address emergency food needs, HCPs were an essential part of the support network, working with food banks, core service agencies, county officials, and others. As clinical partners, they networked with other partners to learn about the range of existing and new safety net resources available. Some existing programs had modifications or expansion of eligibility requirements, while new programs were established.

Given the plethora of information, HCPs leveraged in-person clinical interactions, telehealth visits, and automated phone calls and clinic-wide text messaging to disseminate community-level information to patients. As trusted messengers, they dispersed consistent and accurate information obtained from credible sources in a language-specific and culturally relevant manner (Brochier et al., 2022; Escobar et al., 2021).

Finally, the pandemic offered numerous opportunities for HCPs to engage in advocacy efforts to promote systems and policy solutions aimed at increasing utilization of key programs and public benefits. Healthcare providers knew well about the extant and exacerbated barriers that families faced, bearing witness to the harsh realities of the pandemic. As such, they were well positioned to advocate on behalf of their patients and families, working alongside community and policy partners to advocate for programs (e.g., rental/mortgage moratoriums, financial assistance, and expansion of federal and state benefits) and elevate the needs of patients and families through testimonials and formal story banking. Civic engagement and incorporation of clinician voice to advocacy efforts elevated the needs of children and families and the realities of their lived experiences during the pandemic.

Institutional Level Strategies

Educational institutions were already part of the critical safety net for children and families, ready to respond to the unforeseen needs that arose at the start of the pandemic. By March 2020, schools across the country closed, prompting massive losses in the number of school breakfasts and lunches available to children. At the peak, it is estimated that approximately 169.6 million meals were missed in 1 week (Kinsey et al., 2020b).

School systems, given their experience serving meals, were quick to adapt programming based on COVID-19 safety requirements and parent/guardian needs (Jowell et al., 2021; Kinsey et al., 2020b; McLoughlin et al., 2020). They capitalized on important pandemic-specific USDA nutrition waivers which allowed for greater flexibility in meal provision (e.g., added eligible meal locations, removed requirement for children to eat meals on site, allowed for parents to pick-up single or batched grab-and-go meals without a child present, relaxed nutrition requirements) (Jowell et al., 2021; Kinsey et al., 2020b). At the start of the pandemic, the number of children eligible for free or reduced-price meals was about 30 million, and grab-and-go meals went out to an estimated 8.0 million children (27%) (Kenney et al., 2022).

Schools also innovated in many other ways to increase participation and reduce access barriers. Namely, they designated centrally located pick-up sites (e.g., parking lots, social service agencies, community centers, bus stops, libraries, apartment complexes, and churches), co-locating some sites with food pantries to reach the highest concentrations of students and limit transportation barriers. Schools dispensed meals beyond lunch (e.g., breakfast and dinner), offered meals on select days of the week, operated mobile distribution via buses, supplied food to the community, provided home deliveries when resources allowed (Jablonski et al., 2020), and distributed backpacks filled with food. In some cases, districts with greater capacity supplied food to students in other nearby districts not able to provide meals due to staffing shortages, economic constraints, and other barriers. Schools developed external cross-collaborations to further strengthen their ability to serve meals given the many unprecedented constraints poised by the pandemic (Jowell et al., 2021; Kinsey et al., 2020b).

Intersection of Clinical Care

Pediatric HCPs have a long history of developing partnerships with schools at many levels to support optimal health, development, and educational outcomes for children (Harrison et al., 2021). As schools scrambled to adapt to pandemic-related constraints, pediatric HCPs became a channel for disseminating information to families regarding availability of food through schools and child care centers.

In some cases, schools looked to pediatric partners to get up-to-date information on COVID-19 rates in children, health implications, and vaccine safety. The bi-directional information exchange and collaboration between these two critical safety net systems were essential to maintain communication and connection to the most under-resourced hard-to-reach populations.

Federal Level Policy Strategies

At the start of the pandemic, eligible children and families utilized federal safety programs such as SNAP and WIC for supplemental food support (Akseer et al., 2020; Sharma et al., 2022). The SNAP program rose from a monthly average of 35.7 million participants pre-pandemic (FY 2019) (Cronquist, 2021), to 43 million by June 2020 (Center on Budget and Policy Priorities, 2022). Despite the widespread availability of these programs, barriers to participation persisted and were heightened during the pandemic (e.g., structural barriers, immigration fears, worries of public charge). For example, only 50% of eligible families were enrolled in SNAP and WIC, leaving available benefits on the table for many families (Stenmark et al., 2023).

In 2020, the Families First Coronavirus Response Act approved state waivers to request SNAP emergency allotments, which increased household benefits to the maximum allotment allowed through the SNAP program, helping additional households formerly ineligible for the maximum allotment. In late 2020, the President signed the Consolidated Appropriation Act (COVID-19 relief bill), which temporarily increased SNAP maximum allotments by an additional 15% for January through June 2021. This increased benefits to the lowest-income households already receiving close to or the maximum allotment. Families in this category received roughly an additional $95 per month for a new monthly total of $218 per person (Center on Budget and Policy Priorities, 2022). The American Rescue Plan Act of 2021 further extended the maximum benefit increase through October 2021 (Center on Budget and Policy Priorities, 2022) and provided additional funding for fruits and vegetables for SNAP and WIC recipients (Stenmark et al., 2023).

The Families First Coronavirus Response Act also provided emergency funding for Pandemic-EBT (P-EBT), a new federal child nutrition program operated through SNAP and utilizing the existing electronic benefit transfer (EBT) system, which adds benefits onto individual debit cards for participants' ease of use. The P-ETB program was designed to give states emergency funds to support children who, if not for pandemic closures and distance learning, would have received free or reduced-price school breakfasts and lunches (Kinsey et al., 2020b; Reimold et al., 2021; Waxman et al., 2020; Wolfson & Leung, 2020). Benefits ranged from $250 to $450 per child during the 2020 spring closure. To facilitate access, benefits were loaded onto new or existing SNAP EBT debit cards, obscuring the difference between P-EBT and SNAP funds.

P-EBT funding was initially set to cover the spring of 2020; however, this was extended multiple times to ultimately include the entire 2020–2021 school year. Later additions to the P-EBT program included provision of benefits to children aged 6 years and under in child care who had similarly lost access to meals in the child care setting due to widespread closures, and summer benefits for school aged and children in child care facilities beginning in 2021 (Waxman et al., 2021). Benefits extended through May 2023 for children under 6 years in child care (USDA Food and Nutrition Service, 2023). In the first few months of the pandemic from March to June 2020, it is estimated that the P-EBT program reach 26.9 million children, distributing $3.2 billion in monthly cash benefits (Kenney et al., 2022).

Critical changes to and expansion of SNAP benefits, and enactment of P-EBT greatly expanded children's access to food during the pandemic, removing some administrative barriers to enrollment, streamlined access to cash benefits, and allowed for greater operational flexibility (Balasuriya et al., 2021). However, despite efforts to reduce barriers, old barriers persisted, and new barriers arose. For example, caregivers of children newly eligible for benefits during the pandemic didn't always know about such changes. Families reported receiving EBT cards in the mail that they didn't recognize, and consequently threw them in the trash before realizing the cash value. Other caregivers aware of benefit increases waited for cards that never arrived or did not have the accurate amount for their eligible children (Cadenhead et al., 2022).

In addition to policies in support of federal nutrition programs, other critical federal programs supported families during the pandemic. They included, but were not limited to, Temporary Assistance for Needy Families, Child Tax Credit (CTC) in 2021 (Marr et al., 2021), housing subsidies and payment deferrals, and other tax breaks (Stenmark et al., 2023). Unlike the Great Recession, the swift policy response and innovations reinforced benefits to already eligible children in need, expanded benefits to children newly impacted by the pandemic and previously ineligible, and eased some of the existing barriers preventing marginalized groups from accessing public resources. Despite the federal policy breakthroughs, operation of economic safety net programs during the pandemic was fraught with strict eligibility requirements and barriers to participation. Allowable benefit amounts provided through SNAP and P-EBT were not enough to support families' food and economic resource needs given dramatic changes to employment that resulted due to shelter in place mandates, business closures, evictions, and other hardships. Emergency expansion of existing safety net programs aimed to expand benefits, remediate participation barriers, and address urgent economic needs, but gaps remained (Akseer et al., 2020; Dunn et al., 2020; Kinsey et al., 2020b).

The COVID Public Health Emergency ended in May 2023. This marked the end of important pandemic-era programs (e.g., CTC, SNAP emergency allotments, stimulus payments). The expansion of the CTC expired at the end of 2021, which reverted to credit amounts based on President Trump's 2017 tax law (Cox et al., 2023). The number of individuals living below the poverty line rose dramatically in 2022 to 37.9 million, compared to 34 million people in 2019 (U.S. Census Bureau, 2020). The child poverty rate more than doubled from a historic low of 5.2% in 2021 to 12.4% in 2022 (based on the Supplemental Poverty Measure). Policy analysts from the Center on Budget and Policy Priorities link the rise in poverty to the expiration of pandemic-era relief programs, including the CTC (U.S. Census Bureau, 2023). Further analyses suggest that a continuation of the American Rescue Plan's Child Tax Credit increase in 2022 could have kept approximately three million children out of poverty, preventing much of the recent increase (Parrott, 2023).

Furthermore, with respect to the SNAP program, it is estimated that emergency allotments kept approximately 4.3 million people above the federal poverty line in 2021, reducing overall poverty by 10% and child poverty by 14%. An analysis by the Center on Budget and Policy Priorities estimated that SNAP prevented nearly 3.6 million children from falling into poverty. Such estimated reductions in poverty were highest for Black and Latino participants. The SNAP emergency allotments ended in March 2023, resulting in a return to pre-pandemic benefits amounts (average decrease of $90 per person per month) (Rosenbaum et al., 2023). Subsequently, food insecurity in households with children increased to 8.8% (3.3 million households) in 2022 (Rabbitt, 2022), up from 6.5% (2.4 million households) in 2019 (Coleman-Jensen, 2019). One silver lining to the end of SNAP emergency allotments was the creation of a permanent Summer EBT program, which is projected to supply nearly 30 million children in low-income households with additional benefits during the summer months when they have decreased access to school meals (Rosenbaum et al., 2023).

Intersection of Clinical Care

The health care sector and pediatric HCPs were important conveyors of information related to available federal and state programs for patients and families. Their awareness of expanded program benefits allowed them to not only share critical program updates but also share positive health impacts of utilizing benefits, dispelling myths and fears associated with program participation. Healthcare providers helped alleviate access barriers by encouraging families to claim all of the benefits for which they were eligible (Stenmark et al., 2023). Increasing families' access to programs aimed at addressing food insecurity and economic hardship help reduce parent and caregiver stress, further promoting the overall health and well-being of children.

As children and families' needs increased during the pandemic, pediatric HCPs strengthened or developed relationships with community and policy partners to advocate for sound food and nutrition policies.

Lessons Learned

The pandemic showed the depths of inequities in social and financial needs, health outcomes, technology access, and more. Compared to white children, Black and Latino children experienced higher rates of poverty as a result of the pandemic, as their parents were more likely to lose jobs and have fewer financial resources to fall back, thus resulting cascade of negative effects on their household social and economic well-being (Parolin, 2021; USDA Food and Nutrition Service, 2023). The pandemic's impact on all US households prompted the country to take notice of inequities in a way that hadn't occurred for many years. Our nation was better able to comprehend the struggles of low-income and marginalized populations.

Sufficient access to nutritionally adequate and safe foods and the ability to acquire them in socially acceptable ways were one of the first significant social needs to be elevated during the pandemic, given the acute needs that quickly arose. Community, institutional, and federal level innovations addressed the complexity of food access required to support the needs of children and families during the pandemic. The multi-level response staved off what could have been far greater increases in food and housing insecurity, poverty, and poor child health outcomes (Rosenbaum et al., 2023). As community organizations, HCPs, policy makers, and advocates at each of these levels responded to the pressing needs of individuals and families, and elevated the importance of equitable distribution of food resources as a social determinant of health (Santilli et al., 2022).

Pediatric HCPs played an important role in increasing children and families' access to food and nutrition across all levels, given their status as trusted messengers and proximity to the most marginalized and hard-to-reach communities. They are a critical part of the safety net for children, with strong ties to community partners, institutions, and policy makers essential for serving and protecting children.

The expiration of pandemic-era benefits reversed important gains to the stability and well-being of households with children. Lessons learned from food security innovations demonstrate how we can and should do better by our nation's greatest asset, our children. It is likely that we won't know the full impact of the pandemic for many years to come, but hopefully we can learn from these efforts in the event that our nation faces a similar crisis—we will be ready to respond quickly, strategically, collaboratively, and most importantly with a lens of health equity.

Calls to Action
- Pediatric HCPs are trusted messengers who build important partnerships and collaborations with community and policy partners to ensure children and families are met. The breadth of collaborative engagement is diverse, with opportunities to develop and strengthen cross-sector efforts in advance of national emergencies to ensure a swift response.
- Pediatric HCPs inherit the results of poor social policies. They can and should bear witness to the inequitable lived experiences of under-resources and marginalized populations, sharing stories, and experiences with community partners and policy makers to inform needs systems and policy changes.

References

Abrams, E. M., Greenhawt, M., Shaker, M., Pinto, A. D., Sinha, I., & Singer, A. (2022). The COVID-19 pandemic. *Annals of Allergy, Asthma & Immunology, 128*(1), 19–25.

Akseer, N., Kandru, G., Keats, E. C., & Bhutta, Z. A. (2020). COVID-19 pandemic and mitigation strategies: Implications for maternal and child health and nutrition. *The American Journal of Clinical Nutrition, 112*(2), 251–256.

Alaimo, K., Briefel, R. R., Frongillo, E. A., Jr., & Olson, C. M. (1998). Food insufficiency exists in the United States: Results from the third National Health and nutrition examination survey (NHANES III). *American Journal of Public Health, 88*(3), 419–426.

Ambrose, A. J. H. (2020). Inequities during COVID-19. *Pediatrics, 146*(2), e20201501.

Ashikkali, L., Carroll, W., & Johnson, C. (2020). The indirect impact of COVID-19 on child health. *Paediatrics & Child Health, 30*(12), 430–437.

Balasuriya, L., Berkowitz, S. A., & Seligman, H. K. (2021). Federal Nutrition Programs after the pandemic: Learning from P-EBT and SNAP to create the next generation of food safety net programs. *Inquiry, 58*, 004695802110051.

Bartholomew, A., Adedze, P., Soto, V., Funanich, C., Newman, T., & MacNeil, P. (2017). Historical perspective of the WIC program and its breastfeeding promotion and support efforts. *Journal of Nutrition Education and Behavior, 49*(7), S139–S143.e1.

Berman, R. S., Patel, M. R., Belamarich, P. F., & Gross, R. S. (2018). Screening for poverty and poverty-related social determinants of health. *Pediatrics in Review, 39*(5), 235–246.

Bowen, S., Elliott, S., & Hardison-Moody, A. (2021). The structural roots of food insecurity: How racism is a fundamental cause of food insecurity. *Sociology Compass, 15*(7), e12846. https://doi.org/10.1111/soc4.12846

Brochier, A., Garg, A., & Peltz, A. (2022). Clinical and public policy interventions to address food insecurity among children. *Current Opinion in Pediatrics, 34*(1), 2–7.

Cadenas, G. A., Cerezo, A., Carlos Chavez, F. L., Capielo Rosario, C., Torres, L., Suro, B., et al. (2022). The citizenship shield: Mediated and moderated links between immigration status, discrimination, food insecurity, and negative health outcomes for Latinx immigrants during the COVID-19 pandemic. *Journal of Community Psychology, 51*, 2355.

Cadenhead, J. W., McCarthy, J. E., Nguyen, T. T. T., Rodriguez, M., & Koch, P. A. (2022). Qualitative study of participation facilitators and barriers for emergency school meals and pandemic electronic benefits (P-EBT) in an urban setting during COVID-19. *Nutrients, 14*(16), 3358.

Caswell, J. A., & Yaktine, A. L. (Eds.). (2013). *Committee on examination of the adequacy of food resources and SNAP allotments*. The National Academies Press. https://www-ncbi-nlm-nih-gov.laneproxy.stanford.edu/books/NBK206911/pdf/Bookshelf_NBK206911.pdf

Center on Budget and Policy Priorities. (2022). *Policy basics: The supplemental nutrition assistance program (SNAP)*. Center on Budget and Policy Priorities. https://www.cbpp.org/research/food-assistance/the-supplemental-nutrition-assistance-program-snap

Chilton, M., Black, M. M., Berkowitz, C., Casey, P. H., Cook, J., Cutts, D., et al. (2009). Food insecurity and risk of poor health among US-born children of immigrants. *American Journal of Public Health, 99*(3), 556–562.

Chilton, M., & Booth, S. (2007). Hunger of the body and hunger of the mind: African American women's perceptions of food insecurity, health and violence. *Journal of Nutrition Education and Behavior, 39*(3), 116–125.

Chung, E. K., Siegel, B. S., Garg, A., Conroy, K., Gross, R. S., Long, D. A., et al. (2016). Screening for social determinants of health among children and families living in poverty: A guide for clinicians. *Current Problems in Pediatric and Adolescent Health Care, 46*(5), 135–153.

Coleman-Jensen, A. (2019). *Household food security in the United States in 2019* (Economic Research Report No. ERR-275). U.S. Department of Agriculture, Economic Research Service.

Coleman-Jensen, A., McFall, W., & Nord, M. (2013). *Food insecurity in households with children: Prevalence, severity, and household characteristics, 2010–11* (Economic Research Report).

Coleman-Jensen, A., Rabbitt, M. P., Gregory, C. A., & Sing, A. (2016). *Household food security in the United States in 2015* (Economic Research Report No. ERR-215). U.S. Department of Agriculture, Economic Research Service. https://www.ers.usda.gov/webdocs/publications/79761/err215_summary.pdf?v=4

Coleman-Jensen, A., Rabbitt, M. P., Gregory, C. A., & Singh, A. (2018). *Household food security in the United States in 2017* (Economic Research Report No. ERR-256). U.S. Department of Agriculture, Economic Research Service. https://www.ers.usda.gov/webdocs/publications/90023/err256_summary.pdf?v=0

Cook, J. T., Frank, D. A., Berkowitz, C., Black, M. M., Casey, P. H., Cutts, D. B., et al. (2004). Food insecurity is associated with adverse health outcomes among human infants and toddlers. *The Journal of Nutrition, 134*(6), 1432–1438.

Council on Community Pediatrics; Committee on Nutrition. (2015). Promoting food security for all children. *Pediatrics, 136*(5), e1431–e1438.

Council on Community Pediatrics, Gorski, P. A., Kuo, A. A., Granado-Villar, D. C., Gitterman, B. A., Brown, J. M., et al. (2013). Community pediatrics: Navigating the intersection of medicine, public health, and social determinants of children's health. *Pediatrics, 131*(3), 623–628.

Cox, K., Marr, C., Calame, S., & Hingtgen, S. (2023). *Top tax priority: Expanding the child tax credit in upcoming economic legislation*. Center on Budget and Policy Priorities. https://www.cbpp.org/sites/default/files/6-7-23tax.pdf

Cronquist, K. (2021). *Characteristics of supplemental nutrition assistance program households: Fiscal year 2019* (Supplemental Nutrition Assistance Program Nutrition Assistance Program Report Series Report No. SNAP-20-CHAR). U.S. Department of Agriculture, Food and Nutrition Service, Office of Policy Support. https://fns-prod.azureedge.us/sites/default/files/resource-files/Characteristics2019.pdf

Defeyter, M. A., Graham, P. L., & Russo, R. (2015). More than just a meal: Breakfast club attendance and children's social relationships. *Frontiers in Public Health, 3*, 183. https://doi.org/10.3389/fpubh.2015.00183

Dunn, C. G., Kenney, E., Fleischhacker, S. E., & Bleich, S. N. (2020). Feeding low-income children during the COVID-19 pandemic. *The New England Journal of Medicine, 382*(18), e40.

Elder, J. P., Ayala, G. X., Parra-Medina, D., & Talavera, G. A. (2009). Health communication in the Latino community: Issues and approaches. *Annual Review of Public Health, 30*(1), 227–251.

Escobar, M., Mendez, A. D., Encinas, M. R., Villagomez, S., & Wojcicki, J. M. (2021). High food insecurity in Latinx families and associated COVID-19 infection in the Greater Bay Area, California. *BMC Nutrition, 7*(1), 23.

Garba, N. A., Sacca, L., Clarke, R. D., Bhoite, P., Buschman, J., Oller, V., et al. (2022). Addressing food insecurity during the COVID-19 pandemic: Intervention outcomes and lessons learned from a collaborative food delivery response in South Florida's underserved households. *International Journal of Environmental Research and Public Health, 19*(13), 8130.

Garcini, L. M., Domenech Rodríguez, M. M., Mercado, A., & Paris, M. (2020). A tale of two crises: The compounded effect of COVID-19 and anti-immigration policy in the United States. *Psychological Trauma Theory Research Practice and Policy, 12*(S1), S230–S232.

Gitterman, B. A., Chilton, L. A., Cotton, W. H., Duffee, J. H., Flanagan, P., Keane, V. A., et al. (2015). Promoting food security for all children. *Pediatrics, 136*(5), e1431–e1438.

Goldman, N., Sheward, R., Ettinger de Cuba, S., Black, M. M., Sandel, M., Cooke, J., et al. (2014). *The hunger vital sign: A new standard of care for preventive health (Policy action brief).* Children's Health Watch.

Gundersen, C. (2013). Food insecurity is an ongoing national concern. *Advances in Nutrition: An International Review Journal, 4*(1), 36–41.

Gundersen, C., Kreider, B., & Pepper, J. (2012). The impact of the National School Lunch Program on child health: A nonparametric bounds analysis. *Journal of Econometrics, 166*(1), 79–91.

Gundersen, C., & Ver Ploeg, M. (2015). Food assistance programs and child health. *The Future of Children, 25*(1), 91.

Gundersen, C., & Ziliak, J. P. (2014). Childhood food insecurity in the US: Trends, causes, and policy options. *The Future of Children, 24*(2), 1–19.

Hager, E. R., Quigg, A. M., Black, M. M., Coleman, S. M., Heeren, T., Rose-Jacobs, R., et al. (2010). Development and validity of a 2-item screen to identify families at risk for food insecurity. *Pediatrics, 126*(1), e26–e32.

Harrison, E., Garbutt, J., Sterkel, R., Dodd, S., Wang, R., Newland, J., et al. (2021). Collaborating to advocate in primary care for children during COVID-19. *Pediatrics, 148*(4), e2021052106.

Hetrick, R. L., Rodrigo, O. D., & Bocchini, C. E. (2020). Addressing pandemic-intensified food insecurity. *Pediatrics, 146*(4), e2020006924.

Jablonski, B. B. R., Casnovsky, J., Clark, J. K., Cleary, R., Feingold, B., Freedman, D., et al. (2020). Emergency food provision for children and families during the COVID—19 pandemic: Examples from five U.S. cities. *Applied Economic Perspectives and Policy, 43*, 169.

Jowell, A. H., Bruce, J. S., Escobar, G. V., Ordonez, V. M., Hecht, C. A., & Patel, A. I. (2021). Mitigating childhood food insecurity during COVID-19: A qualitative study of how school districts in California's San Joaquin Valley responded to growing needs. *Public Health Nutrition, 30*, 1–11.

Kenney, E. L., Walkinshaw, L. P., Shen, Y., Fleischhacker, S. E., Jones-Smith, J., Bleich, S. N., et al. (2022). Costs, reach, and benefits of COVID-19 pandemic electronic benefit transfer and grab-and-go school meals for ensuring youths' access to food during school closures. *JAMA Network Open, 5*(8), e2229514.

Kinsey, E. W., Kinsey, D., & Rundle, A. G. (2020a). COVID-19 and food insecurity: An uneven patchwork of responses. *Journal of Urban Health, 97*(3), 332–335.

Kinsey, E. W., Hecht, A. A., Dunn, C. G., Levi, R., Read, M. A., Smith, C., et al. (2020b). School closures during COVID-19: Opportunities for innovation in meal service. *American Journal of Public Health, 110*(11), 1635–1643.

Lofton, S., Kersten, M., Simonovich, S. D., & Martin, A. (2022). Mutual aid organisations and their role in reducing food insecurity in Chicago's urban communities during COVID-19. *Public Health Nutrition, 25*(1), 119–122.

Loomba, S., De Figueiredo, A., Piatek, S. J., De Graaf, K., & Larson, H. J. (2021). Measuring the impact of COVID-19 vaccine misinformation on vaccination intent in the UK and USA. *Nature Human Behaviour, 5*(3), 337–348.

Lozoff, B., Jimenez, E., Hagen, J., Mollen, E., & Wolf, A. W. (2000). Poorer behavioral and developmental outcome more than 10 years after treatment for iron deficiency in infancy. *Pediatrics, 105*(4), e51.

Marr, C., Cox, K., Hingtgen, S., Windham, K., & Sherman, A. (2021). *American rescue plan act includes critical expansions of child tax credit and EITC.* Center on Budget and Policy Priorities.

Martínez, M. E., Nodora, J. N., & Carvajal-Carmona, L. G. (2021). The dual pandemic of COVID-19 and systemic inequities in US Latino communities. *Cancer, 127*(10), 1548–1550.

McLeroy, K. R., Bibeau, D., Steckler, A., & Glanz, K. (1988). An ecological perspective on health promotion programs. *Health Education Quarterly, 15*(4), 351–377.

McLoughlin, G. M., McCarthy, J. A., McGuirt, J. T., Singleton, C. R., Dunn, C. G., & Gadhoke, P. (2020). Addressing food insecurity through a health equity lens: A case study of large Urban School districts during the COVID-19 pandemic. *Journal of Urban Health, 97*(6), 759–775.

Merchant, R. M., South, E. C., & Lurie, N. (2021). Public health messaging in an era of social Media. *JAMA, 325*(3), 223.

Montiel, G. I., Cantero, P. J., Montiel, I., Moon, K., & Nawaz, S. (2021). Commentary: Rebuilding with impacted communities at the center: The case for a civic engagement approach to COVID-19 response and recovery. *Family & Community Health, 44*(2), 81–83.

Morales, D. X., Morales, S. A., & Beltran, T. F. (2021). Racial/ethnic disparities in household food insecurity during the COVID-19 pandemic: A nationally representative study. *Journal of Racial and Ethnic Health Disparities, 8*(5), 1300–1314.

Murphy, J. M., Wehler, C. A., Pagano, M. E., Little, M., Kleinman, R. E., & Jellinek, M. S. (1998). Relationship between hunger and psychosocial functioning in low-income American children. *Journal of the American Academy of Child and Adolescent Psychiatry, 37*(2), 163–170.

Oberg, C. N. (2011). The great Recession's impact on children. *Maternal and Child Health Journal, 15*(5), 553–554.

Parolin, Z. (2021). What the COVID-19 pandemic reveals about racial differences in child welfare and child Well-being: An introduction to the special issue. *Race and Social Problems, 13*(1), 1–5.

Parrott, S. (2023). *Record rise in poverty highlights importance of child tax credit; health coverage marks a high point before pandemic safeguards ended* (CBPP statement). Center on Budget and Policy Priorities. https://www.cbpp.org/press/statements/record-rise-in-poverty-highlights-importance-of-child-tax-credit-health-coverage

Peretz, P. J., Islam, N., & Matiz, L. A. (2020). Community health workers and Covid-19—Addressing social determinants of health in times of crisis and beyond. *The New England Journal of Medicine, 383*(19), e108.

Petterson, S. M., & Albers, A. B. (2001). Effects of poverty and maternal depression on early child development. *Child Development, 72*(6), 1794–1813.

Rabbitt, M. P. (2022). *Household food security in the United States in 2022* (Economic research report). U.S. Department of Agriculture, Economic Research Service. https://www.ers.usda.gov/webdocs/publications/107703/err-325.pdf?v=9779

Ralston, K., Treen, K., Coleman-Jensen, A., & Guthrie, J.. (2017). *Children's Food Security and USDA Child Nutrition Programs* (Report No. EIB-174). USDA, Economic Research Service. https://www.ers.usda.gov/webdocs/publications/84003/eib-174.pdf?v=0

Reimold, A. E., Grummon, A. H., Taillie, L. S., Brewer, N. T., Rimm, E. B., & Hall, M. G. (2021). Barriers and facilitators to achieving food security during the COVID-19 pandemic. *Preventive Medical Reports, 23*, 101500.

Rose, D. (1999). Economic determinants and dietary consequences of food insecurity in the United States. *The Journal of Nutrition, 129*(2), 517S–520S.

Rose, D., & Oliveira, V. (1997). Nutrient intakes of individuals from food-insufficient households in the United States. *American Journal of Public Health, 87*(12), 1956–1961.

Rose-Jacobs, R., Black, M. M., Casey, P. H., Cook, J. T., Cutts, D. B., Chilton, M., et al. (2008). Household food insecurity: Associations with at-risk infant and toddler development. *Pediatrics, 121*(1), 65–72.

Rosenbaum, D., Bergh, K., & Hall, L. (2023). *Temporary pandemic SNAP benefits will end in remaining 35 states in March 2023*. Center on Budget and Policy Priorities. https://www.cbpp.org/research/food-assistance/temporary-pandemic-snap-benefits-will-end-in-remaining-35-states-in-march

Rosenthal, E. L., Brownstein, J. N., Rush, C. H., Hirsch, G. R., Willaert, A. M., Scott, J. R., et al. (2010). Community health workers: Part of the solution. *Health Affairs (Millwood), 29*(7), 1338–1342.

Santilli, A., Lin-Schweitzer, A., Morales, S. I., Werlin, S., Hart, K., Cramer, J., et al. (2022). Coalition building and food insecurity: How an equity and justice framework guided a viable food assistance network. *International Journal of Environmental Research and Public Health, 19*(18), 11666.

Scott, K., Beckham, S. W., Gross, M., Pariyo, G., Rao, K. D., Cometto, G., et al. (2018). What do we know about community-based health worker programs? A systematic review of existing reviews on community health workers. *Human Resources for Health, 16*(1), 39.

Sharma, A., Lin, M., Okumus, B., Kesa, H., Jeyakumar, A., & Impellitteri, K. (2022). Adopting a systems view of disrupting crisis-driven food insecurity. *Public Health, 211*, 72–74.

Sinha, I. P., Lee, A. R., Bennett, D., McGeehan, L., Abrams, E. M., Mayell, S. J., et al. (2020). Child poverty, food insecurity, and respiratory health during the COVID-19 pandemic. *The Lancet Respiratory Medicine, 8*(8), 762–763.

Stenmark, S. H., Sheward, R. S., Marcil, L. E., Bovell-Ammon, A. R., Bruce, C. O., & Cuba, S. A. E. (2023). The American Rescue Plan Act, a critical opportunity to improve child and family health. *Health Affairs Forefront*. https://doi.org/10.1377/forefront.20210804.897720/full/

Stuff, J. E., Casey, P. H., Szeto, K. L., Gossett, J. M., Robbins, J. M., Simpson, P. M., et al. (2004). Household food insecurity is associated with adult health status. *The Journal of Nutrition, 134*(9), 2330–2335.

Tester, J. M., Rosas, L. G., & Leung, C. W. (2020). Food insecurity and pediatric obesity: A double whammy in the era of COVID-19. *Current Obesity Reports, 9*(4), 442–450.

Tsao, S. F., Chen, H., Tisseverasinghe, T., Yang, Y., Li, L., & Butt, Z. A. (2021). What social media told us in the time of COVID-19: A scoping review. *Lancet Digit Health, 3*(3), e175–e194.

U. S. Department of Agriculture Food and Nutrition Service. (2017). *The national school lunch program*. United States Department of Agriculture Food and Nutrition Service. https://fns-prod.azureedge.us/sites/default/files/resource-files/NSLPFactSheet.pdf

U.S. Census Bureau. (2020). *Income, poverty and health insurance coverage in the United States: 2019*. Census.gov. https://www.census.gov/newsroom/press-releases/2020/income-poverty.html

U.S. Census Bureau. (2023). *Income, poverty and health insurance coverage in the United States: 2022*. Census.gov. https://www.census.gov/newsroom/press-releases/2023/income-poverty-health-insurance-coverage.html

U.S. Department of Agriculture. (2023). *National level annual summary tables: FY 1969–2022*. https://www.fns.usda.gov/pd/child-nutrition-tables

U.S. Department of Agriculture Food and Nutrition Service. (2019). *Summer food service program history*. https://www.fns.usda.gov/sfsp/program-history

USDA Food and Nutrition Service. (2023). *State guidance on pandemic EBT*. Food and Nutrition Service. https://www.fns.usda.gov/snap/state-guidance-coronavirus-pandemic-ebt-pebt

Waxman, E., Gupta, P., & Gonzalez, D. (2020). *Food insecurity edged back up after COVID-19 relief expired*. The Urban Institute and Robert Wood Johnson Foundation.

Waxman, E., Gupta, P., & Pratt, E. (2021). *Documenting pandemic EBT for the 2020–21 school year: State perspectives on implementation challenges and lessons for the future*. The Urban Institute and Robert Wood Johnson Foundation.

Whitaker, R. C., Phillips, S. M., & Orzol, S. M. (2006). Food insecurity and the risks of depression and anxiety in mothers and behavior problems in their preschool-aged children. *Pediatrics, 118*(3), e859–e868.

Willems, S. J., Castells, M. C., & Baptist, A. P. (2022). The magnification of health disparities during the COVID-19 pandemic. *The Journal of Allergy and Clinical Immunology. In Practice, 10*(4), 903–908.

Wise, P. H. (2009). Children of the recession. *Archives of Pediatrics & Adolescent Medicine, 163*(11), 1063–1064.

Wolfson, J. A., & Leung, C. W. (2020). Food insecurity during COVID-19: An acute crisis with long-term health implications. *American Journal of Public Health, 110*(12), 1763–1765.

Access to Care: Assessment of Financial, Structural, Political, and Social Barriers

Rajashree Koppolu and April Kapu

Improving health equity requires a holistic approach. Change is needed everywhere-from the bedside to the boardroom to how payers pay for care to health policy changes.

—National Academy of Medicine

Introduction and Background

At the beginning of the COVID-19 pandemic, a public narrative rapidly emerged that children were not impacted and were spared severe burdens of morbidity and mortality. While the latter is generally true when compared to adult populations, the infrastructure of pediatric care delivery systems was radically disrupted. Primary care clinics had limited visits or were closed. Parents had significant fears of viral transmission and avoided seeking preventive or routine care. Once friendly, bustling pediatric offices with smiling staff now had closed waiting rooms and staff masked with personal protective equipment that was unfamiliar and frightening to their patients. Children's health centers delayed surgical procedures, halted services for children with chronic illness, and worked to convert pediatric units into care environments for adults. Parents and other caregivers lost their jobs and subsequently their children's insurance coverage, further decreasing access to care. Political divisiveness inflamed parental fears and unprecedented mistrust of healthcare providers (HCPs) ensued (Bartek et al., 2021; Koppolu, 2021; Peck, 2020). All of these factors deeply influenced access to pediatric care, the impacts of which will likely be studied for generations to come.

R. Koppolu
Stanford Medicine Children's Health, Palo Alto, CA, USA
e-mail: rkoppolu@stanfordchildrens.org

A. Kapu (✉)
Vanderbilt University School of Nursing, Nashville, TN, USA
e-mail: april.n.kapu@vanderbilt.edu

J. L. Peck (ed.), *COVID-19 Impacts on Child Health*,
https://doi.org/10.1007/978-3-031-80369-7_14

257

Points of Care

Access to Care: Assessment of Economic Barriers

COVID-19 presented stressful economic challenges for families with children, limiting their ability to access basic healthcare needs. Beginning in February 2020, a rapidly unfolding economic recession created extremely high rates of unemployment and lowered household income. The Kaiser Family Foundation estimates that between March 1st and May 2nd, 2020, over 20 million children were in a family in which someone experienced loss of employment (Garfield & Chidambaram, 2020). In a household survey from June 29, 2021 to July 11, 2022, adults living with children reported more difficulty in paying for daily household expenses, providing food, and making housing payments when compared to households without children. Household income is connected to children's health outcomes, education access, and cognitive and social development (Drake & Williams, 2022). While many federal relief efforts such as direct stimulus payments and unemployment benefits greatly helped during the peak of the pandemic, rising inflation and expiration of some of these credits threaten a family's ability to pay for daily costs of living. Benefits from programs like the Supplemental Nutrition Assistance Program (SNAP) could not keep up with the rising costs families incurred in the wake of the pandemic. The economic impact of food shortages and insecurity are covered more in-depth in this chapter.

In June 2022, supply chain challenges led to a baby formula shortage, which limited the formula availability for many families and increased the cost of available of formula, which women, infants, and children (WIC) could not fully cover. This shortage was severely compounded by a massive large scale product recall following reports of compromised formula quality related to contamination. Retailers reported stock shortages of 74% nationally and over 90% in selected states. Consumers responded with panic buying and reported experiencing price gouging. The shortages disproportionately impacted communities of color and families who relied upon financial assistance programs. Guidance from professional organizations and government entities was insufficient in assuaging consumer concerns, who turned to widely shared recommendations on social media for homemade, inexpensive recipes (Kalaitzandonakes et al., 2023).

There were substantial changes to the funding of public health insurance programs during the pandemic. About half of all children in the United States (40 million) are insured through Medicaid and the Children's Health Insurance Program (CHIP). From February 2020 to June 2021, children's enrollment increased by 11%. This was largely due to parental or caregiver unemployment and income loss as well as federal provisions requiring that adults and children are continuously covered during the public health emergency. While many children maintained or gained access to Medicaid coverage during the pandemic, it is estimated that 6.7 million children are likely to lose coverage and are at risk for becoming uninsured for a period of time (Alker & Brooks, 2022). In addition, there are a number of children who are eligible for Medicaid or CHIP, but experience difficulty in completing the application or possess a lack of understanding regarding eligibility, making it difficult for more children to receive adequate coverage (Garfield & Chidambaram, 2020). Lack of coverage coupled with physical barriers to care environments resulting from social distancing policies greatly affected children's access to care. Even for those who did have coverage, early data analysis from the Centers for Medicare and Medicaid Services (CMS) shows a substantial decline in the use of preventative care such as vaccination, child screening, dental services, and outpatient mental health services for Medicaid and CHIP beneficiaries between January and May 2020. With time, society will bear witness to both the short- and long-term health outcomes of children who were in families unable to access not only basic healthcare needs, but also adequate insurance coverage to provide essential services related to well child care and preventive health.

It's evident that while some relief funding provided assistance to families during the pandemic, the economic hardships may be magnified as federal assistance funds are decreased or end. As the public health emergency was declared over on May 11, 2023, many policies which supported access to public insurance programs will be lifted. For example, state fiscal relief, increased nutrition assistance, Medicaid funding, and Child Tax Credit (CTC) and Earned Incomes Tac Credit (EITC) could be impacted (Drake & Williams, 2022). States will be faced with challenges in processing referrals and managing transitions of children and families to new public coverage courses. Most concerning is the potential that many children and families will lose coverage together.

Access to Care: Assessment of Structural Barriers

Early in 2020, structural barriers were identified as health systems and clinical leaders struggled to implement new modes of care delivery to address challenges arising from the pandemic. Long-standing challenges in access to care and staffing flexibility were exacerbated, resulting in new and innovative solutions being quickly introduced and discussed in hospitals and clinics across the United States. Not only were health systems and professionals leaning in to new ideas to recruit and retain staff to meet the rising volume of patients within the unique circumstances of the COVID-19 pandemic, there were efforts to create more efficient and flexible staffing models to assure children were served in every community, both within and beyond the doors of established clinics and hospitals. The need to question traditional structures and modalities for patient care to assure families had access to care was quickly recognized by pandemic leaders (Agency for Healthcare Research and Quality, 2021).

Alarming structural barriers presented at institutional, local, state, and federal levels. In the face of rising public demand for care, staffing shortages, and physical barriers required for infection control that decreased access to care facilities, states adopted the use of convention and conference facilities, stadiums, community centers, city parks, and other non-traditional venues to set up temporary field hospitals and immunization administration sites (Jeffery, 2020). Community and faith leaders played an important role in providing venues and dialogue to encourage access to care (Sklar & Goldman, 2023). Institutionally, there were shifts in staffing needs, particularly between adult and pediatric patient volumes. In many hospitals and clinics, healthcare experts in pediatric care, representing multiple professions including respiratory therapists, physicians, pharmacists, nurses, nurse practitioners, and many others, were called upon to care for adult patients. This required an intense review of hospital and clinic policies, established norms, and reworking of on-the-job training and orientation, along with a keener understanding of how experts could be leveraged to assist with patient volumes while still working within their educational and professional scope of practice (Lulgjuraj et al., 2021). The impacts of this are discussed in further detail in chapter one "*Acute Care Implications: Principles of Inpatient Management*". The volume of patients needing care in one area often required reaching deep into existing staffing pools from other areas while requiring intense reworking of traditional orientation and competency verification programs within a much shorter period of time. Existing policies, programs, clinical orientation tracks, and other existing healthcare entities stressed traditional boundaries and pushed toward new sets of norms, much of which would continue as innovative and flexible staffing structures. It was a time of rapid cycle implementation and improvement of novel staffing modalities to prioritize both accessible and quality care (Conlon et al., 2021; Jain et al., 2020; Penwill et al., 2021).

Local barriers were identified and addressed rapidly as there was increased urgency to meet patients where they were. In the past, movement was slow to adopt newer care modalities such as mobile clinics, community center clinics, and home visits and telehealth for pediatric care delivery. However, during the pandemic, these structures and systems were leveraged to increase access to care in an efficient and safe manner, particularly given barrier constructs presented by the COVID-19 virus. This systematic improvement happened quickly out of necessity. For example, processes and systems were built to evaluate and care for pediatric patients more effectively within the home. Every step from identifying the need for visit to preparing for the visit (supplies, equipment, documentation, and training) to implementing and evaluating the visit was considered. It was necessary to determine and ascertain costs for the visit and qualified staff needed to complete the visit. These collective factors pushed the boundaries of usual structures for care and allowed for innovation and technological advancements (Agency for Healthcare Research and Quality, 2021).

Meanwhile, more traditional methods of care were challenged because they were less accessible during the pandemic (Nunez et al., 2021). Schools, for example, transitioned to virtual education delivery. This limited accessibility of school-based healthcare, which for many children is the most frequently accessed route for their healthcare needs. Immunizations, health screenings, and physicals, often required to attend school or participate in school-based activities or sports, were delayed (Gallardo et al., 2022). This highlighted the need for creative solutions to continue provision of essential healthcare services through different means of access. Healthcare needs, such as mental health services, were intensified given pandemic-related circumstances such as lack of social interaction, general feelings of uncertainty about the future, and experiencing traumatic events in the sequelae of a global crisis.

States needed to examine and improve healthcare delivery structures to increase access to care. Structural barriers by way of outdated laws and regulations were amplified. Onerous occupational licensing requirements diminished HCP flexibility for geographic transition and relocation (Timmons & Norris, 2022). Questions arose about regulatory issues such as time required to apply for and obtain a healthcare license to practice in a different state, and regulatory requirements to see multiple HCPs for redundant care because of restrictions related to licensing and reimbursement. State licensure requirements often had outdated parameters and unnecessary barriers contributing to delay of licensure and subsequently hands-on provision of care. Nurse Practitioners (NPs) in some states were required to acquire a contract with a physician for licensure in a different state. However, they were often needed in several areas of the state, and at times had to manage multiple physician agreements that were not required at all in other states. This required paperwork and verification to add or change contracts and meet contractual obligations such as fees for physician contracts and non-disclosure agreements, delaying hands-on care delivery (Kleinpell et al., 2021). A 2021 national survey of advanced practice registered nurses (APRNs) ($n = 7467$) found that 84.8% ($n = 6334$) reported practice barriers that impeded their ability to provide quality care in a timely manner (Kleinpell et al., 2021). Alternative, flexible, and expedited licensing requirements that maintain quality of care while promoting access to care are essential in times of disaster or emergency (Timmons & Norris, 2022). A 2023 study of APRNs ($n = 16,699$) found that practice waivers in states that temporarily lifted licensure restrictions had the most positive impact in private outpatient clinics, health provider shortage areas, and rural geographic areas. APRNs also noted the waivers gave them more time with their patients, ability to take on new patients in a wider geographic area, increased telehealth practice, and resulted in no increased reports of adverse legal outcomes such as malpractice (Martin et al., 2023). During a time, physicians were needed in full force to meet patient needs and amidst unprecedented rates of burnout (Berg, 2022), they were at times burdened with arbitrary oversight of paperwork (rarely including direct oversight of clinical care provision) related to NP practice (Kleinpell et al., 2021). Some state laws were outdated and limited access to care and on-site availability for provision of healthcare services. In response, CMS temporarily waived the requirement of physicians to supervise NPs in Federally Qualified Health Centers and Rural Health Centers, allowing NPs to practice to the greatest extent allowable in state law (O'Reilly-Jacob et al., 2022). While state waivers allowed more flexibility in care provision, effectiveness was limited by lack of change in correlating organizational policies, NPs who remained in states with less regulatory restriction, and perceptions of the NP role as disposable as waivers expired despite evidence of effectiveness in increasing access to care (O'Reilly-Jacob et al., 2022).

Federal laws were reviewed, and new programs enacted to augment access to care throughout the pandemic and some continued to set new norms for the future. One such initiative was the Coronavirus Aid, Relief, and Economic Security (CARES) Act, which provided immediate relief to health systems and businesses to mitigate economic challenges related to the pandemic, especially in creating new forms of access to care. As staffing was a critical challenge to assure access to care, a significant portion of the CARES Act pertained specifically to keeping healthcare workers employed, benefited, and with several programs to reduce debt burden (US Department of Treasury, 2020).

Access to Care: Assessment of Political Barriers

Politics played a major role throughout the pandemic and on many levels, created unprecedented barriers to access to healthcare. Political polarization ensued with sharply divided political party leadership amid public fears informed and inflamed by misinformation and disinformation. Public trust in the healthcare system and in long established institutions such as the Centers for Disease Control and Prevention and Prevention (CDC) and the Federal Food and Drug Administration (FDA) was questioned. More than ever before, political decisions, affiliations, and directives heavily influenced public trust in healthcare and HCPs, magnified healthcare disparities, and shaped the future for healthcare access. Political disagreements in many states slowed access to vital healthcare services, spanning access to supplies, vital prevention measures, immunizations, and treatments for illness. Political commentary dominated news coverage of topics including universal access to care, affordability of care, and systems influencing social determinants of health. This profoundly shaped narratives on health-seeking behaviors, health disparities, and health outcomes in access to care. When considering the significant political impact, Albrecht (Albrecht, 2022) emphasized "Moving forward, it is critical to find ways to overcome political division and rebuild trust in science and health professionals."

The need to form effective, equitable, and representative governing processes was highlighted amid a healthcare crisis generating disagreement over the role of government and influence of political engagement. For example, state governors enacted executive orders to allow for healthcare affiliated waivers to allow for provision of services in a more streamlined, expedited manner. However, political influence on expiration and continuance of these waivers was profound despite evidence supporting increased access to high quality care. When discussing the need to maintain momentum made in updating licensure authority laws, Yuanhong et al. (Yuanhong et al., 2020) stated that practice authority should be based on outcomes such as access, quality, and cost of care and that the return to practice restrictions must align with empirical evidence. Although this seems reasonable, political influence remained the most impactful force in efforts to modernize healthcare law during the COVID-19 pandemic.

Access to Care: Assessment of Social Barriers

There were a number of social barriers which arose for children during the pandemic which disproportionately affected marginalized and underrepresented populations. Health disparities represent differences in health outcomes due to racial, ethnic, immigration status, or other marginalizing characteristics (Menon & Belcher, 2020). Prior to the pandemic, the healthcare community continued to address these differences in healthcare outcomes by focusing efforts through a lens of considering social determinants of health as directed in the Future of Nursing Report 2020–2030: Charting A Path to Achieve Health Equity, authored by the National Academy of Medicine (National Academy of Medicine and National Academies of Science, Engineering, and Medicine, 2021). However, health disparities worsened during the pandemic as more children were increasingly dependent on their adult caregivers who may have experienced unemployment and potential loss of insurance coverage. Children experienced significant hardship during the pandemic due to food and housing insecurity and lack of access to healthcare coverage. Overrepresentation of Black and Hispanic individuals among essential workers influenced ability to socially distance or work remotely from home and subsequently increased exposure to COVID-19 and furthering of health inequities. In addition, disparities extended to inadequate access to COVID-19 testing and/or vaccination, lack of transportation, and insurance coverage. Hospitalization, mortality rates, and disease severity were higher among Black, indigenous, Latin, Hispanic, and Asian populations (Menon & Belcher, 2020).

Social determinants of health such as food and housing insecurity impact health outcomes by affecting a child's access to care (Romain et al., 2022). Before the COVID-19 pandemic, children experiencing unstable housing situations such as frequent moving or eviction at age 2 years were at higher risk of experiencing gaps in health insurance coverage between the ages of 2 and 4 years of age (Carroll et al., 2017). These gaps then led to more limited interactions with the healthcare system. In addition, there were alarming levels of food insecurity seen among young adults with greater impact on Black and Hispanic youth (Daniels & Morton, 2022). Between August 19, 2020 and June 7, 2021, 12.8% of young adults reported often or always having little to eat in the prior week (Daniels & Morton, 2022). There continued to be a strong connection between low income and job loss with food insecurity. Many children didn't have access to low-cost or free meals as provided by programs such as the National School Lunch Program. This was somewhat mitigated by direct cash transfers, eviction moratoriums, and support from the Supplemental Nutrition Assistance Program (SNAP). However, there is a need to expand these programs, especially given the connection between food insecurity and physical and mental health (Daniels & Morton, 2022).

Disparities in testing rates have been reported across the United States with a disproportionate impact to not only racial and ethnic minorities but also low-income and rural communities (Vicetti Miguel et al., 2022). In the early stages of the pandemic, priority was given to those who were symptomatic. Therefore, those under the age of 18 who were more likely to be asymptomatic or have mild symptoms may have not met criteria for testing (Tan et al., 2020). Barriers for children to have access to SARS-CoV-2 testing include an insufficient number of testing sites, lack of access to transportation, lack of accurate information on testing criteria, lack of testing availability, and prohibitive associated costs (Tan et al., 2020). Undertesting of populations makes it difficult to accurately determine the number of children who were impacted by COVID-19. As the pandemic continued, innovative testing sites such as schools, community centers, and others were utilized for children to have access to prompt testing.

Telehealth services became a primary mode of care provision during the pandemic. However, as demand for telehealth exponentially increased, so did prior challenges and disparities, which made adoption of telehealth challenging before the pandemic. This included inequitable access to care, unsustainable costs in a fee-for-service model, and lack of quality metrics (Curfman et al., 2021). For example, children with complex medical conditions benefited from telehealth by decreasing parental burden through limiting time needed to be off from work and eliminating distance travelled to seek care (Menon & Belcher, 2020). However, research identified disparities in access to telehealth services in underserved communities (Vicetti Miguel et al., 2022). Access to the internet, smartphone devices, limited English proficiency, and digital literacy are barriers that unfairly prevent children from being able to access telehealth services (Curfman et al., 2021). Going forward, telehealth is fast becoming a normative form of care access in pediatric healthcare provision. There is opportunity to learn lessons from the pandemic as it relates to providing equitable access to these services to have a sustainable impact.

While children were at lower risk for severe disease from COVID-19, they still required access to therapeutic treatments. Treatment options often required pediatric patients to have access to a major pediatric hospital or healthcare systems (Vicetti Miguel et al., 2022). Unfortunately, data on these disparities and parental acceptance of various therapies remains limited in the pediatric population (Vicetti Miguel et al., 2022). Access to vaccinations also is disparate based not only on race and ethnicity but also on rural and urban populations. Moreover, maintenance of routine immunizations and care were challenging especially in the early stages of the pandemic. This led to creative options for vaccination access such as the use of community centers, EDs, and pharmacies (Wagh et al., 2022).

Barriers and Breakthroughs

Barriers and breakthroughs are best examined through a lens considering holistic health impacts in children, recognizing that children's health outcomes are largely directed by adult decisions.

Social

The pandemic amplified social barriers related to health disparities in housing and food insecurity and COVID-19 testing and treatment options. However, increasing access to these vital resources through innovative community centers and expanded access to care through telehealth were important breakthroughs to support improved child health outcomes.

Political

Political barriers were a significant factor in children's access to COVID-19 testing and treatment, leading to disparities in healthcare, particularly among vulnerable populations. Addressing these barriers required a multifaceted approach that included transparent communication, equitable resource allocation, and interprofessional collaboration among healthcare providers, policymakers, health systems and community leaders.

Economic

While the pandemic presented many financial barriers to children and families such as increasing unemployment and changes in funding for public health insurance programs, there were many breakthroughs in the development of federal relief efforts to support children and families respond to these dynamic economic changes.

Structural

Structural barriers, such as limited access to healthcare services, transportation, and language barriers, significantly impacted children's ability to receive timely treatment. Targeted interventions addressing specific needs of each community, such as mobile testing units, culturally sensitive outreach programs, homecare services, and telehealth were substantial breakthroughs in improving access to care.

Lessons Learned

- The benefit of investing in pediatric and family-focused social support services during the COVID-19 pandemic was essential to addressing important social determinants of health.
- High functioning, high-effective teams/mutual respect for interprofessional roles are essential for optimizing access to pediatric care.
- Innovation, adaptability, and flexibility are critical to improvement efforts at the institutional, local, regional, and national level.
- Children in marginalized and underrepresented populations were disproportionately affected by the dynamic changes which occurred during the pandemic. These disparities contribute greatly to a child's physical, mental, cognitive, and emotional development.

Calls to Action
- Advocacy is needed at the state and federal levels for sustained funding for children's hospitals and public insurance programs such as Medicaid and CHIP and expansion of Medicaid eligibility for those who lose employer-based insurance during a public health emergency.
- Further research and data collection are needed to explore health disparities related to COVID-19 and access to care, with appropriate response from park child health advocates and public health stakeholders.
- Advanced contingency planning and public health infrastructure development are urgently needed and should be addressed by health care organizations and communities to be able to respond rapidly in the setting of a potential future public health emergency.

Health disparity has been highlighted in the pandemic and this will need to be addressed so all children can get access to equal care.
—Pei-Ni Jone, MD

References

Agency for Healthcare Research and Quality. (2021). *2021 National healthcare quality and disparities report.* https://www.ncbi.nlm.nih.gov/books/NBK578526/

Albrecht, D. (2022). Vaccination, politics, and COVID-19 impacts. *BMC Public Health, 22,* 96. https://doi.org/10.1186/s12889-021-12432-x

Alker, J., & Brooks, T. (2022, February 17). *Millions of children may lose Medicaid: What can be done to help prevent them from becoming uninsured.* https://ccf.georgetown.edu/2022/02/17/millions-of-children-may-lose-medicaid-what-can-be-done-to-help-prevent-them-from-becoming-uninsured/

Bartek, N., VanCleve, S., Garzon, D., & Peck, J. (2021). Addressing the clinical impact of COVID-19 on pediatric mental health. *Journal of Pediatric Health Care, 35*(4), 377–386. https://doi.org/10.1016/j.pedhc.2021.03.006

Berg, S. (2022). *Pandemic pushes U.S. doctor burnout to all-time high of 63%.* American Medical Association. https://www.ama-assn.org/practice-management/physician-health/pandemic-pushes-us-doctor-burnout-all-time-high-63

Carroll, A., Corman, H., Curtis, M. A., Noonan, K., & Reichman, N. E. (2017). Housing instability and children's health insurance gaps. *Academic Pediatrics, 17*(7), 732–738. https://doi.org/10.1016/j.acap.2017.02.007

Conlon, C., McDonnell, T., Barrett, M., Cummins, F., Deasy, C., Hensey, C., McAuliffe, E., & Nicholson, E. (2021). The impact of the COVID-19 pandemic on child health and the provision of care in pediatric emergency departments: A qualitative study of frontline emergency staff. *BMC Health Services Research, 21,* 279. https://doi.org/10.1186/s12913-021-06284-9

Curfman, A., McSwain, S. D., Chuo, J., Yeager-McSwain, B., Schinasi, D. A., Marcin, J., Herendeen, N., Chung, S. L., Rheuban, K., & Olson, C. A. (2021). Pediatric telehealth in the COVID-19 pandemic era and beyond. *Pediatrics, 148*(3), e2020047795. https://doi.org/10.1542/peds.2020-047795

Daniels, G. E., & Morton, M. H. (2022). COVID-19 recession: Young-adult food insecurity, racial disparities, and correlates. *The Journal of Adolescent Health, 72,* 237–245.

Drake, P., & Williams, E. (2022, August 5). *A look at the economic effects of the pandemic for children*. Kaiser Family Foundation. https://www.kff.org/coronavirus-covid-19/issue-brief/a-look-at-the-economic-effects-of-the-pandemic-for-children/

Gallardo, M., Zepeda, A., Biely, C., Jackson, N., Puffer, M., Anton, P., & Dudovitz, R. (2022). School-based health center utilization during COVID-19 pandemic-related school closures. *The Journal of School Health, 92*(11), 1045–1050. https://doi.org/10.1111/josh.13226

Garfield, R., & Chidambaram, P. (2020, September 24). *Children's health and well being during the coronavirus pandemic*. Kaiser Family Foundation. https://www.kff.org/coronavirus-covid-19/issue-brief/childrens-health-and-well-being-during-the-coronavirus-pandemic/

Jain, P. N., Finger, L., Schieffelin, J. S., Zerr, D. M., & Hametz, P. A. (2020). Responses of three urban children's hospitals to COVID-19: Seattle, New York, and New Orleans. *Paediatric Respiratory Reviews, 35*, 15–19. https://doi.org/10.1016/j.prrv.2020.06.002

Jeffery, A. (2020). *Photos of field hospitals set up around the world to treat coronavirus patients*. CNBC. https://www.cnbc.com/2020/04/03/photos-of-field-hospitals-set-up-around-the-world-to-treat-coronavirus-patients.html

Kalaitzandonakes, M., Ellison, B., & Coppess, J. (2023). Coping with the 2022 infant formula shortage. *Preventive Medical Reports, 32*, 1012123. https://doi.org/10.1016/j.pmedr.2023.102123

Kleinpell, R., Myers, C. R., Schorn, M., & Likes, W. (2021). Impact of COVID-19 pandemic on APRN practice: A national survey. *Nursing Outlook, 69*(5), 784–792. https://doi.org/10.1016/j.outlook.2021.05.002

Koppolu, R. (2021). Children's hospitals and impact of COVID-19. *Journal of Pediatric Health Care, 35*(2), 239–241. https://doi.org/10.1016/j.pedhc.2020.12.001

Lulgjuraj, D., Hubner, T., Radzinski, N., & Hopkins, U. (2021). Everyone is someone's child: The experiences of pediatric nurses caring for adult COVID-19 patients. *Journal of Pediatric Nursing, 60*, 198–206. https://doi.org/10.1016/j.pedn.2021.06.015

Martin, B., Buck, M., & Zhong, E. (2023). Evaluating the impact of executive orders lifting restrictions on advanced practice registered nurses during the COVID-19 pandemic. *Journal of Nursing Regulation, 14*(1), 50–58. https://doi.org/10.1016/S2155-8256(23)00068-6

Menon, D. U., & Belcher, H. M. E. (2020). COVID-19 pandemic health disparities and pediatric healthcare-the promise of telehealth. *JAMA Pediatrics, 175*(4), 345–346.

National Academy of Medicine and National Academies of Science, Engineering, and Medicine. (2021). *The future of nursing 2020–2030: Charting a path to achieve health equity*. Wakefield, M. K., Williams, D. R., Le Menestrel, S., & Flaubert, J. L. (Eds.). https://nap.nationalacademies.org/catalog/25982/the-future-of-nursing-2020-2030-charting-a-path-to

Nunez, A., Sreeganga, S. D., & Ramaprasad, A. (2021). Access to care during COVID-19. *International Journal of Environmental Research and Public Health, 18*(6), 2980. https://doi.org/10.3390/ijerph18062980

O'Reilly-Jacob, M., Perloff, J., Sherafat-Kazemzadeh, R., & Flanagan, J. (2022). Nurse practitioners' perception of full practice authority during a COVID-19 surge: A qualitative study. *International Journal of Nursing Studies, 126*, 104141. https://doi.org/10.1016/j.ijnurstu.2021.104141

Peck, J. (2020). COVID-19: Impacts and implications for pediatric practice. *Journal of Pediatric Health Care, 34*(6), 619–629. https://doi.org/10.1016/j.pedhc.2020.07.004

Penwill, N. Y., De Angulo, N. R., Pathak, P. R., Ja, C., Elster, M. J., Hocreiter, D., Newton, J. M., Wilson, K. M., & Kaiser, S. V. (2021). Changes in pediatric hospital care during the COVID-19 pandemic: A national qualitative study. *BMC Health Services Research, 21*, 953. https://doi.org/10.1186/s12913-021-06947-7

Romain, C. V., Trinidad, S., & Kotagal, M. (2022). The effect of social determinants of health on telemedicine access during the COVID-19 pandemic. *Pediatric Annals, 51*(8), e311–e315. https://doi.org/10.3928/19382359-20220606-04

Sklar, R. P., & Goldman, R. E. (2023). The first person they came to is their pastor: The role of New York City faith leaders in supporting their congregation's health and well-being during COVID-19. *Journal of Religion and Health, 62*, 2861–2880. https://doi.org/10.1007/s10943-023-01789-5

Tan, T. Q., Kullar, R., Swartz, T. H., et al. (2020). Location matters: Geographic disparities and impact of coronavirus disease 2019. *The Journal of Infectious Diseases, 222*, 1951–1954.

Timmons, E., & Norris, C. (2022). Potential licensing reforms in light of COVID-19. *Health Policy Open, 3*, 100062. https://doi.org/10.1016/j.hpopen.2021.100062

US Department of Treasury. (2020). *About the CARES act and the consolidated appropriations act.* https://home.treasury.gov/policy-issues/coronavirus/about-the-cares-act

Vicetti Miguel, C. P., Dasgupta-Tsinikas, S., Lamb, G. S., Olarte, L., & Santos, R. P. (2022). Race, ethnicity, and health disparities in US children with COVID-19: A review of the evidence and recommendations for the future. *Journal of the Pediatric Infectious Diseases Society, 11*(Suppl_4), S132–S140. https://doi.org/10.1093/jpids/piac099

Wagh, A., Pan, S., Gordon, S., Hellerova, L., Ji, Y., Park, H., & Tsai, S. L. (2022). Pediatric health care use during the COVID-19 pandemic: Lessons learned from the initial 2020 wave. *Journal of the American College of Emergency Physicians Open, 3*(5), e12814. https://doi.org/10.1002/emp2.12814

Yuanhong, A., Skillman, S. M., & Frogner, B. K. (2020). *Is it fair? How to approach professional scope-of-practice policy after the COVID-19 pandemic.* Health Affairs Blog. https://doi.org/10.1377/hblog20200624.983306/full

Racism: Assessment of the Impact on Pediatric Holistic Health

Jaytoya Manget, Theiline Gborkorquellie, Elizabeth Ireson,
Yolanda Lewis-Ragland, Francisco Cerda, Maria Trent, Aisha Barber,
Olanrewaju Falusi, and Danielle Dooley

> *Of all the forms of inequality, injustice in health is the most shocking and inhuman.*
>
> —Martin Luther King Jr. (1966)

Introduction

Disparities that already existed in mental health for racially minoritized youth have worsened throughout the pandemic. Within the first 6 months of the pandemic, increased rates of anxiety, depression, aggression, and sleep problems were seen in the adolescent Hispanic and Latinx communities. Youth who reported a greater impact from the COVID-19 pandemic also experienced more psychiatric symptoms (Kuhlman et al., 2023). Minoritized patients also experienced decreased access to tele-mental health visits during the pandemic, compared to White patients (Williams et al., 2023).

School engagement, academic performance, and attendance plunged during the pandemic. National academic benchmarks demonstrated racial disparities in performance with Black, Hispanic, and American Indian/Alaskan Native students showing the worst outcomes (https://www.edweek.org/leadership/two-decades-of-progress-nearly-gone-national-math-reading-scores-hit-historic-lows/2022/10). Rates of chronic absenteeism also soared to unprecedented levels, reaching close to

J. Manget (✉) · T. Gborkorquellie · E. Ireson · Y. Lewis-Ragland · F. Cerda · A. Barber
O. Falusi · D. Dooley
Children's National, Washington, DC, USA
e-mail: Jmanget@childrensnational.org; tgborkorq@childrensnational.org;
eireson@childrensnational.org; FCERDA@childrensnational.org;
aisha.barber@childrensnational.org; OOFALUSI@childrensnational.org;
dgdooley@childrensnational.org

M. Trent
Johns Hopkins, Baltimore, MD, USA
e-mail: mtrent2@jhmi.edu

J. L. Peck (ed.), *COVID-19 Impacts on Child Health*,
https://doi.org/10.1007/978-3-031-80369-7_15

50% in some jurisdictions (https://www.dcpolicycenter.org/publications/schools-21-22/).

The COVID-19 pandemic also caused significant disruptions in the family systems affecting pediatric health and well-being. Children of minoritized families were more likely to be affected by caregiver infection and death (https://publications.aap.org/pediatrics/article/148/6/e2021053760/183446/COVID-19-Associated-Orphanhood-and-Caregiver-Death?autologincheck=redirected). Families that experienced historical racism and health disparities were also more likely to be financially impacted by the pandemic (https://www.kff.org/coronavirus-covid-19/issue-brief/communities-of-color-at-higher-risk-for-health-and-economic-challenges-due-to-covid-19/). There was also a significant impact on the health of immigrant children and families. State-level data showed higher death rates among foreign-born residents compared to their US-born counterparts (Douglas et al., 2022; Horner et al., 2022). Additionally, immigrant families were impacted by a lack of emergency services and employment opportunities (Gelatt & Muzaffar, 2022).

Despite the many challenges experienced throughout the pandemic, there were substantial breakthroughs made toward equity. There was increased awareness of health disparities existing in communities of color that were disproportionately affected by the virus due to a lack of resources and support systems in place. This awareness began a trend of hospitals, academic medical centers, and institutions adding resources and programs that help support equity, encouraging all to embrace inclusion, and developing metrics that could help measure progress toward improving disparities (https://www.nih.gov/covid-19-brings-health-disparities-research-forefront). Nevertheless, because many of these challenges persist, efforts to address them should prioritize equitable access to healthcare, culturally responsive care, and community engagement to reduce disparities in pediatric healthcare.

Cultural responsiveness is well studied among primary care practitioners (PCPs) and is essential for providing effective care to historically marginalized populations (Xavier et al., 2023). Culturally responsive communication in primary care involves PCPs engaging with patients "based on views of culturally diverse patients rather than the views of health care professionals" (Tucker et al., 2011). Cultural responsiveness emphasizes the importance of acknowledging and respecting patients' unique experiences and perspectives on health, recognizing clinician biases, and fostering collaboration with patients whose viewpoints may be underrepresented or may not align with the norms of Western medicine. This approach entails an ability to integrate principles of diversity, equity, inclusion, and justice (DEIJ) into patient care through self-reflection and a shared power dynamic between healthcare professionals and patients within the context of racism. Cultural responsiveness at an institutional level encompasses DEIJ-based protocols, policies, and systems that promote appreciation of cultural diversity along with empathetic, unbiased, and anti-racist care (Curtis et al., 2019; Metzl & Hansen, 2014; Ring et al., 2009). Overall, this approach enables healthcare providers (HCPs) to drive equitable outcomes for all patients. By contrast, the term cultural competence has fallen out of favor due to a significant limitation in the notion that one can master culture through knowledge about specific practices, attitudes, standards, and policies of groups of people. While cultural competence has a discrete endpoint, in reality, culture is dynamic and ever changing (https://npin.cdc.gov/pages/cultural-competence). Cultural responsiveness is a patient-centered approach involving self-reflection, whereas cultural competence is based on generalizations about the culture of an individual or group of people (Curtis et al., 2019).

Background

Over half a century ago, Dr. Martin Luther King Jr. made an impactful observation about the state of racism and inequalities in healthcare. Sadly, these injustices have continued to be evident time and time again in disadvantaged, minoritized communities within the United States. The COVID-19 pandemic took the nation by surprise on the verge of Spring 2020. The impact on the health of the whole child was unimaginable to anyone. The long lasting impact of the pandemic on pediatric health was not immediately known; it continues to be revealed in the years following the pandemic's peak. However, the manifestations of COVID-19 on the physical and mental health of children were not the only thing that would become apparent during the pandemic. The long-standing impacts of racism would soon come to light. The pandemic allowed an opportunity for the world to see what many communities have known as their truth for many generations as disparities in health became undeniable by the effects of yet another disease—COVID-19.

This novel disease would go on to jeopardize the holistic health of America's most under-resourced youth by impacting their access to healthcare and vaccines, disrupt their family systems and supports, decimate school engagement, performance, and attendance, and perpetuate barriers to health and healthcare access for children and families who have immigrated. While this is not an exhaustive list of the impact of historical, structural, and contemporary racism during the COVID-19 pandemic, by the end of this chapter, readers should have a better understanding of the detrimental impact of the pandemic on minoritized communities and work that remains to be done.

Points of Care

Access to Healthcare

The COVID-19 pandemic upended the way patients could access healthcare. At the outset of the pandemic, the focus was on emergency care and many primary and preventive care services were deferred. As the pandemic persisted, the healthcare system developed workforce shortages, further impeding access to care at all levels, from primary care to hospital-based specialty care, emergency room care, and inpatient care. Not all groups of patients were affected in the same manner; patients from communities that have been historically and structurally excluded from healthcare services experienced the most substantial impact. Access to primary and preventive pediatric care was severely disrupted; communities that have been historically marginalized due to racism continued to face the greatest disparities and inequities in accessing services.

In the earliest stages of the pandemic, the focus was on diversion of resources to inpatient and emergency settings, particularly adult settings given the impact of COVID-19 disease on adult populations. Almost immediately, pediatric emergency department (ED) visits declined, with larger declines for minoritized youth compared to non-Hispanic white youth, creating disparities in access to care (https:// sma.org/southern-medical-journal/article/disruption-of-pediatric-emergency-department-use-during-the-covid-19-pandemic/). The Centers for Medicare and Medicaid Services issued guidance in April 2020 that recommended postponing routine primary, preventive, and specialty care and listed pediatric vaccinations as intermediate acuity, recommending initial visits via telehealth and in-person visits only as necessary (https://www.cms.gov/files/document/cms-non-emergent-elective-medical-recommendations.pdf). In this ecosystem focused on conservation of healthcare resources and reducing COVID-19 exposures for patients and providers, pediatric practices experienced a precipitous drop in patient visits for preventive care. Shelter in place and lockdown orders, combined with caregiver concerns about exposure to COVID-19, resulted in a perfect storm that impacted pediatric care access. By May 2020, the US Centers for Disease Control and Prevention (CDC) reported a decrease in vaccine ordering and administration in children (Santoli et al., 2020). By September 2020, CMMS released data on healthcare utilization by children covered by Medicaid and the Children's Health Insurance Program (CHIP), which together covered approximately 40 million children in the United States. The CMMS reported that "When compared to data from the same time period last year (March through May 2019), preliminary data for 2020 shows 1.7 million (22%) fewer vaccinations for beneficiaries up to age 2, 3.2 million (44%) fewer child screening services, 6.9 million (44%) fewer outpatient mental health services even after accounting for increased telehealth services, and 7.6 million (69%) fewer dental services" (https://www.cms.gov/newsroom/fact-sheets/fact-sheet-service-use-among-medicaid-chip-beneficiaries-age-18-and-under-during-covid-19). Difficulties in accessing care such as well-child visits and immunizations were not experienced equally across populations. Disruptions in access to care were the most pronounced in Black and Latinx households (Phan et al., 2023). Even a year later, a survey of households with children showed that ¼ had missed or delayed preventive care, and the most common reasons were limited appointment availability, closed practices, and concerns about contracting COVID-19 (https://journals.stfm.org/ familymedicine/2022/may/nguyen-2021-0392/). Further research identified racial disparities, with Asian or Pacific Islander, Hispanic, and multiracial groups more likely to have delayed or missed preventive care (https://jamanetwork.com/journals/ jamanetworkopen/fullarticle/2807109#:~:text=Overall%2C%2027.6%25%20 of%20children%20had,32.1%25%20of%20multiracial%20children).   Research also showed disparities in immunizations, with Black children experiencing lower rates of routine childhood vaccinations compared to other groups (https://jamanetwork.com/journals/jamapediatrics/fullarticle/2784888). These disparities are rooted in inequities that stem from structural racism, including payment and insurance coverage, access to healthcare facilities, access to employment that provides time off for medical appointments, and historical and current-day mistrust of the medical system by minoritized communities due to historical and contemporary mistreatment (https://www.kff.org/racial-equity-and-health-policy/issue-brief/addressing-racial-equity-vaccine-distribution/). Even as practices gradually returned to pre-pandemic demand for services, they were faced with another challenge due to workforce shortages. Multiple waves of COVID-19 and other respiratory viruses in pediatric populations, combined with the demand for appointments due to deferred preventive care and pediatric workforce shortages, have led to prolonged access issues for pediatric patients, including a decline in kindergarten vaccination rates from 95% pre-pandemic to 93% in 2021–2022 (https://www.kff.org/coronavirus-covid-19/issue-brief/headed-back-to-school-in-2023-a-look-at-childrens-routine-vaccination-trends/#:~:text=Specifically%2C%20the%20share%20of%20kindergarteners,and%20then%20declining%20again%20to).

As practices faced challenges with delivering in-person care, there was a rapid adoption of telehealth services or the delivery of healthcare remotely. Telehealth can be an important tool for delivering medical care and can potentially overcome obstacles including transportation barriers, economic costs of missed employment time (see chapter "Institutional Care Settings: Principles of Systems-Based Support"), and provider shortages, especially in rural areas. However, there are also disparities in access to telehealth services. A study at two large pediatric hospitals during the pandemic showed that minoritized patients experienced decreased access to tele-mental health visits during the pandemic, compared to white patients (Williams et al., 2023). Similarly, an adolescent medicine clinic also demonstrated that during a rapid scale-up to telehealth during the pandemic, non-white patients had decreased visit completion rates (Wood et al., 2020). A large study in New York illustrated that Black patients and those who lived in areas with lower mean incomes and higher average household sizes were less likely to access telemedicine for care (Chunara et al., 2021). Disparities in access to and the utilization of telehealth services are informed by a variety of factors, including racial disparities in access to broadband service, with Black and Hispanic adults reporting less access to high-speed internet at home (https://www.pewresearch.org/internet/fact-sheet/internet-broadband/?tabId=tab-3109350c-8dba-4b7f-ad52-a3e976ab8c8f). The American Academy of Pediatrics (AAP) Policy Statement on Telehealth: Improving Access to and Quality of Pediatric Health Care, states "The availability of telehealth care enabled greater access to care for many children and adolescents, but gaps in digital infrastructure continue to persist because of poverty, systemic racism, and other inequities, which were a barrier to equitable technology-enabled care" (https://publications.aap.org/pediatrics/article/148/3/e2021053129/181044/Telehealth-Improving-Access-to-and-Quality-of?autologincheck=redirected).

The COVID-19 pandemic placed unprecedented strain on the healthcare delivery system, magnifying disparities and inequities that already existed. As this burden is addressed going forward, access to healthcare must be viewed through a racial health equity lens, with programs, practices, and policies deliberately designed to eliminate disparities. Important features include continually monitoring pediatric preventive care, screening and immunization data to identify racial disparities, co-creating strategies by partnering with trusted messengers in the community to encourage immunization and well-child visits, and promoting policies that support enhanced broadband access for groups that have historically been marginalized due to racism.

Vaccine Access

In December 2020, the United States Food & Drug Administration (FDA) issued emergency use authorizations (EUAs) for the first two mRNA-based COVID-19 vaccines for adults (https://www.immunize.org/timeline/). Initial administration of the vaccine included healthcare workers and residents of long-term care facilities, mostly older adults. The EUAs were subsequently expanded to include adolescents 12 to 15 years old (May 2021), children 5 to 11 years old (October 2021), and young children 6 months through 4 years old (June 2022) (https://www.immunize.org/timeline/). The COVID-19 vaccine has demonstrated efficacy in preventing COVID-19 infections as well as mitigating severity of symptoms and complications such as multisystem inflammatory syndrome in children or MIS-C (a serious and sometimes deadly condition where organs such as the heart, lungs, kidneys, and brain become inflamed) (Fowlkes et al., 2022; Oliveira et al., 2022). Despite these promising findings, uptake of the vaccine has been limited among pediatric patients. A National Survey of parents in February 2021 identified high levels of parental hesitancy for COVID-19 vaccines in their children, with many reporting they would like to "wait and see" further information that becomes available about the vaccine over time (Szilagyi et al., 2021). In July 2022, 1 month after the vaccine became available to young children, only 3.5% of children 6 months through 4 years of age were vaccinated (https://www.cdc.gov/mmwr/volumes/71/wr/mm7146a3.htm).

In addition to vaccine hesitancy, COVID-19 vaccine distribution and uptake highlight key racial and ethnic inequities in healthcare. Racial and ethnic disparities in COVID-19 infections and deaths were identified early in the pandemic (https://www.cdc.gov/mmwr/volumes/70/wr/mm7011e1.htm) yet when initial COVID-19 vaccines became available, distribution efforts focused on predominantly white and wealthy communities (Anderson et al., 2022) with lower distribution in counties with higher Black composition (Hernandez et al., 2022).

Recognition of these disparities in access to and uptake of the COVID-19 vaccine among minoritized populations led to efforts to better understand barriers. Research demonstrates that vaccine hesitancy was prominent and often focused on potential side effects, vaccine effectiveness, speed of vaccine development, and vaccine ingredients. Participants described confusing messages from the media and public health agencies. They also cited structural racism and historical mistrust in the healthcare system as contributing to reduced engagement in health behaviors (Kenworthy et al., 2022).

It is important for HCPs to recognize the impact of pervasive, structural racism, and the historical abuse of minoritized populations by the healthcare system (Laurencin, 2021). To combat this and to address vaccine hesitancy, HCPs should strive to develop a healthcare workforce whose demographics represent those of the population they serve; to prioritize public health messaging that is transparent, consistent, and developed in partnership with trusted community leaders; and to mitigate socioeconomic barriers to vaccine access including, but not limited to, timing and location of vaccine distribution (Anderson et al., 2022).

Across the country, various efforts sought to uplift the voices of minoritized populations to build trust and to combat mis- and dis-information. The *Vaccine Voices* program asked a diverse group of artists to share why they got vaccinated and the positive impact of vaccination on their communities (https://www.arts.gov/about/nea-on-covid-19/vaccine-voices). Black healthcare providers formed *The Black Coalition Against COVID* to provide trustworthy and reliable COVID-19 information to minoritized communities (https://blackcoalitionagainstcovid.org/about/). The CDC developed a *Rapid Community Assessment Guide* to help local and state health departments efficiently gather community insights surrounding a public health issue (https://www.cdc.gov/vaccines/covid-19/vaccinate-with-confidence/rca-guide/index.html) as well as *A Guide for Community Partners* to increase COVID-19 vaccination among racially and ethnically minoritized communities (https://www.cdc.gov/vaccines/covid-19/downloads/guide-community-partners.pdf). Many communities developed local vaccine awareness campaigns and offered rides to vaccination sites. These examples highlight some of the work that has helped to decrease the racial and ethnic disparities in COVID-19 vaccine uptake (https://www.kff.org/coronavirus-covid-19/issue-brief/latest-data-on-covid-19-vaccinations-by-race-ethnicity/).

Vaccine uptake in the pediatric community continues to be subpar, especially in children of color. As of June 2023, 32.2% of U.S. children (age 6 months to 17 years) had completed the primary COVID-19 vaccination series (32.7% of white, non-Hispanic children; 28.2% of Black, non-Hispanic children). Only 7.1% were up to date with the bivalent booster (7.9% of white, non-Hispanic children; 4% of Black, non-Hispanic children) (https://www.cdc.gov/vaccines/imz-managers/coverage/covidvaxview/interactive/children.html). Although racial disparities in COVID-19 vaccination have decreased, there is still work to be done to encourage vaccination in all pediatric patients and ensure it is accessible in all communities. Future efforts to increase COVID-19 vaccination series completion in children should focus on developing trust in the patient–provider relationship, partnering with trusted community leaders to share consistent messaging, and addressing socioeconomic barriers to accessing the healthcare system.

Mental Health

The COVID-19 pandemic continues to have a substantial impact on the mental health of youth, doubling the rates of depression, suicidal ideation, and anxiety. It is estimated that one in five youth suffer from mental illness (Hawks, 2023). As a result of these alarming statistics, the American Academy of Pediatrics, the American Academy of Child and Adolescent Psychiatry, the Children's Hospital Association, and the US Surgeon General all declared a national state of emergency in child and adolescent mental health (see chapter "Mental Health: Assessment of Risk, Clinical Manifestations, and Access to Care") (Hawks, 2023; Office of the Surgeon General, 2021; Shim et al., 2022).

The pandemic has led to poor mental health outcomes in racially minoritized youth, worsening the existing racial disparities in mental health care. Disparities in mental health care access for racially minoritized youth have been a long-standing public health concern, associated with barriers such as racial discrimination, insurance coverage, language, health literacy, transportation, scheduling, and childcare (Hawks, 2023). Although telehealth was offered as a viable solution to address the gaps in mental health service accessibility during the pandemic, one study found that racial disparities in mental health service use were magnified following telemedicine transition. The cause for this widening gap was likely due to multiple factors including the digital divide, and temporary suspension of new patient visits during the initial telehealth transition mandated by some practices (Williams et al., 2023).

Because childhood is an important period for social and emotional development, many children experienced excessive fear and worry during the pandemic. These fears were further exacerbated by social stressors such as lifestyle modifications, school closures, and social isolation. One longitudinal study investigated the effect of the COVID-19 pandemic on the mental health of a majority Black American youth sample of 7–10-year-old children in an urban setting. Lower socioeconomic status (SES) families were found to have an elevated risk of mental health sequelae. The study showed a correlation between SES and internalizing symptoms in Black youth (Bhogal et al., 2021). Internalizing symptoms are characterized by emotional and peer problems experienced by the individual, including social withdrawal, anxiety, and depression, whereas externalizing symptoms involve conduct problems, such as hyperactivity, anger, and aggression (Vacaru et al., 2022). Higher current internalizing symptoms were linked to greater perceived impact of the pandemic and reduced COVID-19 preventive behaviors such as hand sanitizer use and mask-wearing. Fears of social distancing and illness were more likely to be reported in lower SES Black American youth than higher SES youth. These fears increased over time and were possibly attributed to uncertainty and stressors related to the pandemic's effect on family pressures, school, and social life. This study underscored that COVID-19 impacted lower SES households differently, with lower SES conditions being linked to heightened fears about social distancing, likely because of scarce resources, barriers to healthcare access, and decreased ability to social distance (Bhogal et al., 2021).

The COVID-19 pandemic significantly disrupted the lives of adolescents, resulting in decreased in-person interactions, transitions in schooling, and a drastic increase in time spent at home. Adolescents, who are in a critical developmental period, were particularly susceptible to the stressors of the pandemic which impacted their peer relationships, independence, and brain maturation. In one study of Hispanic and Latinx youth, deleterious effects on adolescent mental health became apparent within the first 6 months of the pandemic as evidenced by increased rates of anxiety, depression, aggression, and sleep problems. Youth who reported a greater impact from the COVID-19 pandemic also experienced more psychiatric symptoms. Mental health issues among this population persisted into 2021 with an increased prevalence of suicidal ideation as youth struggled with ongoing challenges related to the chronic stress of the pandemic. Social support, emotion regulation, optimism, and humor were found to be protective against pandemic-related mental illness in Hispanic and Latinx adolescents (Kuhlman et al., 2023). One study examined racial and ethnic differences in suicidal behavior encounters among children and adolescents with Medicaid coverage during the COVID-19 pandemic and found that suicide attempt and intentional self-harm encounters increased for all racial and ethnic groups throughout the pandemic. The study sample included youth aged 3 to 17 years in the US who were enrolled in Medicaid or Children's Health Insurance Program (CHIP). American Indians or Alaska Native youth were found to have significantly higher rates of encounters related to suicidal behavior compared to youth from other racial and ethnic groups. However, further research is warranted to elucidate the underlying causes in these subgroups of youth (Ali et al., 2023). To avoid further disparities and inequities, it is critical that society prioritizes funding and resources for this important research to identify more supports and bolster protective factors.

The COVID-19 pandemic has disproportionately impacted low-income Black and Latinx families, particularly undocumented and first-generation immigrants, due to structural inequities. Structural inequities, such as chronic poverty, barriers to public benefits, lack of employer-sponsored insurance, and limited linguistically and culturally effective services, have made Latinx children especially vulnerable to the psychological effects of the pandemic. In the US, more Latinx children experience poverty than any other groups. COVID-19 hospitalization and mortality rates are higher among Latinx and Black Americans compared to non-Latinx Whites, resulting in increased mental health needs among Latinx children. Consequently, Latinx youth have experienced elevated rates of depression, anxiety, suicidal ideation, and substance abuse during the pandemic; these rates are significantly higher compared to their non-Latinx white counterparts. Economic factors, such as limited government support for immigrants and minimum-wage jobs, exacerbate mental health challenges. The devastating emotional toll of the pandemic on Latinx children highlights the importance of trauma-informed care, increased advocacy for public benefits, and improved resource allocation for Latinx families (Rothe et al., 2021).

School Engagement and Performance

As school engagement took an immediate plunge, school systems had to quickly shift to virtual learning. For many districts, there were not any existing platforms in place to assist with the transition. As it became apparent that return to the classroom would take more than the originally anticipated 2 weeks, it became necessary to continue education of the Nation's youth. For many students, the stress of the quick transition was too much to bear. Some were disengaged from the beginning. Many were affected by caregiver and family stressors. Some were unable to engage due to limited or no access to a computer or reliable internet. Others quickly grew tired of online classes—commonly called "Zoom fatigue" (https://www.mckinsey.com/industries/education/our-insights/covid-19-and-education-the-lingering-effects-of-unfinished-learning).

Although some of these stressors were addressed later in the pandemic as school districts and families received supplemental funding, there continued to be disparities in the affected communities throughout the duration of the pandemic. An analysis of elementary school operating statuses showed that school districts with higher representation of Black and Hispanic children were more likely to be virtual in Fall 2020 compared to predominately white school districts (https://read.dukeupress.edu/demography/article/59/1/1/286878/Research-Note-School-Reopenings-During-the-COVID). Students of districts with higher Black and Hispanic children were already at an academic and social disadvantage prior to the COVID-19 pandemic and included districts with lower math scores, higher numbers of multilingual learners, higher rates of students experiencing homelessness, and higher rates of students eligible for free and reduced meals (https://www.nature.com/articles/s41562-021-01087-8). Therefore, these minoritized youth from under-resourced communities had an increased susceptibility to academic decline and risk of limited resources to support the virtual environment.

Not only did engagement in school decline during the era of virtual learning, but academic performance also deteriorated. International studies of schools in countries with the highest performance and test scores pre-pandemic have shown that there was little to no progress made during the months and years of virtual learning (https://osf.io/preprints/socarxiv/ve4z7/). In education, "unfinished learning" is a term that is often used to capture the deficiencies that occurred during the pandemic virtual learning years. It most often refers to the academic learning that students missed during the virtual years in comparison to the typical in-person school year. However, it is important to note that students also failed to learn social skills, behaviors, and mindsets that come with in-person learning (https://www.mckinsey.com/industries/education/our-insights/covid-19-and-education-the-lingering-effects-of-unfinished-learning).

As of the 2023–2024 academic year, school systems are continuing to recover from the academic setbacks that occurred during the pandemic's peak. The National Assessment of Academic Progress taken in Spring 2022 showed significant drops in the reading and math score of fourth and eighth grade students; the largest decline in over 30 years. Results of this assessment also demonstrated racial disparities in performance with Black, Hispanic, and American Indian/Alaskan Native students showing the worst outcomes. Among fourth grade students, 45% of Black, 41% of American Indian/Alaskan Native, and 36% of Hispanic students did not meet the national benchmarks for math. This is compared to only 14% of white and 10% of Asian/Pacific Islander students showing deficiencies. A similar trend in racial disparities persisted at the eighth grade math level where 63% of Black, 55% of American Indian/Alaskan Native, and 51% of Hispanic students did not meet the benchmarks compared to 26% of white and 16% of Asian/Pacific Islander students. With regard to reading, 37% of all students failed to meet the fourth grade benchmark. When further broken down into racial and ethnic groups, 56% of Black, 57% of American Indian/Alaskan Native, and 50% of Hispanic students did not reach the national goal compared to only 27% of white students and 19% of Asian/Pacific Islander students. At the eighth grade reading level, 30% of all students are below the benchmark; results stratified by racial and ethnic group show 47% of Black students, 45% of American Indian/Alaskan Native, and 39% of Hispanics are below the national benchmark compared to 22% of white and 15% of Asian/Pacific Islander students (https://www.edweek.org/leadership/two-decades-of-progress-nearly-gone-national-math-reading-scores-hit-historic-lows/2022/10).

Chronic absenteeism—defined as missing 10% or more of the school year—was a national epidemic that was on the rise before the introduction of COVID-19. During the COVID-19 pandemic, the rates of chronic absenteeism skyrocketed to unprecedented levels. In the 2021–2022 school year, over 30% of students met the definition of chronic absenteeism in many states. For some jurisdictions, rates of chronic absenteeism rose to nearly 50% during the 2021–2022 school year (https://osse.dc.gov/sites/default/files/dc/sites/osse/publication/attachments/2021-22%20Attendance%20Report%20%28Nov%2028%202022%29.pdf). As with other indicators, there were already racial and ethnic disparities that existed pre-pandemic in the rates of chronic absenteeism. These disparities have only worsened in recent years (https://www.whitehouse.gov/cea/written-materials/2023/09/13/chronic-absenteeism-and-disrupted-learning-require-an-all-hands-on-deck-approach/). The most impacted students include students of color and students from low-income families. Other social factors, which minoritized populations disproportionately experience due to structural racism, are also leading risk factors for chronic absenteeism. Among these are food insecurity, housing and transportation instability, bullying, and fear of violence (https://files.eric.ed.gov/fulltext/ED592870.pdf).

There are short- and long-term effects associated with school disengagement. Chronic absenteeism is directly tied to learning loss, grades, and performance on standardized tests and ultimately affects high school graduation. Students who are chronically absent are also at higher risk of adverse health outcomes as adults, less favorable job prospects, and increased involvement in the criminal justice system (https://www.whitehouse.gov/cea/written-materials/2023/09/13/chronic-absenteeism-and-disrupted-learning-require-an-all-hands-on-deck-approach/). In September 2023, the White House publicly recognized chronic absenteeism as an extensive problem and called for a "all hand on deck" approach. Their goal is to help get students reengaged in well-resourced schools with effective teachers and improve the learning disruptions that have occurred since 2020 (https://www.white-house.gov/cea/written-materials/2023/09/13/chronic-absenteeism-and-disrupted-learning-require-an-all-hands-on-deck-approach/).

Family Systems and Supports

Historically, extended family and intergenerational care have played a large role in communities of color. However, in the setting of the pandemic, families received messages to stay apart to decrease the spread of COVID-19 and many remained segregated to minimize infection. But this was not possible for all. Many families did not have the luxury of ample space to spread out and open air to retreat to. Minoritized families are more likely to live in urban, crowded, and/or multi-unit living areas. Families of color make up over half (56%) of the population in urban counties, while white families account for the majority in suburban (68%) and rural (79%) counties (https://www.kff.org/coronavirus-covid-19/issue-brief/communities-of-color-at-higher-risk-for-health-and-economic-challenges-due-to-covid-19/). Initially, COVID-19 outbreak concerns were concentrated in more urban areas, increasing fears in families who lived in close living quarters.

Children of minoritized families were also more likely to be affected by care-giver infection or death. Hispanic, Native Hawaiian, or Other Pacific Islander and American Indian or Alaska Native groups had a 1.5 increased risk of obtaining COVID-19 infections compared to white counterpart. These minoritized groups as well as Black residents were two times more likely to die from COVID-19 infections (https://www.kff.org/racial-equity-and-health-policy/issue-brief/covid-19-cases-and-deaths-by-race-ethnicity-current-data-and-changes-over-time/#:~:text=Age%2Dstandardized%20data%20show%20that,White%20counterparts%20(Figure%201). Analysis of caregiver deaths in the first 15 months of the pandemic showed that children of minoritized racial and ethnic groups were up to 4.5 more likely to be orphaned by the loss of parent or grandparent caregiver to COVID-19 compared to non-Hispanic white children (https://publications.aap.org/pediatrics/article/148/6/e2021053760/183446/COVID-19-Associated-Orphanhood-and-Caregiver-Death?autologincheck=redirected).

The economic implications for minoritized families during the pandemic should not be overlooked. Families that were already experiencing historical racism and health disparities were also more likely to be financially impacted by the pandemic. Prior to the pandemic onset, Black, Hispanic, and American Indian and Alaskan Native families were more likely to experience food insecurity and report concerns about paying housing expenses and monthly bills. Almost 25% of families of color were employed in service industries pre-pandemic compared to 16% of white families (https://www.kff.org/coronavirus-covid-19/issue-brief/communities-of-color-at-higher-risk-for-health-and-economic-challenges-due-to-covid-1). Many of these industries cut hours or closed completely during the pandemic. For those that remained open, the workers faced other challenges when they were forced to choose between making money to support their family or placing themselves at higher risk of an infection that was already disproportionately affecting them.

In addition, families of color are more likely to be headed by a single parent. As of 2021, 64% of Black children, 49% of American Indian, and 42% of Hispanic children were in single-family homes compared to only 24% of non-Hispanic white children. When parents—especially those in single-headed households—returned to work, securing childcare and supervising virtual learning for school-aged children created additional challenges. This combined with the increased risk of death in these minoritized families, left many households vulnerable. Nevertheless, leaning on extended family members during the COVID-19 pandemic was the only way many survived. These systems provided emotional as well as caretaking support.

Immigrant Health

The COVID-19 pandemic was a stark example of challenges and inequities faced by millions of immigrant families living in the United States. In fact, one in four children (over 18 million) in the United States live in an immigrant family, while additional seven million children live in mixed status families, meaning that at least one parent or household member is not a US citizen (Ayalew et al., 2021). Health disparities were present prior to the pandemic, with children in immigrant families (CIF) facing baseline increased health risks, less access and utilization of the health care system, and higher poverty rates. Non-citizen immigrants are more susceptible to discrimination and food insecurity (Cadenas et al., 2023). The combination of these factors during an ill-prepared pandemic response exacerbated health disparities. Despite a lack of national data on the COVID-19 mortality rates for immigrants, state-level data has shown higher death rates among foreign-born residents compared to their US-born counterparts (Douglas et al., 2022; Horner et al., 2022).

Systemic failures and structural violence potentially caused an increase in mortality rates. Research demonstrates that families who preferred a language other than English (PLOE) had high rates of COVID-19 infections during the infection peaks of 2020–2021 (Otto et al., 2021). This may be attributed to poor initial non-English public health messaging, difficulty with stay-at-home orders for CIF who shared multi-generational and sometimes multi-family homes, and immigrants working in essential jobs. These challenges were illustrated by the outbreaks in agriculture and meat processing plants that disproportionately affected immigrant workers (Cholera et al., 2020).

Additionally, immigrant families were hit hard with a lack of emergency services and employment opportunities. Immigrant workers, particularly women, had the highest rates of unemployment during the COVID-19 pandemic, creating a vulnerable state of limited income with potentially high-risk jobs deemed as essential (Gelatt & Muzaffar, 2022). Existing political fear and discourse regarding essential social services greatly impacted CIF. Even when children qualified for services based on their US citizenship or permanent residency status, their immigrant parents often reported avoiding services such as federal food and cash assistance due to fear of retaliation through the Public Charge policy (Iraheta & Morey, 2023). Over 14 million immigrants were excluded from government stimulus payments distributed throughout the COVID-19 pandemic (Gelatt & Muzaffar, 2022).

As we delve further into the ramifications of COVID-19 and the health of CIF, it is important to evaluate what effects the pandemic had on the socioecological model. Gaps in safety net services noted above further drive the rates of food insecurity and poor nutrition. Compounding levels of stress due to economic, social, and health burdens on immigrant families may affect the overall health of these children, especially their mental health (Rothe et al., 2021). Telehealth is another stark example of a gap in service. Many immigrant families were unable to access telemedicine due to the digital divide, a lack of technical knowledge, and/or health/ English literacy (Rothe et al., 2021). There are future ramifications for CIF as they are exposed to high-risk circumstances for toxic stress and adverse childhood experiences (ACEs).

Despite the adversities in immigrant communities, it is important to observe the resiliency and strengths that immigrant communities provide for their children. Immigrant families have demonstrated higher rates of COVID-19 vaccination when compared to US-born citizens despite having persistent barriers to care (Gelatt & Muzaffar, 2022). Local and private groups have partnered with immigrant communities to create mutual aid groups to provide funding to immigrants who were not eligible for federal government relief funds. Further, these groups have advocated and secured state-level relief for undocumented immigrants in states such as California, Washington, Oregon, and New York (Roels et al., 2022). A growing amount of literature demonstrates the impact of youth empowerment in immigrant and refugee communities during the COVID-19 pandemic, which provides opportunities for CIF to enact change through civil engagement (King et al., 2023; Roels et al., 2022).

Barriers and Breakthroughs

The intersection of the combined trauma imposed by historic and institutionalized racism and the devastation of the novel COVID-19 virus illuminated various successes and challenges that uniquely impacted pediatric healthcare in America both then and now. As with any disaster, as the pandemic unfolded, it became evident that those who were most marginalized and under-resourced were the most adversely affected and that meant caring for our children would require innovative and extensive effort.

As the United States grappled with various COVID-19 challenges and changes, there were substantial breakthroughs made toward equity. With the onset of the COVID-19 virus came an increased awareness of health disparities existing in communities of color that were disproportionately affected by the virus due to a lack of resources and ineffective support systems. This awareness helped open dialogue and began a trend of hospitals, academic medical centers, and institutions adding resources and programs that would allow those who were willing and require those who were less eager to embrace equity and inclusion to monitor metrics that could indicate whether they were effectively addressing disparities and closing the gaps (https://www.nih.gov/covid-19-brings-health-disparities-research-forefront).

Another contribution of the pandemic was the universal embrace of isolation of infected individuals. This isolation not only helped decrease transmission of the virus, but it emphasized our need to be innovative in healthcare, which helped increase resources toward making telemedicine accessible to many more communities. This effort to digitize healthcare was another step toward equity for communities of color who have been historically marginalized and disproportionately affected by healthcare deserts where they have had little to no direct access to primary care or specialty physicians, advanced practice clinicians, and mental health providers (https://www.ncbi.nlm.nih.gov/pmc/articles/PMC9035352/#:~:text=A%20national%20study%20including%2036,interactions%20in%20the%20same%20period).

As our knowledge of the virus grew, so did our understanding of ways to best protect ourselves from it. In August 2021, the first COVID-19 vaccine was approved by the FDA for use in adults, which was shortly followed by a vaccine approved for children ages 5–11 years in October 2021. Although it would be another full year before a COVID vaccine would be approved for children 6 months and above, the need to effectively and efficiently disseminate these new vaccines was instrumental in increasing community outreach for immunization information. Widespread efforts were made to improve access through local pharmacies, community and civic centers, public libraries, and more. This had a positive impact on equity because the provision of vaccines at no cost and with no need to set appointments allowed local pharmacies, community centers, and public libraries in communities of color to help close the gap in providing vaccine coverage in communities that were often marginalized and under-immunized with most other childhood vaccines due to various barriers (www.immunize.org).

On the other hand, the COVID-19 pandemic also illuminated challenges in the healthcare system. Many of those that were unique to the pediatric population were even more detrimental for children in communities of color who have been impacted by historic and institutionalized racism. Although there was some increased awareness of health disparities among racialized groups in America, studies demonstrated that disparities in COVID-19 outcomes were worse than expected and continue to persist. Early data showed that Black and Hispanic children received less testing, faced higher infection rates, were hospitalized more often, and were more likely to suffer from the complication, including multisystem inflammatory syndrome in children or MIS-C (https://covid.cdc.gov/covid-data-tracker/#mis-national-surveillance). Likewise, a collaborative commissioned report entitled "Hidden Pain" revealed that in high-income nations like the United States, ethnic minoritized children were more likely to lose both parents to the COVID-19 virus. The report stated that American Indian, Alaska Native, Native Hawaiian, and Pacific Islander children were four times more likely to have been orphaned than their white counterparts, with Black and Hispanic children two and a half times more likely (https://www.covidcollaborative.us/).

The COVID-19 pandemic also highlighted the phenomenon of "silent" or occult hypoxia, whereby individuals can have dangerously low oxygen levels without experiencing typical symptoms such as shortness of breath (McGuire et al., 2020). Pulse oximeters, devices commonly used to measure blood oxygen saturation levels (SpO_2), have reduced accuracy for patients with darker skin pigmentation. Although overestimation of blood oxygenation by pulse oximeters in individuals with darker skin has been evident since the 1970s, the clinical implications of this inaccuracy have not been well understood (Sudat et al., 2023). Oxygen saturation levels impact treatment decisions and are critical indicators of disease severity, particularly for COVID-19 patients. Consequently, underestimation of disease severity due to discrepancies in pulse oximeter readings between racial groups may result in delayed care, exacerbating health disparities. Studies have shown that errors in pulse oximeter measurements may influence the timing of treatment decisions such as hospital admission and administration of remdesivir, dexamethasone, and supplemental oxygen therapies in COVID-19 patients (Fawzy et al., 2022; Sudat et al., 2023). One study found that pulse oximetry consistently overestimated blood oxygen saturation in Black, Hispanic, and Asian patients compared to non-Hispanic white patients. Black and Hispanic patients also had an increased likelihood of experiencing unrecognized or delayed recognition of COVID-19 therapy eligibility, which could be associated with adverse outcomes (Fawzy et al., 2022). Racial bias in pulse oximetry may lead to disparities in healthcare delivery. Regulatory bodies such as the FDA and NIH should prioritize efforts to foster diversity in clinical trials and improve pulse oximeter standards (Plaisime, 2023).

For many reasons, the pandemic's racial disparities also greatly contributed to increased stress and mental health issues among pediatric patients of color. According to research conducted among primary healthcare providers in pediatric health centers in the nation's capital, children of color experienced higher rates of ADHD (Anxiety/Depression and Sleep Disorders) (Everett et al., 2020; Nguyen et al., 2023). With these communities also experiencing mental health care deserts, the added stress from the pandemic caused damage that is likely to be felt in these communities for generations.

Furthermore, although there were increased resources poured into telemedicine to help connect communities to healthcare providers during the COVID pandemic, in communities of color, there continues to be limited access to technology and the infrastructure to support technology. This is due to institutionalized and systemic racism resulting in redlining policies and underinvestment in communities which contribute to their marginalization from accessing healthcare for preventive, urgent, or emergent care (Everett et al., 2020; Nguyen et al., 2023).

And lastly, but equally important, there remains the phenomenon of vaccine hesitancy that challenges healthcare facilities that have been tasked with immunizing children and families in communities of color. Although this was not as widespread as first reported, communities of color often have trust issues regarding the scientific community which are rooted in the historical exploitation perpetrated by many "highly esteemed" medical institutions and healthcare agencies (McClenny et al., 2022).

Lessons Learned

To address the disparities noted during the COVID-19 pandemic, the nation must get to the source of a problem that has been present since long before the pandemic began: racial inequities. Decade after decade, disease after disease, the same marginalized racial and ethnic groups continue to experience injustices. While there have been short-term band-aids applied to many of the problems, what our nation needs now is a long-term, permanent solution. It is understood that historic racism is a deeply rooted, multilayered problem that will take many years to resolve. However, there must be movement forward.

During the COVID-19 pandemic, marginalized communities experienced limited access to healthcare as many in-person facilities closed. There was a swift shift to telehealth; however, many families and children of color experienced decreased access and utilization of these platforms. Once routine preventive care resumed, non-white families continued to have lower access and fell further behind on preventive visits and routine immunizations. Likewise, once the COVID-19 vaccine became available, there was initial resistance due to historical mistrust and structural racism. Although minoritized communities were initially impacted by more severe illnesses, vaccine distribution was not initially offered in these communities, thus exacerbating the inequities.

Minoritized families were more likely to be living in urban, crowded conditions where COVID-19 was initially more likely to be contracted. Nevertheless, family and extended family support during the pandemic was instrumental for the well-being of working minoritized parents. Already at an economic disadvantage, many Black and Hispanic families had to make hard decisions about placing their family at an increased risk of infection versus earning needed income.

The COVID-19 pandemic has underscored and exacerbated systemic inequalities in the United States, including disparities in mental health care access among racially minoritized youth. Addressing these disparities will require a multi-faceted and comprehensive approach that incorporates public policy reform, reduction of socioeconomic barriers, and addressing structural racism (Williams et al., 2023). The pandemic has resulted in poor mental health outcomes in racially minoritized youth, worsening the existing racial disparities in mental health care.

The academic engagement and performance of students during the pandemic were less than ideal. Historically students of color already experienced disparities in learning outcomes, and during the pandemic, these disparities were amplified. National benchmarks for reading and math are at a historic low for Black, Hispanic, American Indian, and Alaska Native students (https://www.edweek.org/leadership/

two-decades-of-progress-nearly-gone-national-math-reading-scores-hit-historic-lows/2022/10). Rates of chronic absenteeism, particularly for students from minoritized communities, worsened. Switching to virtual school was not equitably achieved across districts, and minoritized students did not always have equal access to the necessary environment to make virtual learning optimal, including a computer and high-speed internet (https://read.dukeupress.edu/demography/article/59/1/1/286878/Research-Note-School-Reopenings-During-the-COVID). However, the Biden-Harris administration committed to tackling the increasing rates of chronic absenteeism and reversing learning loss in schools (https://www.whitehouse.gov/cea/written-materials/2023/09/13/chronic-absenteeism-and-disrupted-learning-require-an-all-hands-on-deck-approach/).

Immigrants also faced historical disparities which were amplified throughout the pandemic, including lack of employment, lack of resources for assistance, and fear of political retaliation. Similar to other minoritized populations, rates of infection were high among this group and immigrants were more likely to be working in high-risk occupations including agriculture and meat processing.

Although there were many barriers that were present during the height of the COVID-19 pandemic, there were also some breakthroughs in healthcare that occurred. The development of the vaccine offered an opportunity to understand the science behind vaccine development and distribution. Minoritized communities, while initially hesitant about governmental intentions and general vaccine mistrust, worked together to help educate each other about the vaccine benefits. Many grassroots community agencies were established and amplified, thus allowing many residents to have their voices heard.

Calls to Action
- Health, economic, and educational disparities in minoritized communities existed prior to the COVID-19 pandemic and exacerbated the stress faced by children and families during the pandemic. Efforts to stabilize our public health and clinical workforce and facilities to deliver pediatric care to all communities in a crisis are warranted with more attention to restorative justice in marginalized communities that are underserved.
- During the COVID-19 pandemic, racial/ethnic and immigration disparities appeared in infection rates and severity, healthcare access, academic achievement, mental health disorders, and vaccine access and uptake. Leaning into lessons learned, improving educational outcomes, access to care, and vaccine hesitancy are critically important.
- Economic, educational, and social policies are needed to optimize recovery from the pandemic, particularly for racial and ethnic groups historically affected by racism and other intersectional forms of discrimination.

References

Ali, M. M., West, K. D., Dubenitz, J., et al. (2023). Racial and ethnic differences in encounters related to suicidal behavior among children and adolescents with Medicaid coverage during the COVID-19 pandemic. *JAMA Pediatrics, 177*(8), 864–865. https://doi.org/10.1001/jamapediatrics.2023.1934

Anderson, R. E., Heard-Garris, N., & DeLapp, R. C. T. (2022). Future directions for vaccinating children against the American endemic: Treating racism as a virus. *Journal of Clinical Child & Adolescent Psychology, 51*(1), 127–142. https://doi.org/10.1080/15374416.2021.1969940

Ayalew, B., Dawson-Hahn, E., Cholera, R., et al. (2021). The health of children in immigrant families: Key drivers and research gaps through an equity lens. *Academic Pediatrics, 21*(5), 777–792. https://doi.org/10.1016/j.acap.2021.01.008

Bhogal, A., Borg, B., Jovanovic, T., & Marusak, H. A. (2021). Are the kids really alright? Impact of COVID-19 on mental health in a majority Black American sample of schoolchildren. *Psychiatry Research, 304*, 114146. https://doi.org/10.1016/j.psychres.2021.114146

Cadenas, G. A., Cerezo, A., Carlos Chavez, F. L., et al. (2023). The citizenship shield: Mediated and moderated links between immigration status, discrimination, food insecurity, and negative health outcomes for latinx immigrants during the COVID-19 pandemic. *Journal of Community Psychology, 51*(6), 2355–2371. https://doi.org/10.1002/jcop.22831

Cholera, R., Falusi, O. O., & Linton, J. M. (2020). Sheltering in place in a xenophobic climate: COVID-19 and children in immigrant families. *Pediatrics, 146*(1), e20201094. https://doi.org/10.1542/peds.2020-1094

Chunara, R., Zhao, Y., Chen, J., Lawrence, K., Testa, P. A., Nov, O., & Mann, D. M. (2021). Telemedicine and healthcare disparities: A cohort study in a large healthcare system in New York City during COVID-19. *Journal of the American Medical Informatics Association, 28*(1), 33–41. https://doi.org/10.1093/jamia/ocaa217

Curtis, E., Jones, R., Tipene-Leach, D., et al. (2019). Why cultural safety rather than cultural competency is required to achieve health equity: A literature review and recommended definition. *International Journal for Equity in Health, 18*, 174. https://doi.org/10.1186/s12939-019-1082-3

Douglas, J. A., Bostean, G., Miles Nash, A., John, E. B., Brown, L. M., & Subica, A. M. (2022). Citizenship matters: Non-citizen COVID-19 mortality disparities in New York and Los Angeles. *International Journal of Environmental Research and Public Health, 19*(9), 5066. https://doi.org/10.3390/ijerph19095066

Everett, K., Kelley, F., Sharma, S., Gborkorquellie, T., & Lewis-Ragland, Y. (2020). Closing the mental health gap for primary care physicians in pediatric community health centers. *Journal of the National Medical Association, 112*(5), S41–S42.

Fawzy, A., Wu, T. D., Wang, K., Robinson, M. L., Farha, J., Bradke, A., Golden, S. H., Xu, Y., & Garibaldi, B. T. (2022). Racial and ethnic discrepancy in pulse oximetry and delayed identification of treatment eligibility among patients with COVID-19. *JAMA Internal Medicine, 182*(7), 730–738. https://doi.org/10.1001/jamainternmed.2022.1906

Fowlkes, A. L., Yoon, S. K., Lutrick, K., et al. (2022). Effectiveness of 2-dose BNT162b2 (Pfizer BioNTech) mRNA vaccine in preventing SARS-CoV-2 infection among children aged 5–11 years and adolescents aged 12–15 years—PROTECT Cohort, July 2021–February 2022. *Morbidity and Mortality Weekly Report, 71*(11), 422–428. https://doi.org/10.15585/mmwr.mm7111e1

Gelatt, J., & Muzaffar, C. (2022). *COVID-19's effects on U.S. immigration and immigrant communities, two years on.* Migration Policy Institute. https://www.migrationpolicy.org/research/covid19-effects-us-immigration

Hawks, J. L. (2023). Editorial: The impact of the COVID-19 pandemic on racial disparities in pediatric mental health. *Journal of the American Academy of Child and Adolescent Psychiatry, 62*(4), 398–399. https://doi.org/10.1016/j.jaac.2022.12.015

Hernandez, I., Dickson, S., Tang, S., Gabriel, N., Berenbrok, L. A., & Guo, J. (2022). Disparities in distribution of COVID-19 vaccines across US counties: A geographic information system–

based cross-sectional study. *PLoS Medicine, 19*(7), e1004069. https://doi.org/10.1371/journal. pmed.1004069

Horner, K. M., Wrigley-Field, E., & Leider, J. P. (2022). A first look: Disparities in COVID-19 mortality among US-born and foreign-born Minnesota residents. *Population Research and Policy Review, 41*(2), 465–478. https://doi.org/10.1007/s11113-021-09668-1

Iraheta, S., & Morey, B. N. (2023). Mixed-immigration status families during the COVID-19 pandemic. *Health Equity, 7*(1), 243–250. https://doi.org/10.1089/heq.2022.0141

Kenworthy, T., Harmon, S. L., Delouche, A., Abugattas, N., Zwiebel, H., Martinez, J., Sauvigné, K. C., Nelson, C. M., Horigian, V. E., Gwynn, L., & Pulgaron, E. R. (2022). Community voices on factors influencing COVID-19 concerns and health decisions among racial and ethnic minorities in the school setting. *Frontiers in Public Health, 10*, 1002209. https://doi.org/10.3389/fpubh.2022.1002209

King, J., Kam, J. A., Cornejo, M., & Mendez Murillo, R. (2023). Enacting resilience at multiple levels during the COVID-19 pandemic: Exploring communication theory of resilience for U.S. undocumented college students. *Journal of Applied Communication Research, 51*, 539. https://doi.org/10.1080/00909882.2023.2178855

Kuhlman, K. R., Antici, E., Tan, E., Tran, M. L., Rodgers-Romero, E. L., & Restrepo, N. (2023). Predictors of adolescent resilience during the COVID-19 pandemic in a community sample of Hispanic and Latinx youth: Expressive suppression and social support. *Research on Child and Adolescent Psychopathology, 51*(5), 639–651. https://doi.org/10.1007/s10802-022-01019-8

Laurencin, C. T. (2021). Addressing justified vaccine hesitancy in the black community. *Journal of Racial and Ethnic Health Disparities, 8*(3), 543–546. https://doi.org/10.1007/s40615-021-01025-4

McClenny, A., Gelin, D., Rucker, E., Olowojesiku, R., Quarles-Fisher, A., Gborkorquellie, T., & Lewis-Ragland, Y. (2022). Navigating COVID-19 vaccine hesitancy among Black, indigenous and people of color (BIPOC) communities in 2021. *Journal of the National Medical Association, 114*(3), S47.

McGuire, C., Macnaughton, J., & Carel, H. (2020). The color of breath. *Literature and Medicine, 38*(2), 233–238. https://doi.org/10.1353/lm.2020.0015

Metzl, J. M., & Hansen, H. (2014). Structural competency: Theorizing a new medical engagement with stigma and inequality. *Social Science & Medicine, 103*, 126–133. https://doi.org/10.1016/j.socscimed.2013.06.032

Nguyen, V., Gborkorquellie, T., & Lewis-Ragland, Y. (2023). Closing the mental health gap for primary care physicians in pediatric community health centers. In: *Children's National Hospital 13th annual research, education, and innovation (REI) week abstract book* (pp. 252–253). Washington, DC.

Office of the Surgeon General. (2021). *Protecting youth mental health: The U.S. Surgeon General's Advisory*. US Department of Health and Human Services. https://www.hhs.gov/sites/default/files/surgeon-general-youth-mental-healthadvisory.pdf

Oliveira, C. R., Niccolai, L. M., Sheikha, H., Elmansy, L., Kalinich, C. C., Grubaugh, N. D., Shapiro, E. D., & Yale SARS-CoV-2 Genomic Surveillance Initiative. (2022). Assessment of clinical effectiveness of BNT162b2 COVID-19 vaccine in US adolescents. *JAMA Network Open, 5*(3), e220935. https://doi.org/10.1001/jamanetworkopen.2022.0935

Otto, W. R., Grundmeier, R. W., Montoya-Williams, D., et al. (2021). Association between preferred language and risk of severe acute respiratory syndrome coronavirus 2 infection in children in the United States. *The American Journal of Tropical Medicine and Hygiene, 105*(5), 1261–1264. https://doi.org/10.4269/ajtmh.21-0779

Phan, T. T., Enlow, P. T., Lewis, A. M., Arasteh, K., Hildenbrand, A. K., Price, J., Schultz, C. L., Reynolds, V., Kazak, A. E., & Alderfer, M. A. (2023). Persistent disparities in pediatric health care engagement during the COVID-19 pandemic. *Public Health Reports, 138*(4), 633–644. https://doi.org/10.1177/00333549231163527

Plaisime, M. V. (2023). Invited commentary: Undiagnosed and undertreated-the suffocating consequences of the use of racially biased medical devices during the COVID-19 pandemic. *American Journal of Epidemiology, 192*(5), 714–719. https://doi.org/10.1093/aje/kwad019

Ring, J., Nyquist, J., & Mitchell, S. (2009). *Curriculum for culturally responsive health care: The step- by-step guide for cultural competence training.* CRC Press.

Roels, N. I., Estrella, A., Maldonado-Salcedo, M., Rapp, R., Hansen, H., & Hardon, A. (2022). Confident futures: Community-based organizations as first responders and agents of change in the face of the Covid-19 pandemic. *Social Science & Medicine, 294*, 114639. https://doi.org/10.1016/j.socscimed.2021.114639

Rothe, E. M., Fortuna, L. R., Tobon, A. L., Postlethwaite, A., Sanchez-Lacay, J. A., & Anglero, Y. L. (2021). Structural inequities and the impact of COVID-19 on Latinx children: Implications for child and adolescent mental health practice. *Journal of the American Academy of Child and Adolescent Psychiatry, 60*(6), 669–671. https://doi.org/10.1016/j.jaac.2021.02.013

Santoli, J. M., Lindley, M. C., DeSilva, M. B., et al. (2020). Effects of the COVID-19 pandemic on routine pediatric vaccine ordering and administration—United States, 2020. *MMWR. Morbidity and Mortality Weekly Report, 69*, 591–593. https://doi.org/10.15585/mmwr.mm6919e2

Shim, R., Szilagyi, M., & Perrin, J. M. (2022). Epidemic rates of child and adolescent mental health disorders require an urgent response. *Pediatrics, 149*(5), e2022056611. https://doi.org/10.1542/peds.2022-056611

Sudat, S. E. K., Wesson, P., Rhoads, K. F., Brown, S., Aboelata, N., Pressman, A. R., Mani, A., & Azar, K. M. J. (2023). Racial disparities in pulse oximeter device inaccuracy and estimated clinical impact on COVID-19 treatment course. *American Journal of Epidemiology, 192*(5), 703–713. https://doi.org/10.1093/aje/kwac164

Szilagyi, P. G., Shah, M. D., Delgado, J. R., Thomas, K., Vizueta, N., Cui, Y., Vangala, S., Shetgiri, R., & Kapteyn, A. (2021). Parents' intentions and perceptions about COVID-19 vaccination for their children: Results from a national survey. *Pediatrics, 148*(4), e2021052335. https://doi.org/10.1542/peds.2021-052335

Tucker, C. M., Marsiske, M., Rice, K. G., Nielson, J. J., & Herman, K. (2011). Patient-centered culturally sensitive health care: Model testing and refinement. *Health Psychology, 30*(3), 342–350. https://doi.org/10.1037/a0022967

Vacaru, S. V., Beijers, R., & de Weerth, C. (2022). Internalizing symptoms and family functioning predict adolescent depressive symptoms during COVID-19: A longitudinal study in a community sample. *PLoS One, 17*(3), e0264962. https://doi.org/10.1371/journal.pone.0264962

Williams, J. C., Ball, M., Roscoe, N., Harowitz, J., Hobbs, R. J., Raman, H. N., Seltzer, M. K., Vo, L. C., Cagande, C. C., Alexander-Bloch, A. F., Glahn, D. C., & Morrow, L. (2023). Widening racial disparities during COVID-19 telemedicine transition: A study of child mental health services at two large children's hospitals. *Journal of the American Academy of Child and Adolescent Psychiatry, 62*(4), 447–456. https://doi.org/10.1016/j.jaac.2022.07.848

Wood, S. M., White, K., Peebles, R., Pickel, J., Alausa, M., Mehringer, J., & Dowshen, N. (2020). Outcomes of a rapid adolescent telehealth scale-up during the COVID-19 pandemic. *Journal of Adolescent Health, 67*(2), 172–178. https://doi.org/10.1016/j.jadohealth.2020.05.025

Xavier, J., Ward, M. C., Corr, P. G., Kalita, N., & McDonald, P. (2023). Identifying the barriers and facilitators to culturally responsive HIV and PrEP screening for racial, ethnic, sexual, and gender minoritized patients: A scoping review protocol. *PLoS One, 18*(5), e0281173. https://doi.org/10.1371/journal.pone.0281173

Social Media and Adolescents: Assessment of Risk, Clinical Manifestations, and Prevention

Morgan E. PettyJohn ⓘ**, Angela J. Calvin** ⓘ**, Ellen M. Selkie** ⓘ**, and Jeff Temple**

> *COVID-era research largely echoes what the field already knew about the relationship between adolescent social media use and well-being. In short, it's complicated.*
>
> —Morgan E. Petty John, PhD

Introduction and Background

During the COVID-19 pandemic, rates of social media use increased around the world as people used these platforms to stay connected, follow the news, and combat boredom (Cauberghe et al., 2021; Luo et al., 2021; Rosen et al., 2022). Adolescents in the United States were no exception, with data signaling significant increases in the amount of time spent on social media during the pandemic compared to pre-COVID rates (Burke et al., 2021; Drouin et al., 2020; Rideout et al., 2022). The rise in usage has reiterated ongoing questions about the long-term impacts of social media use for adolescents, particularly for "Gen Z" (those born

M. E. PettyJohn (✉)
School of Social Work, The University of Texas at Arlington, Arlington, TX, USA
e-mail: morgan.pettyjohn@uta.edu

A. J. Calvin
Common Sense Media, San Francisco, CA, USA
e-mail: acalvin@commonsense.org

E. M. Selkie
Division of General Pediatrics and Adolescent Medicine, University of Wisconsin-Madison, Madison, WI, USA
e-mail: selkie@wisc.edu

J. Temple
School of Behavioral Health Sciences, The University of Texas Health Science Center at Houston, Houston, TX, USA
e-mail: jeffrey.r.temple@uth.tmc.edu

© The Author(s), under exclusive license to Springer Nature Switzerland AG 2025
J. L. Peck (ed.), *COVID-19 Impacts on Child Health*,
https://doi.org/10.1007/978-3-031-80369-7_16

between 1997 and 2012) (Dimock, 2019), whose development has been shaped by these unprecedented contexts. While forthcoming research will continue shaping our understanding of this phenomenon, current COVID-era literature largely echoes what the field already knew about the relationship between adolescent social media use and well-being. In short, it's complicated. The dualistic nature of social media use, offering both benefits and potential for harm, was laid bare under the unique circumstance of widespread social isolation (Drouin et al., 2020; Hamilton et al., 2023).

> COVID-era research supports the notion that outcomes are more strongly associated with the *way social media are being used* rather than the *amount of time spent* on these platforms (Hamilton et al., 2022; Marciano et al., 2022).

It should be noted that, while adolescent social media use has returned to pre-COVID baseline rates for certain platforms, others have seen sustained increases coming out of the pandemic. According to a nationally representative survey of U.S. teens (age 13–18), overall screentime increased 17% pre—to post-pandemic (from spring 2019 to fall 2021), but rates of daily use for platforms such as Snapchat, Instagram, and Facebook did not change (63% vs. 62%, respectively) (Rideout et al., 2022). However, consumption of online videos from platforms like YouTube and TikTok (which include social media components) significantly increased and endured after pandemic restrictions lifted, with daily use rising from 69% to 77% and daily time spent increasing by 23 min (Rideout et al., 2022). Additionally, the pandemic seems to have spurred first-time and earlier engagement with online platforms among youth (Hamilton et al., 2023). Significant increases were observed in both social media usage (13–18%) and online video consumption (56% to 64%) among 8- to 12-year-olds from 2019 to 2022 (Rideout et al., 2022). Notably, it is difficult to disentangle whether this increase was a consequence of the pandemic or the growing ubiquity of smartphone ownership among younger populations.

The current chapter focuses on the impacts of social media during COVID-19 among adolescents, primarily from 12 to 25 years old. We draw on extant empirical and theoretical literature to discuss potential cohort effects extending beyond the pandemic and provide practice recommendations for monitoring adolescent social media users' development, health, and well-being. Given recent data suggesting an increased uptake of social media use among pre-teens, we recommend integrating social media assessment, psychoeducation, and parent engagement with children as young as 8. It should be specified that this review and these practice recommendations are focused on social media use specifically, distinct from the broader constructs of overall screentime or problematic internet use, and not inclusive of video games or other types of media consumption (e.g., television/streaming services). In this context, social media refer to internet-based platforms or applications ("apps") which facilitate communication between users, inclusive of social networking sites (e.g., Instagram, Snapchat), direct messaging platforms (e.g., WhatsApp), community discussion boards and forums (e.g., Reddit), and interactive video sharing platforms (e.g., YouTube, TikTok). To ensure precision when communicating empirical findings, we use "teens" to describe samples composed of 13 to 18-year-olds and "young adults" to describe 18 to 25-year-olds.

General State of Social Media Research

Before examining adolescent social media use during COVID-19, we must first review the general state of social media research. In the grand scheme of scientific inquiry, social media research is still in its infancy; however, we will discuss what is currently known about trends in adolescent social media use, how social media may impact adolescent developmental processes, and outcome research evaluating adolescent well-being in relation to social media use.

Adolescent Social Media Use Trends

Since their emergence in the early 2000s, uptake of social media among adolescents has been swift and escalated with access to smart phones. Smart phone ownership rose from 73% in 2014–2015 to 95% in 2022 (Vogels et al., 2022). Presently, 95% of U.S. teens report using social media, with YouTube (95%), TikTok (67%), Instagram (62%), Snapchat (59%), and Facebook (32%) being the most popular platforms (Vogels et al., 2022). Overall, teens spend an average of 1.5 h on social media each day (Rideout et al., 2022), though more than a third (35%) report being on at least one of these platforms "almost constantly" (Vogels et al., 2022).

The landscape of available social media and popular use trends among teens are constantly shifting. For example, while 71% of U.S. teens used Facebook in 2014–2015, by 2022 that number dropped to 32% (Vogels et al., 2022). Conversely, TikTok was only brought to the U.S. market in 2018 and is already the second most popular platform among teens (Vogels et al., 2022). Trends in social media use vary demographically as well. Teenage girls spend more time on social media (around 2 h each day) and are more likely to use highly visual social media platforms such as TikTok, Instagram, and Snapchat, while boys more often use sites that overlap with videogaming, such as YouTube, Twitch, and Reddit (Nesi et al., 2023; Vogels et al., 2022). Sexual and gender minority (SGM) youth use certain social media platforms, namely Discord, Among Us, Twitch, and Omegle, at higher rates than their cisgender-heterosexual counterparts (Thorn, 2023). SGM adolescents are also more likely to interact with people they do not know from offline contexts and are twice as likely to have secondary social media accounts to allow privacy from their parents (Thorn, 2023). Moreover, Black and Hispanic teens are more likely than white teens to report being online "almost constantly," and use certain platforms (TikTok, Instagram, Twitter, and WhatsApp) at higher rates (Vogels et al., 2022).

Despite its commonality, teens report mixed feelings about social media usage. Recent national data show that only a third (34%) of teens enjoy traditional social media sites "a lot" (e.g., Facebook, Instagram), though this number jumps to 62% when asked about sites focused on video sharing (e.g., YouTube, TikTok) (Rideout et al., 2022). A slight majority (55%) of American teens think they spend an appropriate amount of time on social media, though more than a third (36%) believe they spend too much time on these platforms (Vogels et al., 2022). Indeed, nearly half (45%) of young teen girls in the USA (age 11 to 15) feel "addicted" to social media (Nesi et al., 2023). Many adolescent social media users report "digital stress" from pressures to gain digital approval from peers and to be constantly available for online interactions (Hamilton et al., 2023; Nesi et al., 2023). Despite reservations and challenges, about half of teens report it would be difficult to give up social media, with more (58%) girls and older teens (age 15 to 17) stating this would be a challenge (Vogels et al., 2022).

Adolescent Development in the Social Media Era

Social media have become a normative component of adolescence, garnering intense interest from practitioners, researchers, parents, and policymakers to identify the impacts of these platforms. The co-construction model explains how, due to the interactive nature of social media compared to traditional media outlets (e.g., TV), adolescents' offline and online worlds are closely interrelated, reciprocally shaping developmental trajectories in ways not experienced by previous generations (Subrahmanyam et al., 2006; Vannucci et al., 2020). These platforms have altered the social ecologies of young people by allowing users to connect with people they know from offline contexts (e.g., family, friends) as well as strangers, organizations, and information sources from around the world. The ability to access vast digital networks is particularly appealing to adolescents whose primary developmental tasks include forming social connections, especially with peers (Gerwin et al., 2018). Beyond socializing opportunities, these sites uniquely contribute to numerous other developmental milestones for adolescents such as self-expression, identity exploration, accessing information, gaining independence from caretakers, pursuing romantic interests, and seeking approval and gratification from peers (Gerwin et al., 2018; Hamilton et al., 2023).

Social Media Use and Adolescent Well-Being

As social media use has proliferated, so has research aiming to understand its impact on adolescent safety and well-being. This interest has been intensified by the simultaneous rise in mental health disorders and suicidality among children and adolescents over the past decade, which was recently declared a national emergency by the American Academy of Pediatrics (American Academy of Pediatrics, 2021). In 2023, the U.S. Surgeon General took this a step further by issuing a specific advisory tying adolescent mental health to social media use (U.S. Department of Health and Human Services, 2023). Adolescents, compared to older social media users, are considered at unique risk for outcomes such as addiction, negative peer influences, and mental health disturbances due to their developmental stage and underdeveloped prefrontal cortex (Sugaya et al., 2019; Vannucci et al., 2020). Moreover, social media provide novel avenues for exposure to harmful content (e.g., violence, graphic pornography), cyberbullying, and abuse (e.g., harassment, sexual exploitation) (Nesi et al., 2023).

Meta-analytic studies have indeed identified small to medium, positive associations between adolescents' general social media use and a variety of negative outcomes (i.e., depression, anxiety, psychological distress, risk behaviors, substance use, and self-injurious thoughts and behaviors) (Curtis et al., 2018; Ivie et al., 2020; Keles et al., 2020; Nesi et al., 2021; Vannucci et al., 2020). Importantly however, the researchers who conducted these meta-analyses emphasize caution in interpreting these relationships due to limitations in social media research methodologies. Most extant research has used cross-sectional, self-report surveys, primarily using total time spent on social media as the independent variable. Until more rigorous longitudinal studies are conducted, it is impossible to determine the directionality of the relationship between social media use and negative dimensions of well-being (Parry et al., 2022). Moreover, there are substantial differences in findings between studies looking at the same outcomes which suggest that associations between social media use and well-being are influenced by other salient variables that may vary between study samples (Ivie et al., 2020).

The Differential Susceptibility to Media Effects Model (See Fig. 1) emerged in the last decade and emphasizes that an individual's disposition, developmental stage, and social milieu shape susceptibility to positive or negative effects of media, which can account for some of the discrepant findings in population studies of social media and well-being among adolescents (Valkenburg & Peter, 2013). In

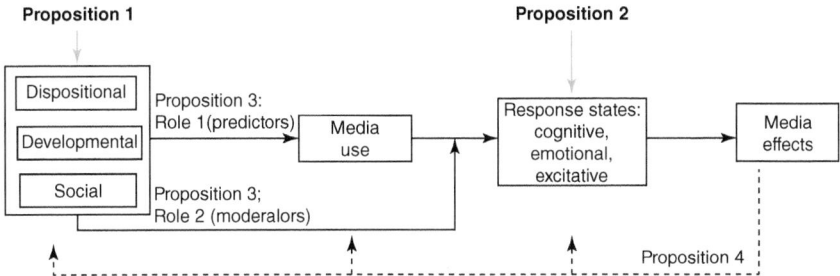

Proposition 1: Media effects depend on three types of differential susceptibility variables.
Proposition 2: Three media response states mediate the relationship between media use and effects.
Proposition 3: The differential susceptibility variables have two roles; they act as predictors and moderators.
Proposition 4: Media effects are transactional.

Fig. 1 The Differential Susceptibility to Media Effects Model. (With permission from Valkenburg PM. Differential susceptibility to media effects model. In Bulck J, editor. The International Encyclopedia of Media Psychology. 2020. https://doi.org/10.1002/9781119011071.iemp0122)

other words, within-person variables, nuances in how adolescents are using social media, and what content they are exposed to appear to drive differences in outcome; however, person-level research in this area remains underdeveloped. Some factors that have been found to impact the relationship between social media use and well-being across adolescent samples include sleep disruption (Becker & Lienesch, 2018; Woods & Scott, 2016), increases in sedentary activity (Iannotti et al., 2009), individual trait differences among users (O'Dea & Campbell, 2011; Wang et al., 2018), number of platforms used (Primack et al., 2017), negative versus supportive online experiences (Frison & Eggermont, 2016; Kırcaburun et al., 2019), and motivations for use (Barry et al., 2017; Nesi & Prinstein, 2019).

Because social media use has become normative, there is a push from researchers to focus on problematic social media use in relation to adolescent well-being; however, problematic use has not been consistently operationalized in the field, and often conflates "addictive use" with simply higher rates of use (Nesi et al., 2021; Sun & Zhang, 2021). In sum, there is justification for investigating the links between social media use and adolescent well-being. However, there is a growing consensus in the field that the amount of time spent on social media is not inherently related to negative outcomes; rather, nuances in the way adolescents engage with social media likely explains disparate impacts (Odgers & Jensen, 2020; Orben, 2020). Continued research using more sophisticated research methods is needed to help clarify these relationships. This contention should be kept in mind while reviewing research on social media use during COVID-19.

Impacts of Social Media Use During COVID-19

COVID-19 caused systemic disruptions to adolescents' lives, contributing to adverse, interrelated social, physical, and mental health outcomes. Within this context, social media shaped adolescent experiences and outcomes in various ways, both positively and negatively. Here we summarize currently published, peer-reviewed literature on this topic. It should be noted that social media behaviors vary between countries based on a variety of factors such as internet and technology access, availability of different social media platforms, and cultural differences (Fumagalli et al., 2021). As such, adolescents' experiences and outcomes may vary based on country of origin. To date, less COVID-19 specific social media research has been published from U.S. samples compared to other regions (e.g., Asia and Europe). We will include all available literature in our review, with the caveat that practitioners should think critically about how their cultural contexts may influence the patients they are treating.

Sociodevelopmental Impacts

The pandemic interrupted typical adolescent sociodevelopmental processes by forcing separation from peers and requiring more time spent within the home. Adolescence is typically a transition period in which youth switch from spending most of their time with family to spending most of their time with peers with little adult oversight. Peer relationships are immensely important for adolescents' identity, brain, and social development, as well as their overall well-being (Brown & Larson, 2009; Odgers et al., 2020). Indeed, evidence has shown high quality peer relationships to be protective against mental health issues and improve resiliency (Van Harmelen et al., 2017). Unfortunately, social distancing measures and school closures translated into feelings of isolation; indeed, 42% of teens felt lonelier than usual during the first year of COVID-19 (Common Sense Media, 2020). This likely drove many adolescents to social media to satisfy their need for peer connection (Hamilton et al., 2023). During this period, two-thirds (66%) of U.S. teens reported using social media to connect with friends and family outside the home every day (Common Sense Media, 2020) and nearly half (44%) of U.S. parents reported teens' use of technology to socialize increased "a lot" (Drouin et al., 2020). Data from Australia suggests that SGM adolescents used social media most often during the pandemic, followed by cisgender girls, then cisgender boys (Bailey et al., 2022).

Research suggests a complicated relationship between social media use and loneliness during the pandemic. A multi-country study found social media use to be positively associated with loneliness; however, this relationship was fully mediated by users' reported level of FOMO ("fear of missing out") (Fumagalli et al., 2021). Interestingly, despite social distancing measures eliminating opportunity for most offline activities, FOMO levels were found to persist among European young adults during the pandemic, as they worried about missing out on virtual events and other digital content (Hayran & Anik, 2021). In the United States, compared to teen boys, teen girls reported both higher levels of loneliness and FOMO during the pandemic (Common Sense Media, 2020; Mousavi et al., 2023). Meta-analytic work suggests that loneliness was diminished for adolescents who used social media in specific ways, including direct messaging for one-to-one conversations, providing self-disclosures to trusted peers, and having positive and funny experiences online (Marciano et al., 2022). In other words, loneliness and other indicators of negative well-being (e.g., depression and stress) were mitigated when adolescents used social media to foster close online relationships, while poorer outcomes were observed for users who simply spent a lot of time on these platforms without these type of engagements (Boursier et al., 2023).

Social media became even more central to the adolescent developmental tasks of identity formation and self-expression during COVID-19, as these digital platforms were one of the only ways young people were able to explore the outside world and share pieces of themselves with others (Hamilton et al., 2023). As in non-pandemic times (Thorn, 2023), these sites were particularly important for identity development and connection among SGM youth. The pandemic forced many SGM adolescents to stay at home with unaware or unsupportive caretakers (Fish et al., 2020).

Indeed, transgender and gender non-conforming adolescents reported significantly lower satisfaction with peer connection during the pandemic compared to their cisgender peers (Cingel et al., 2022). However, for some SGM adolescents, the pandemic provided perceptions of time to reflect on and gain a deeper understanding of their gender and sexuality identity through engagement with online queer communities (Hanckel & Chandra, 2021).

Both related and unrelated to COVID-19, the pandemic-era also fostered a surge in civic engagement and digital activism among adolescents. In the aftermath of George Floyd's murder, the resurgence of the #BlackLivesMatter movement, disparities in COVID-19 outcomes among communities of color, and rise in Anti-Asian sentiments, many adolescents (70%) turned to social media to participate in digital conversations about racial justice (Hamilton et al., 2023; Yazdani et al., 2022). Participation in offline activism is associated with generally positive impacts on adolescent development and adult outcomes (e.g., higher income and education level) (Ballard et al., 2019). However, participation in digital activism increases exposure to discrimination, as racist content is common on social media sites (Nesi et al., 2023; Nguyen et al., 2020). Indeed, Tao and Fisher found that youth who participated in online racial civic engagement during COVID-19 were more likely to experience social media discrimination which in turn increased the risk for depressive symptoms and alcohol misuse. Vicarious social media racial discrimination (observing these interactions secondhand) also mediated the relationship between online civic engagement and negative outcomes (Tao & Fisher, 2022). Alongside harmful by-products of engagement, youth have described positive aspects of these experiences as well. Adolescents reported expressing themselves by telling personal stories or challenging dominant narratives related to these discourses. Still, others described feeling a sense of community and using social media as a tool to take collective action (Keles et al., 2023; Wilf & Wray-Lake, 2021).

Mental Health Impacts

Adolescent mental health greatly suffered within the context of COVID-19 (see Chapter "Mental Health: Assessment of Risk, Clinical Manifestations, and Access to Care"). Efforts to understand how social media use interacted with this broader phenomenon have identified both harms (e.g., heavy, passive use associated with adverse outcomes) and benefits (e.g., using as a tool for coping and support seeking) (Bailey et al., 2022). Similar to non-pandemic contexts, a meta-analysis of 30 COVID-era studies identified a small, positive correlation ($r = 0.171$, $p = 0.011$) between time spent on social media and negative mental health indicators (i.e., symptoms of anxiety, depression, mood disorders, and ruminative thinking) (Marciano et al., 2022). In comparison, measures of media addiction (inclusive of social media and other types of screen addiction) demonstrated a much stronger association ($r = 0.434$, $p = 0.024$) to negative mental health (Marciano et al., 2022). While benefits to certain types of social media use have been identified in relation to positive outcomes such as decreased loneliness and increased social support, meta-analytic work shows no associations between time spent on social media and overall well-being (i.e., life satisfaction, optimism, and happiness) (Marciano et al., 2022). Taken together, the literature supports that general social media use during the pandemic was weakly associated with negative mental health outcomes for adolescents; though, this relationship is best explained by examining the level of use (e.g., at risk for addiction or not) and types of online behaviors users engaged in. Here we will briefly unpack these distinctions.

Risk of media addiction during the pandemic appeared to be greater among younger users, possibly due to poorer self-control and gratification management from underdeveloped prefrontal cortexes (Marciano et al., 2022). Moreover, certain platforms appeared to confer greater risk for addiction. While WhatsApp (a one-to-one chat application) and YouTube (a video streaming site) were associated with low addiction risk, use of TikTok was the strongest predictor of high addiction risk (Marengo et al., 2022). Passive social media use during COVID-19 was associated with poorer well-being, such as increased anxiety, depression, and loneliness (Hudimova et al., 2021; Marciano et al., 2022). Other factors which increased risk of poor outcomes included greater engagement in social comparison, higher levels of FOMO, and more exposure to negative content (e.g., cyber victimization) (Marciano et al., 2022). Notably, preliminary data from U.S. teens suggests that increases in social media use were not significantly related to cyber victimization during the pandemic (Burke et al., 2021). Research among adolescent and young women in Spain identified significant increases in passively following appearance-focused Instagram accounts during the pandemic, with these changes associated with lower self-esteem, greater body dissatisfaction, and drive for thinness (Vall-Roque et al., 2021). These trends are consistent with pre-pandemic literature on appearance-focused social media content and may help explain significant increases in disordered eating among adolescents in the context of greater social media use during COVID-19 (Gilsbach et al., 2022; Hartman-Munick et al., 2022), though further research is required to clarify this relationship.

Social media also served as a coping tool for many adolescents during this unprecedented period of stress and separation. Using social media to foster close interpersonal relationships via one-to-one communication tools, self-disclosure to trusted groups of friends, and positive online experiences helped buffer negative outcomes during COVID-19 (Marciano et al., 2022). These platforms were particularly important for those experiencing higher levels of distress, those with pre-existing mental health concerns, and among sexual and gender minority youth (Bailey et al., 2022; Drouin et al., 2020; Marciano et al., 2022). Adolescents in Belgium with higher levels of anxiety reported using social media to adapt to the uncertainty and rapid changes brought on by the pandemic, with active social media use significantly mediating the relationship between anxiety level and happiness (Cauberghe et al., 2021). Data from U.S. teens indicate that while increases in social media use were associated with increased anxiety and depression, using social media for coping through social connections significantly moderated the relationship between usage and depressive symptoms (though not anxiety) (Burke et al., 2021). Research in Australia found over one-third (36%) of adolescents used social media during the pandemic to seek peer support for thoughts of suicide or self-harm, and half (50%) had used social media to give this type of support to others (Bailey et al., 2022). Patterns of activity on the community discussion board and forum, Reddit, support that teens with mental health concerns may have more actively sought digital connections during this time. Users on teen mental health and suicidality subreddits posted more frequently than teens in the general teen subreddit communities (Zhang et al., 2021). Increases in activity on these Reddit boards corresponded with both positive and negative COVID-19 events (e.g., lockdowns, vaccines being released) suggesting social media provided an outlet for teens responding to the sociopolitical contexts and associated stressors (Zhang et al., 2021). Most (68%) adolescents who sought support online reported feeling better afterwards, as did half (51%) of users giving online support to their peers (Bailey et al., 2022). Again, the ways in which adolescents used social media for support seeking resulted in variable outcomes. Self-disclosing to smaller networks of peers helped moderate negative impacts of stressors compared to those who casually posted to wide audiences (Zhen et al., 2021). Importantly, though, a quarter (25%) of adolescents who offered support to peers in distress reported feeling worse afterwards, suggesting a potentially negative contagion effect facilitated through social media platforms (Bailey et al., 2022).

Many young people reported COVID-19 related stress during the early phase of the pandemic (Temple et al., 2022), with 61% of U.S. teens worried about family members being exposed to the virus, and 63% concerned about their family's financial situation (Common Sense Media, 2020). Given disparities in how the pandemic affected different communities (Mude et al., 2021), teens of color were disproportionately impacted by these stressors. Black teens (71%) were most concerned about family members' health, while Hispanic/Latino teens (87%) were particularly worried about their families' financial status (Common Sense Media, 2020). In the context of these stressors, adolescents used social media as a source for information and to spread public health messages regarding COVID-19, with seemingly mixed outcomes. In 2020, 44% of surveyed U.S. teens reported seeking news about COVID-19 at least once a day (Mousavi et al., 2023). In this study, teens with accurate COVID-19 knowledge who checked social media less frequently had the lowest levels of anxiety, while teens with less or inaccurate COVID-19 knowledge and who checked social media more frequently had higher levels of anxiety (Mousavi et al., 2023). Among Belgian youth, using social media to seek out guidance on COVID-19 and encourage others to do the same significantly mediated the relationship between anxiety and happiness (Cauberghe et al., 2021). However, research with young adults in China and the UK identified that high levels of social media exposure to COVID-19 information were associated with poor mental health outcomes, and that high levels of COVID-19 stress fostered addictive social media use tendencies (Li et al., 2021; Liu et al., 2021; Zhao & Zhou, 2021). Another study with young adults in China found the relationship between social media exposure and distress to be mediated by individuals' rumination tendencies and that practicing mindfulness helped moderate negative outcomes (Hong et al., 2021). Differences in engagement and associated outcomes regarding COVID-19 information may be attributable to contextual differences among young people (e.g., country of origin, point of time in the pandemic) as well as the types of online behaviors in which they engaged.

Physical Health

As with the other dimensions of health, extant, pre-COVID literature has identified associations between social media use and some physical health outcomes, such as sleep and physical activity. Negative physical health outcomes are thought to stem from what social media use is displacing. In this way, unlike sociodevelopmental processes and mental health, physical health outcomes may be more directly related to the *quantity* of social media use rather than the *quality*. While much COVID-era research has examined changes in adolescent physical health (see earlier chapters), little work has been published examining these changes alongside changes in social media behaviors. Still, drawing from existing literature, we can extrapolate how increased social media use during the pandemic may have influenced changes in certain aspects of adolescent physical health.

Sleep disruption has been consistently associated with excessive social media use (Alonzo et al., 2021; Pagano et al., 2023), and preliminary studies have identified similar patterns during the pandemic (Marciano et al., 2022). Among adolescent girls in the United States, increased social media use during COVID-19 was associated with delayed sleep timing (Hamilton et al., 2022). No changes to duration or quality of sleep were observed, likely due to most adolescents being able to sleep in later than normal during the pandemic (Hamilton et al., 2022). Over half of surveyed teenagers in Sweden reported social media as having the most negative effect on their sleep (compared to other life areas, such as schoolwork, physical activity) both before (55%) and during (57%) the pandemic (Nilsson et al., 2022). Notably, these negative impacts on sleep were reported nearly twice as often for social media as for gaming (34% before COVID-19, 35% during COVID-19), likely due to the accessibility of social media on smartphones and notifications which can grab users' attention any time of day or night (Nilsson et al., 2022). While sleep deprivation was significantly correlated to increased social media use among young adults in Europe, a stronger relationship was identified between sleep disturbances and users' reported levels of FOMO (Hayran & Anik, 2021).

Lockdowns during the pandemic created barriers to physical activity at multiple levels of children and adolescents' social ecologies, including schools, sports programs, and recreation centers being shut down, caretakers having additional COVID-related stressors, and government policies restricting movement outside the home (Rahman & Chandrasekaran, 2021). Simultaneous to these barriers and decreases in physical activity, time spent on social media, digital devices, and other sedentary activities increased significantly (Hamilton et al., 2022). While multiple reviews have noted the promise of increasing physical activity through social media among young people, these interventions were not specifically studied during the pandemic (Goodyear et al., 2021; Günther et al., 2021; Rose et al., 2017). Taken together, much work remains to assess potential long-term cohort effects for children and adolescents' whose normal sleep patterns and physical activity levels were altered, in part by increased social media time, during this key developmental period.

Points of Care

Given the ubiquity of social media among adolescents and known associations between certain types of use and negative outcomes, universal screening during annual teen wellness visits and in clinics serving young adults or college students are warranted. Pediatric clinics should be proactive in providing caregiver guidance for monitoring adolescent social media use following evidence-based, developmentally appropriate tools. Alongside these points of care, it should be noted that clinical guidelines for defining and measuring problematic internet use, particularly on social media, are still under development. In 2013, the Diagnostic and Statistical Manual of Mental Disorders, 5th edition (DSM-5) included internet gaming disorder in an appendix as a condition "warranting more research" (American Psychiatric Association, 2013). Subsequently, the International Statistical Classification of Diseases and Related Health Problems, 11th edition (ICD-11) published in 2019 included online gaming and gambling disorders as the first and only official digital-media related diagnoses (World Health Organization, 2019). Until standardized diagnostic criteria become available, practitioners should use caution in pathologizing social media use among patients. Rather, clinicians should use available tools and guidance to identify individual patterns of use and specific areas of impairment or distress (e.g., a patient losing sleep due to using social media in bed, mood changes related to online harassment, changes in eating behavior or weight after viewing food or fitness accounts on social media) for targeted interventions (Paschke et al., 2021). Moreover, patterns of social media use among adolescents are constantly evolving (e.g., popular platforms, digital tools, and viral trends/challenges) and require practitioners and parents to stay up-to-date on changes for assessment and interventions to be effective.

Assessment Tools

In line with the principles of the American Medical Association's Guidelines for Adolescent Preventive Services, assessing for problematic social media use in relation to behavioral, emotional, and developmental well-being should be a universal practice (Alderman, 1994). Assessment tools can be integrated into the standardized paperwork given at annual well-visits, or during routine physical exams for young adults. To minimize burden on patients and caregivers, assessments should be brief and only provided for adolescents who report using social media platforms.

Table 1 The 9-item SMD scale

Criterion	During the past year, have you …
Preoccupation	… regularly found that you can't think of anything else but the moment that you will be able to use social media again?
Tolerance	… regularly felt dissatisfied because you wanted to spend more time on social media?
Withdrawal	… often felt bad when you could not use social media?
Persistence	… tried to spend less time on social media, but failed?
Displacement	… regularly neglected other activities (e.g., hobbies, sport) because you wanted to use social media?
Problem	… regularly had arguments with others because of your social media use?
Deception	… regularly lied to your parents or friends about the amount of time you spend on social media?
Escape	… often used social media to escape from negative feelings?
Conflict	… had serious conflict with your parents, brother(s) or sister(s) because of your social media use?

With permission from: van den Eijnden RJJM, Lemmens JS, Valkenburg PM. The social media disorder scale. Comput Hum Behav. 2016. https://doi.org/10.1016/j.chb.2016.03.038

Numerous assessment tools are available and have been validated among different age-groups and cultural contexts. Based on available evidence, we suggest using the Social Media Disorder Scale (SMDS) for adolescent patients (van den Eijnden et al., 2016). The SMDS is a self-report, 9-item questionnaire (see Table 1) based on the DSM-5 (American Psychiatric Association, 2013) proposed criteria for internet gaming disorder (i.e., preoccupation with social media, tolerance requiring increased use, withdrawal symptoms, unsuccessful attempts to stop use, loss of interest in other things, continued use despite psychosocial problems, deceiving others about level of use, using as an escape, and jeopardizing relationships or personal opportunities). This scale was developed with samples of Dutch adolescents (10–17 years old) and has since been validated with adolescent samples in dozens of countries (Boer et al., 2020, 2022; Fung, 2019), including the U.S. (Watson et al., 2020). Items are answered using dichotomous (yes/no) responses. In line with proposed DSM-5 criteria for internet gaming disorder, endorsement of 5 or more items alongside clinically significant symptoms of impairment or distress indicates risk for disordered social media use (van den Eijnden et al., 2016). In the original study, between 7.3% and 11.6% of adolescents were identified as at risk for problematic use. Rates of problematic use as indicated by the SMDS vary between countries, with the average prevalence rate across 44 European countries and Canada reported as 12.9% (Boer et al., 2022). To our knowledge, comparable prevalence rates using this scale with American adolescents have not been published. The full SMDS measure is available from the authors' original paper (van den Eijnden et al., 2016).

A complementary tool, the Social Media Disorder Scale—Parental Version (SMDS-P), is available for caretakers as well (Austermann et al., 2021). The SMDS-P consists of 9 yes/no-items that were adapted for caretakers to report their perceptions of their child's social media use. While universal assessment among caretakers whose adolescents use social media is ideal, the SMDS-P is particularly useful when working with younger patients and teens who may deny or minimize problematic behaviors and symptoms (Austermann et al., 2021). A less stringent cut-off point of 4 endorsed items alongside significant impairment or distress is recommended for the SMDS-P. In the original study, this yielded a higher rate (18.6%) of adolescents labeled at risk for problematic usage. This measure was validated among German caretakers with children between 10 and 17 years old and demonstrated strong convergent validity. Psychometric data suggest moderate concordance between SMDS and SMDS-P, highlighting that caregiver input can provide additional, different information for clinical assessment. Both agreement and discrepancies between child and caregiver reports can provide opportunities for valuable clinical discussions and intervention. The full SMDS-P measure is available in the original paper (Austermann et al., 2021).

Information from the SMDS and SMDS-P should be considered in the context of the full battery of physical, psychosocial, and developmental assessments completed by patients. Social media has become so normative for the current generation of adolescents that it may be difficult for patients or their caregivers to identify potential connections between problematic use and adverse health symptoms (e.g., poor sleep, unhealthy eating behaviors). Given known associations between certain types of social media use and mental health disorders, patients identified as at risk for problematic social media use may warrant additional screenings for other concerns. All patients in this context should be screened for depression and anxiety. Based on the client's age and other clinically relevant information, screening for substance misuse, suicidality, and disordered eating may also be warranted.

Guidance for Caretakers

- Understand that increased use of social media during times of isolation (whether in acute circumstances like holiday breaks from school, or in extreme circumstances such as global pandemics) is a developmentally normative response from adolescents and is not inherently harmful if they are actively engaging in meaningful online relationships.
  - Help monitor the social media content adolescents consume during times of high stress (e.g., global pandemics, racial injustice) because accurate information about crises in appropriate (non-excessive) amounts are protective to their well-being (Mousavi et al., 2023).
- Recognize the importance of allowing children space to explore, gain independence, and socialize without close parental supervision, as this is a normal part of adolescence.
- Pay attention to changes in your child's social media use and any associated changes to mood, behaviors, or health.
- Identify excessive or problematic social media use by whether it is interfering with other key adolescent tasks such as school work, offline socializing and

activities, family time, or overall well-being, rather than simply measuring the amount of time.

- Initiate conversations (not interrogations) about social media use to learn why adolescents are drawn to certain platforms, as well as what they like or don't like.
- Provide education and a safe space for adolescents to identify unsafe or unhealthy social media experiences and feel comfortable coming to you for help.
- Avoid using complete bans on social media as a form of punishment, as social media can be a crucial social tool for adolescents.
- Use shared decision-making with adolescents to determine rules about social media use, such as the times when it can be used, device-free times (e.g., bedtime) and zones (e.g., the dinner table), the types of social media content and behavior that are acceptable, and when to tell a trusted adult about any safety concerns.
  - Tools such as the Family Media Plan created by the American Academy of Pediatrics (American Academy of Pediatrics, n.d.), available for free online, can assist with this process.
- Prioritize quality family time and demonstrate support for adolescents, as these were found to buffer negative outcomes during COVID-19 (Ellis et al., 2020; Magis-Weinberg et al., 2021; Zhen et al., 2021).

Lessons Learned

In an unprecedented period of social isolation and crisis, adolescents turned to social media as a tool for coping and to meet a variety of developmental needs. We saw that active, intentional use of social media to foster one-to-one connections during COVID-19 helped buffer negative outcomes. In a context where access to face-to-face support was limited, social media also provided opportunities for seeking and giving support to adolescents experiencing high levels of distress, including suicidal ideation. However, the stress of providing digital social support to peers in distress should not be placed on adolescent shoulders. There is a need for infrastructure on social media platforms, particularly during periods of widespread crisis, to offer enhanced support and service referrals from trained professionals. This is particularly important for adolescents from marginalized communities (e.g., SGM youth, youth of color) facing disparate levels of stress and disconnection from sources of support. We saw that adolescents experienced unique stressors during this period and often became overwhelmed by COVID-19 information on social media, particularly among users without accurate information about the pandemic. In future crises, public health messaging should be tailored to meet the developmental stage of adolescents and disseminated through platforms most likely to reach young people. Ensuring that adolescents receive an appropriate amount (non-excessive) of accurate crisis information will require active participation from social media platforms, pediatricians, and caretakers. We saw negative changes to aspects of adolescents' mental and physical health during the pandemic as social media supplemented, replaced, or interfered with typical offline activities. In a context where every aspect of young people's routines was already disrupted, social media filled the gaps, sometimes to the point of becoming maladaptive and addictive. During future crises, policy decisions regarding how to restrict people's movement and whether to close facilities should consider these data demonstrating that adolescents generally turn to technology in the absence of other outlets. Finally, it is unknown how much pandemic restrictions and associated increases in social media use during a sensitive developmental period will affect the current cohort of adolescents' developmental trajectories in the long term. Policymakers must fund research and practitioners must stay abreast of the most up-to-date empirical evidence on this subject to help these young people have a healthy transition into adulthood.

Calls to Action
- Understand that, both prior to and after the onset of COVID-19, social media have become a normative component of adolescents' social ecology and interact with psychosocial developmental processes in many ways that are still being studied.
- Recognize social media can contribute to positive, prosocial experiences, or adverse outcomes depending on individual-level factors, types and level of engagement, and broader sociocultural factors, such as global pandemics.
- Assess for social media use among adolescents from a non-pathologizing stance and collaborate with patients and caregivers on targeted interventions based on the patients' unique needs and circumstances.

References

Alderman, E. M. (1994). AMA Guidelines for Adolescent Preventive Services (GAPS): Recommendations and rationale. *JAMA, 272*(12), 980–981. https://doi.org/10.1001/jama.1994.03520120090040

Alonzo, R., Hussain, J., Stranges, S., & Anderson, K. K. (2021). Interplay between social media use, sleep quality, and mental health in youth: A systematic review. *Sleep Medicine Reviews, 56*, 101414. https://doi.org/10.1016/j.smrv.2020.101414

American Academy of Pediatrics. (2021, October 19). *AAP-AACAP-CHA Declaration of a national emergency in child and adolescent mental health.* https://www.aap.org/en/advocacy/child-and-adolescent-healthy-mental-development/aap-aacap-cha-declaration-of-a-national-emergency-in-child-and-adolescent-mental-health/

American Academy of Pediatrics. (n.d.). *Family media plan.* https://www.healthychildren.org/English/fmp/Pages/MediaPlan.aspx

American Psychiatric Association. (2013). *Diagnostic and statistical manual of mental disorders* (5th ed.). https://doi.org/10.1176/appi.books.9780890425596

Austermann, M. I., Thomasius, R., & Paschke, K. (2021). Assessing problematic social media use in adolescents by parental ratings: Development and validation of the Social Media Disorder Scale for Parents (SMDS-P). *Journal of Clinical Medicine, 10*(617), 1–15. https://doi.org/10.3390/jcm10040617

Bailey, E., Boland, A., Bell, I., Nicholas, J., La Sala, L., & Robinson, J. (2022). The mental health and social media use of young Australians during the COVID-19 pandemic. *International Journal of Environmental Research and Public Health, 19*(3), 1077. https://doi.org/10.3390/ijerph19031077

Ballard, P. J., Hoyt, L. T., & Pachucki, M. C. (2019). Impacts of adolescent and young adult civic engagement on health and socioeconomic status in adulthood. *Child Development, 90*(4), 1138–1154. https://doi.org/10.1111/cdev.12998

Barry, C. T., Sidoti, C. L., Briggs, S. M., Reiter, S. R., & Lindsey, R. A. (2017). Adolescent social media use and mental health from adolescent and parent perspectives. *Journal of Adolescence, 61*, 1–11. https://doi.org/10.1016/j.adolescence.2017.08.005

Becker, S. P., & Lienesch, J. A. (2018). Nighttime media use in adolescents with ADHD: Links to sleep problems and internalizing symptoms. *Sleep Medicine, 51*, 171–178. https://doi.org/10.1016/j.sleep.2018.06.021

Boer, M., van den Eijnden, R. J. J. M., Boniel-Nissim, M., Wong, S. L., Inchley, J. C., Badura, P., Craig, W. M., Gobina, I., Kleszczewska, D., Klanšček, H. J., & Stevens, G. W. J. M. (2020). Adolescents' intense and problematic social media use and their well-being in 29 countries. *The Journal of Adolescent Health, 66*(6S), S89–S99. https://doi.org/10.1016/j.jadohealth.2020.02.014

Boer, M., van den Eijnden, R. J. J. M., Finkenauer, C., Boniel-Nissim, M., Marino, C., Inchley, J., Cosma, A., Paakkari, L., & Stevens, G. W. J. M. (2022). Cross-national validation of the social media disorder scale: Findings from adolescents from 44 countries. *Addiction, 117*(3), 784–795. https://doi.org/10.1111/add.15709

Boursier, V., Gioia, F., Musetti, A., & Schimmenti, A. (2023). COVID-19-related fears, stress and depression in adolescents: The role of loneliness and relational closeness to online friends. *Journal of Human Behavior in the Social Environment, 33*, 296–318. https://doi.org/10.1080/10911359.2022.2059605

Brown, B. B., & Larson, J. (2009). Peer relationships in adolescence. In R. M. Lerner & L. Steinberg (Eds.), *Handbook of adolescent psychology: Contextual influences on adolescent development* (pp. 74–103). Wiley. https://doi.org/10.1002/9780470479193.adlpsy002004

Burke, T. A., Kutok, E. R., Dunsiger, S., Nugent, N. R., Patena, J. V., Riese, A., & Ranney, M. L. (2021). A national snapshot of U.S. adolescents' mental health and changing technology use during COVID-19. *General Hospital Psychiatry, 71*, 147–148. https://doi.org/10.1016/j.genhosppsych.2021.05.006

Cauberghe, V., Van Wesenbeeck, I., De Jans, S., Hudders, L., & Ponnet, K. (2021). How adolescents use social media to cope with feelings of loneliness and anxiety during COVID-19 lockdown. *Cyberpsychology, Behavior and Social Networking, 24*(4), 250–257. https://doi.org/10.1089/cyber.2020.0478

Cingel, D. P., Lauricella, A. R., Taylor, L. B., Stevens, H. R., Coyne, S. M., & Wartella, E. (2022). US adolescents' attitudes toward school, social connection, media use, and mental health during the COVID-19 pandemic: Differences as a function of gender identity and school context. *PLoS One, 17*(10), e0276737. https://doi.org/10.1371/journal.pone.0276737

Common Sense Media. (2020). *SurveyMonkey poll: How teens are coping and connecting in the time of the coronavirus.* https://www.commonsensemedia.org/sites/default/files/research/report/2020_surveymonkey-key-findings-toplines-teens-and-coronavirus.pdf

Curtis, B. L., Lookatch, S. J., Ramo, D. E., McKay, J. R., Feinn, R. S., & Kranzler, H. R. (2018). Meta-analysis of the association of alcohol-related social media use with alcohol consumption and alcohol-related problems in adolescents and young adults. *Alcoholism, Clinical and Experimental Research, 42*(6), 978–986. https://doi.org/10.1111/acer.13642

Dimock, M. (2019, January 17). *Defining generations: Where millennials end and generation z begins.* Pew Research Center. https://www.pewresearch.org/short-reads/2019/01/17/where-millennials-end-and-generation-z-begins/

Drouin, M., McDaniel, B. T., Pater, J., & Toscos, T. (2020). How parents and their children used social media and technology at the beginning of the COVID-19 pandemic and associations with anxiety. *Cyberpsychology, Behavior and Social Networking, 23*(11), 727–736. https://doi. org/10.1089/cyber.2020.0284

Ellis, W. E., Dumas, T. M., & Forbes, L. M. (2020). Physically isolated but socially connected: Psychological adjustment and stress among adolescents during the initial COVID-19 crisis. *Canadian Journal of Behavioural Science, 52*(3), 177–187. https://doi.org/10.1037/cbs0000215

Fish, J. N., McInroy, L. B., Paceley, M. S., Williams, N. D., Henderson, S., Levine, D. S., & Edsall, R. N. (2020). "I'm kinda stuck at home with unsupportive parents right now": LGBTQ youths' experiences with COVID-19 and the importance of online support. *The Journal of Adolescent Health, 67*(3), 450–452. https://doi.org/10.1016/j.jadohealth.2020.06.002

Frison, E., & Eggermont, S. (2016). Exploring the relationships between different types of Facebook use, perceived online social support, and adolescents' depressed mood. *Social Science Computer Review, 34*(2), 153–171. https://doi.org/10.1177/0894439314567449

Fumagalli, E., Dolmatzian, M. B., & Shrum, L. J. (2021). Centennials, FOMO, and loneliness: An investigation of the impact of social networking and messaging/VoIP apps usage during the initial stage of the coronavirus pandemic. *Frontiers in Psychology, 12*, 620739. https://doi. org/10.3389/fpsyg.2021.620739

Fung, S. (2019). Cross-cultural validation of the social media disorder scale. *Psychology Research and Behavior Management, 12*, 683–690. https://doi.org/10.2147/PRBM.S216788

Gerwin, R. L., Kaliebe, K., & Daigle, M. (2018). The interplay between digital media use and development. *Child and Adolescent Psychiatric Clinics of North America, 27*(2), 345–355. https://doi.org/10.1016/j.chc.2017.11.002

Gilsbach, S., Plana, M. T., Castro-Fornieles, J., Gatta, M., Karlsson, G. P., Flamarique, I., Raynaud, J.-P., Riva, A., Solberg, A.-L., van Elburg, A. A., Wentz, E., Nacinovich, R., & Herpertz-Dahlmann, B. (2022). Increase in admission rates and symptom severity of childhood and adolescent anorexia nervosa in Europe during the COVID-19 pandemic: Data from specialized eating disorder units in different European countries. *Child and Adolescent Psychiatry and Mental Health, 16*(1), 46. https://doi.org/10.1186/s13034-022-00482-x

Goodyear, V. A., Skinner, B., McKeever, J., & Griffiths, M. (2021). The influence of online physical activity interventions on children and young people's engagement with physical activity: A systematic review. *Physical Education and Sport Pedagogy, 28*, 1–15.

Günther, L., Schleberger, S., & Pischke, C. R. (2021). Effectiveness of social media-based interventions for the promotion of physical activity: Scoping review. *International Journal of Environmental Research and Public Health, 18*(24), 13018.

Hamilton, J. L., Nesi, J., & Choukas-Bradley, S. (2022). Reexamining social media and socioemotional well-being among adolescents through the lens of the COVID-19 pandemic: A theoretical review and directions for future research. *Perspectives on Psychological Science, 17*(3), 662–679. https://doi.org/10.1177/17456916211014189

Hamilton, J. L., Dreier, M. J., & Boyd, S. (2023). Social media as a bridge and a window: The changing relationship of adolescents with social media and digital platforms. *Current Opinion in Psychology, 52*, 101633. https://doi.org/10.1016/j.copsyc.2023.101633

Hanckel, B., & Chandra, S. (2021). *Social media insights from sexuality and gender diverse young people during COVID-19.* Western Sydney University. https://doi.org/10.26183/kvg0-7s37

Hartman-Munick, S. M., Lin, J. A., Milliren, C. E., Braverman, P. K., Brigham, K. S., Fisher, M. M., et al. (2022). Association of the COVID-19 pandemic with adolescent and young adult eating disorder care volume. *JAMA Pediatrics, 176*(12), 1225–1232. https://doi.org/10.1001/jamapediatrics.2022.4346

Hayran, C., & Anik, L. (2021). Well-being and fear of missing out (FOMO) on digital content in the time of COVID-19: A correlational analysis among university students. *International Journal of Environmental Research and Public Health, 18*(1974), 1–13. https://doi.org/10.3390/ijerph18041974

Hong, W., Liu, R. D., Ding, Y., Fu, X., Zhen, R., & Sheng, X. (2021). Social media exposure and college students' mental health during the outbreak of CoViD-19: The mediating role of rumination and the moderating role of mindfulness. *Cyberpsychology, Behavior and Social Networking, 24*(4), 282–287. https://doi.org/10.1089/cyber.2020.0387

Hudimova, A., Popovych, I., Baidyk, V., Buriak, O., & Kechyk, O. (2021). The impact of social media on young web users' psychological well-being during the COVID-19 pandemic progression. *Amazonia Investiga, 10*(39), 50–61. https://doi.org/10.34069/AI/2021.39.03.5

Iannotti, R. J., Janssen, I., Haug, E., Kololo, H., Annaheim, B., Borraccino, A., & HBSC Physical Activity Focus Group. (2009). Interrelationships of adolescent physical activity, screen-based sedentary behaviour, and social and psychological health. *International Journal of Public Health, 54*, 191–198. https://doi.org/10.1007/s00038-009-5410-z

Ivie, E. J., Pettitt, A., Moses, L. J., & Allen, N. B. (2020). A meta-analysis of the association between adolescent social media use and depressive symptoms. *Journal of Affective Disorders, 275*, 165–174. https://doi.org/10.1016/j.jad.2020.06.014

Keles, B., McCrae, N., & Grealish, A. (2020). A systematic review: The influence of social media on depression, anxiety and psychological distress in adolescents. *International Journal of Adolescence and Youth, 25*(1), 79–93. https://doi.org/10.1080/02673843.2019.1590851

Keles, B., Graelish, A., & Leamy, M. (2023). The beauty and the beast of social media: An interpretive phenomenological analysis of the impact of adolescents' social media experiences on their mental health during the COVID-19 pandemic. *Current Psychology*. https://doi.org/10.1007/s12144-023-04271-3

Kırcaburun, K., Kokkinos, C. M., Demetrovics, Z., Kiraly, O., Griffiths, M. D., & Colak, T. S. (2019). Problematic online behaviors among adolescents and emerging adults: Associations between cyberbullying perpetration, problematic social media use, and psychosocial factors. *International Journal of Mental Health and Addiction, 17*, 891–908. https://doi.org/10.1007/s11469-018-9894-8

Li, Y., Zhao, J., Ma, Z., McReynolds, L. S., Lin, D., Chen, Z., Wang, T., Wang, D., Zhang, Y., Zhang, J., Fan, F., & Liu, X. (2021). Mental health among college students during the COVID-19 pandemic in China: A 2-wave longitudinal survey. *Journal of Affective Disorders, 281*, 597–604. https://doi.org/10.1016/j.jad.2020.11.109

Liu, H., Liu, W., Yonganthan, V., & Osburg, V.-S. (2021). COVID-19 information overload and generation Z's social media discontinuance intention during the pandemic lockdown. *Technological Forecasting and Social Change, 166*, 120600. https://doi.org/10.1016/j.techfore.2021.120600

Luo, T., Chen, W., & Liao, Y. (2021). Social media use in China before and during COVID-19: Preliminary results from an online retrospective survey. *Journal of Psychiatric Research, 140*, 35–38. https://doi.org/10.1016/j.jpsychires.2021.05.057

Magis-Weinberg, L., Gys, C. L., Berger, E. L., Domoff, S. E., & Dahl, R. E. (2021). Positive and negative online experiences and loneliness in Peruvian adolescents during the COVID-19 lockdown. *Journal of Research on Adolescence, 31*(3), 717–733. https://doi.org/10.1111/jora.12666

Marciano, L., Ostroumova, M., Schulz, P. J., & Camerini, A. (2022). Digital media use and adolescents' mental health during the COVID-19 pandemic: A systematic review and meta-analysis. *Frontiers in Public Health, 9*, 793868. https://doi.org/10.3389/fpubh.2021.793868

Marengo, D., Fabris, M. A., Longobardi, C., & Settanni, M. (2022). Smartphone and social media use contributed to individual tendencies towards social media addiction in Italian adolescents during the COVID-19 pandemic. *Addictive Behaviors, 126*, 107204. https://doi.org/10.1016/j.addbeh.2021.107204

Mousavi, S. Z., Barry, C. T., & Halter, B. M. (2023). Relations of adolescent knowledge of COVID-19, social media engagement, and experiences during quarantine/lockdown with well-being. *Journal of Child and Family Studies, 32*, 110–121. https://doi.org/10.1007/s10826-022-02465-0

Mude, W., Oguoma, V. M., Nyanhanda, T., Mwanri, L., & Njue, C. (2021). Racial disparities in COVID-19 pandemic cases, hospitalisations, and deaths: A systematic review and meta-analysis. *Journal of Global Health, 11*, 05015. https://doi.org/10.7189/jogh.11.05015

Nesi, J., & Prinstein, M. J. (2019). In search of likes: Longitudinal associations between adolescents' digital status seeking and health-risk behaviors. *Journal of Clinical Child and Adolescent Psychology, 48*(5), 740–748. https://doi.org/10.1080/15374416.2018.1437733

Nesi, J., Burke, T. A., Bettis, A. H., Kudinova, A. Y., Thompson, E. C., MacPherson, H. A., Fox, K. A., Lawrence, H. R., Thomas, S. A., Wolff, J. C., Altemus, M. K., Soriano, S., & Liu, R. T. (2021). Social media use and self-injurious thoughts and behaviors: A systematic review and meta-analysis. *Clinical Psychology Review, 87*, 102038. https://doi.org/10.1016/j.cpr.2021.102038

Nesi, J., Mann, S., & Robb, M. B. (2023). *Teens and mental health: How girls really feel about social media*. Common Sense Media.

Nguyen, T. T., Criss, S., Dwivedi, P., Huang, D., Keralis, J., Hsu, E., Phan, L., et al. (2020). Exploring U.S. shifts in anti-Asian sentiment with the emergence of COVID-19. *International Journal of Environmental Research and Public Health, 17*(19), 7032. https://doi.org/10.3390/ijerph17197032

Nilsson, A., Rosendahl, I., & Jayaram-Lindstrom, N. (2022). Gaming and social media use among adolescents in the midst of the COVID-19 pandemic. *Nordic Studies on Alcohol and Drugs, 39*(4), 347–361. https://doi.org/10.1177/14550725221074997

O'Dea, B., & Campbell, A. (2011). Online social networking amongst teens: Friend or foe? *Annual Review of Cybertherapy and Telemedicine, 2011*, 133–138. https://doi.org/10.3233/978-1-60750-766-6-133

Odgers, C. L., & Jensen, M. R. (2020). Annual research review: Adolescent mental health in the digital age: Facts, fears, and future directions. *Journal of Child Psychology and Psychiatry, 61*(3), 336–348. https://doi.org/10.1111/jcpp.13190

Odgers, C. L., Schueller, S. M., & Ito, M. (2020). Screen time, social media use, and adolescent development. *Annual Review of Developmental Psychology, 2*, 485–502. https://doi.org/10.1146/annurev-devpsych-121318-084815

Orben, A. (2020). Teenagers, screens and social media: A narrative review of reviews and key studies. *Social Psychiatry and Psychiatric Epidemiology, 55*, 407–414. https://doi.org/10.1007/s00127-019-01825-4

Pagano, M., Bacaro, V., & Crocetti, E. (2023). "Using digital media or sleeping… that is the question". A meta-analysis on digital media use and unhealthy sleep in adolescence. *Computers in Human Behavior, 146*, 107813. https://doi.org/10.1016/j.chb.2023.107813

Parry, D. A., Fisher, J. T., Mieczkowski, H., Sewall, C. J. R., & Davidson, B. I. (2022). Social media and well-being: A methodological perspective. *Current Opinion in Psychology, 45*, 101285. https://doi.org/10.1016/j.copsyc.2021.11.005

Paschke, K., Austermann, M. I., & Thomasius, R. (2021). ICD-11-based assessment of social media use disorder in adolescents: Development and validation of the social media use disorder scale for adolescents. *Frontiers in Psychiatry, 12*(661483), 1–16. https://doi.org/10.3389/fpsyt.2021.661483

Primack, B. A., Shensa, A., Escobar-Viera, C. G., Barrett, E. L., Sidani, J. E., Colditz, J. B., & James, A. E. (2017). Use of multiple social media platforms and symptoms of depression and anxiety: A nationally-representative study among U.S. young adults. *Computers in Human Behavior, 69*, 1–9. https://doi.org/10.1016/j.chb.2016.11.013

Rahman, A. M., & Chandrasekaran, B. (2021). Estimating the impact of the pandemic on children's physical health: A scoping review. *The Journal of School Health, 91*(11), 936–947. https://doi.org/10.1111/josh.13079

Rideout, V., Peebles, A., Mann, S., & Robb, M. B. (2022). *Common sense census: Media use by tweens and teens, 2021*. Common Sense.

Rose, T., Barker, M., Jacob, C. M., Morrison, L., Lawrence, W., Strömmer, S., Vogel, C., Woods-Townsend, K., Farrell, D., Inskip, H., & Baird, J. (2017). A systematic review of digital interventions for improving the diet and physical activity behaviors of adolescents. *The Journal of Adolescent Health, 61*(6), 669–677.

Rosen, A. O., Holmes, A. L., Balluerka, N., Hidalgo, M. D., Gorostiaga, A., Gomez-Benito, J., & Huedo-Medina, T. B. (2022). Is social media a new type of social support? Social media use in Spain during the COVID-19 pandemic: A mixed methods study. *International Journal of Environmental Research and Public Health, 19*, 3952. https://doi.org/10.3390/ijerph19073952

Subrahmanyam, K., Smahel, D., & Greenfield, P. (2006). Connecting developmental constructions to the Internet: Identity presentation and sexual exploration in online teen chat rooms. *Developmental Psychology, 42*(3), 395–406. https://doi.org/10.1037/0012-1649.42.3.395

Sugaya, N., Shirasaka, T., Takahashi, K., & Kanda, H. (2019). Bio-psychosocial factors of children and adolescents with internet gaming disorder: A systematic review. *BioPsychoSocial Medicine, 13*, 3. https://doi.org/10.1186/s13030-019-0144-5

Sun, Y., & Zhang, Y. (2021). A review of theories and models applied in studies of social media addiction and implications for future research. *Addictive Behaviors, 114*, 106699. https://doi.org/10.1016/j.addbeh.2020.106699

Tao, X., & Fisher, C. B. (2022). Exposure to social media racial discrimination and mental health among adolescents of color. *Journal of Youth and Adolescence, 51*, 30–44. https://doi.org/10.1007/s10964-021-01514-z

Temple, J. R., Baumler, E., Wood, L., Guillot-Wright, S., Torres, L., & Thiel, M. (2022). The impact of the COVID-19 pandemic on adolescent mental health and substance use. *The Journal of Adolescent Health, 71*, 277–284.

Thorn. (2023). *LGBTQ+ youth perspectives: How LGBTQ+ youth are navigating exploration and risks of sexual exploitation online.* https://info.thorn.org/hubfs/Research/Thorn_LGBTQ+YouthPerspectives_June2023_FNL.pdf

U.S. Department of Health and Human Services. (2023, May 23). *Surgeon general issues new advisory about effects social media use has on youth mental health.* https://www.pewresearch.org/internet/2022/08/10/teens-social-media-and-technology-2022/

Valkenburg, P. M., & Peter, J. (2013). The differential susceptibility to media effects model. *The Journal of Communication, 63*(2), 221–243. https://doi.org/10.1111/jcom.12024

Vall-Roque, H., Andres, A., & Saldana, C. (2021). The impact of COVID-19 lockdown on social network sites use, body image disturbances and self-esteem among adolescent and young women. *Progress in Neuro-Psychopharmacology and Biological Psychiatry, 110*, 110293. https://doi.org/10.1016/j.pnpbp.2021.110293

van den Eijnden, R. J. J. M., Lemmens, J. S., & Valkenburg, P. M. (2016). The social media disorder scale: Validity and psychometric properties. *Computers in Human Behavior, 61*, 478–487. https://doi.org/10.1016/j.chb.2016.03.038

Van Harmelen, A. L., Kievit, R. A., Ioannidis, K., Neufeld, S., Jones, P. B., Bullmore, E., Dolan, R., Fonagy, P., & Goodyer, I. (2017). Adolescent friendships predict later resilient functioning across psychosocial domains in a healthy community cohort. *Psychological Medicine, 47*(13), 2312–2322. https://doi.org/10.1017/S0033291717000836

Vannucci, A., Simpson, E. G., Gagnon, S., & Ohannessian, C. M. C. (2020). Social media use and risky behaviors in adolescents: A meta-analysis. *Journal of Adolescence, 79*, 258–274. https://doi.org/10.1016/j.adolescence.2020.01.014

Vogels, E. A., Gelles-Watnick, R., & Massarat, N. (2022). *Teens, social media and technology 2022.* Pew Research Center. https://www.pewresearch.org/internet/2022/08/10/teens-social-media-and-technology-2022/

Wang, P., Wang, X., Wu, Y., Xie, X., Wang, X., Zhao, F., et al. (2018). Social networking sites addiction and adolescent depression: A moderated mediation model of rumination and self-esteem. *Personality and Individual Differences, 127*, 162–167. https://doi.org/10.1016/j.paid.2018.02.008

Watson, J. C., Prosek, E. A., & Giordano, A. L. (2020). Investigating psychometric properties of social media addiction measures among adolescents. *Journal of Counseling and Development, 98*(4), 458–466. https://doi.org/10.1002/jcad.12347

Wilf, S., & Wray-Lake, L. (2021). "That's how revolutions happen": Psychopolitical resistance in youth's online civic engagement. *Journal of Adolescent Research, 39*, 827–860. https://doi.org/10.1177/07435584211062121

Woods, H. C., & Scott, H. (2016). # Sleepyteens: Social media use in adolescence is associated with poor sleep quality, anxiety, depression and low self-esteem. *Journal of Adolescence, 51*, 41–49. https://doi.org/10.1016/j.adolescence.2016.05.008

World Health Organization. (2019). *International statistical classification of diseases and related health problems* (11th ed.). https://icd.who.int/

Yazdani, N., Hoyt, L. T., Castro, E. M., & Cohen, A. K. (2022). Sociopolitical influences in early emerging adult college students' pandemic-related civic engagement. *Emerging Adulthood, 10*(4), 1041–1047. https://doi.org/10.1177/21676968221098296

Zhang, S., Liu, M., Li, Y., & Chung, J. E. (2021). Teen's social media engagement during the COVID-19 pandemic: A time series examination of posting and emotion on Reddit. *International Journal of Environmental Research and Public Health, 18*, 10079. https://doi.org/10.3390/ijerph181910079

Zhao, N., & Zhou, G. (2021). COVID-19 stress and addictive social media use (SMU): Mediating role of active use and social media flow. *Frontiers in Psychiatry, 12*, 635546. https://doi.org/10.3389/fpsyt.2021.635546

Zhen, L., Nan, Y., & Pham, B. (2021). College students coping with COVID-19: Stress-buffering effects of self-disclosure on social media and parental support. *Communication Research Reports, 38*(1), 23–31. https://doi.org/10.1080/08824096.2020.1870445

Disinfodemic: Responding to Rising Misinformation

Jessica L. Peck, Catrin Gagne, and Tara E. Wise

A lie can travel halfway around the world while the truth is still putting on its shoes.

—Mark Twain

Introduction and Background

The COVID-19 pandemic presented extraordinary and unprecedented challenges of communicating information during a time of crisis. Science by its very nature is slow, careful, and regulated while internet communication can be fast, careless, and unregulated. A single scientific research study (excluding longitudinal methodology) generally reflects a moment in time and requires rigorous repetition in seeking trends over time to eventually provide verified information to guide clinical recommendations based on sound science. However, with the declaration of a global public health emergency and subsequent immediate cataclysmic changes to everyday life in the face of fear-laden reports of mass casualties came an overwhelming demand from the public for immediate information. Daily briefings from the United States White House began in March of 2020, quickly followed by divergent interpretations of emerging science from sources previously viewed as generally credible, as health professionals and governmental, organizational, and civic leaders scrambled to make high-stakes decisions with very little information often in a severely compressed time frame while the general public anxiously awaited implementation and impact. While the scientific community had a structure and nomenclature accustomed to nuanced, technical, high-level debate as data emerged and interpretations evolved, the general public perceived this evolving information and contradictory discussions as unstable, unreliable, and untrustworthy.

J. L. Peck (✉) · C. Gagne · T. E. Wise
Louise Herrington School of Nursing, Baylor University, Dallas, TX, USA
e-mail: jessica_peck@baylor.edu

J. L. Peck (ed.), *COVID-19 Impacts on Child Health*,
https://doi.org/10.1007/978-3-031-80369-7_17

313

Information is composed of accurate facts to the best of an individual's current knowledge. It can change over time as researchers and experts discover more about a subject matter. Although understanding of mechanisms underlying the spread of the novel coronavirus disease (COVID-19) was minimal initially, scientific research and data gathering have gradually improved what is known with more certainty. However, as the virus continues to evolve, research, learning, and recommendations must evolve with it to provide credible information in a timely manner. The lack of objective, credible information during the start of the COVID-19 pandemic created ripe opportunities for misinformation and disinformation to flourish as even professional healthcare providers (HCPs) resorted to forming informal social media communication groups to share unverified, boots-on-the-ground kinds of information in real time.

Misinformation is false information but is created without intent to cause harm and is often initiated by someone who desires to understand a topic and aims to protect others from negative impacts (Oswald et al., 2022). Persons believe that they are sharing beneficial information, not realizing the information is false or discredited or can cause harmful results (World Health Organization, 2023). The motivation of misinformation can be individual desire to convey a sense of expertise or a misguided but beneficent intention to be helpful (Posetti & Bontcheva, 2020a, 2020b). Misinformation flourished on social media during a 2022 crisis in which US supply chain disruption and product recalls caused a severe shortage of infant formula. Panic buying ensued accompanied by well-meaning persons on social media who shared viral posts with potentially harmful recipes for homemade formula as well as advice on switching to other forms of animal milk, diluting formula to make it last longer, and other recommendations eschewed by pediatric professional clinicians who voiced frustration at parents' willingness to so easily accept the information as credible while expressing doubt toward more credible, evidence-based recommendations from primary care providers (Holcombe, 2022).

Disinformation is false information intentionally created and/or spread to generate profit or intentionally cause harm to a person, a group of people, an organization, or a country, and generally serves an agenda. Often, disinformation may be rooted in true scientific facts, but distorted, misrepresented, or presented out of context, which makes it harder to discern what is true and what is false (Brennan et al., 2020). Disinformation causes confusion, distrust and negative health impacts and undermines public health efforts. The United States experienced disinformation from both foreign and domestic sources during the COVID-19 pandemic, which inflamed erosion of trust in government and public institutions' response to the pandemic (World Health Organization, 2023). Motivators for disinformation are diverse: earning profit, scoring political advantage, undermining confidence, shifting blame, polarizing people, and undermining institutional or systems-based responses to the pandemic.

The concept behind a **disinfodemic** is not novel, nor is it specific to healthcare. Disinformation is spread on many topics such as politics, social life, finances, and the natural environment. In a well-known prior case, widespread fear and misinformation originated with a small-scale study ($n = 12$) published (1998) in the Lancet medical journal by a British physician and 12 colleagues, suggesting that the measles mumps rubella (MMR) vaccine may predispose children to autism. The study was retracted amidst allegations of scientific misconduct but nevertheless, vaccination for MMR broadly declined. There are still families who adhere to the ensuing recommendations resulting from the study that have been widely discredited throughout scientific and public health communities by subsequent rigorous, credible research (https://journals.plos.org/plosone/article?id=10.1371/journal.pone.0256395; https://pmc.ncbi.nlm.nih.gov/articles/PMC3136032/).

The United Nations Educational Scientific and Cultural Organization (UNESCO) uses the term *disinfodemic* in reference to excessive dimensions of mis- and disinformation driven by the COVID-19 pandemic and its impacts (Posetti & Bontcheva, 2020b). Disinformation regarding diagnosis, treatment, prevention, and cure for COVID-19 was particularly harmful because it threatened the credibility of good-faith clinical practices and partners in their efforts based on medical science to contain the virus, significantly damaging public trust and inflaming public fears (Posetti & Bontcheva, 2020a, 2020b; Zviyita et al., 2022). Additionally, disinformation delayed access to care, negatively affecting health status (Polyzou et al., 2023). The internet is a key distribution mechanism for information, misinformation, and disinformation, easily transporting runaway narratives that capture public sentiment and guide health behavior choices at an astonishingly rapid pace fueled by influencers and like-minded communities that the scientific medical community simply cannot match in scope (Posetti & Bontcheva, 2020a, 2020b). Disinformation can lead to risk-taking behaviors where people endanger themselves by ignoring professional medical advice. It amplifies distrust in policymakers and governments and diverts journalists' efforts toward reactive disproving of falsehoods instead of proactive reporting of new information (Polyzou et al., 2023; Posetti & Bontcheva, 2020a, 2020b). Disinformation can contribute to public confusion and even outrage, vaccine-related fears, and rejection of public health measures proven effective while more easily accepting other unproven treatments. It also contributes to clinician burnout and exhaustion related to the time and energy necessary to calmly, kindly, and professionally respond to patient inquiries about mis- or disinformation when growing numbers of patients then promptly disregard the advice they are given (Peck & Sonney, 2021; https://www.jpedhc.org/article/S0891-5245(23)00214-6/fulltext). In some extreme cases, persons who felt misled, deceived, or coerced or forced into health protective measures harassed and/or committed violence against public health workers, HCPs, airline staff, and other frontline workers tasked with communicating or enforcing evolving public health measures (Polyzou et al., 2023; U.S. Surgeon General, 2021). Before the COVID-19 pandemic, one in four physicians reported being personally attacked on social media, but increased to 60% of physicians after COVID-19 with 15% receiving threats to their lives (Polyzou et al., 2023). Healthcare workers were more likely to be assaulted in the workplace during the pandemic, in the face of already disproportionately high rates of violence prior to the pandemic (Zhang et al., 2023). Emergency medical services workers reported an increase in violence during non-emergent calls correlating with the onset of the COVID-19 pandemic (Ekşi et al., 2022).

The COVID-19 disinfodemic has been grouped into format types and are characterized by themes. Disinformation format types are the platforms or avenues for spreading misinformation, while themes are the ideas and practices within the format. There are four main disinfodemic format types that generate content driven by feelings and beliefs (Posetti & Bontcheva, 2020a, 2020b).

- **Emotive narrative:** Emotional language with incomplete information or opinions expressed with minimal basis for truth
- **False sources:** Fake government and institutional websites that may appear to be plausible information within the news genre
- **Misleading media:** Fabricated or decontextualized images and videos, such as memes, that create mistrust
- **Disinformation campaigns:** Orchestrated campaigns of disinformation agents infiltrate online communities to cause chaos and advance geopolitical agendas

Themes of the disinfodemic are ideas or practices implemented through the four formats above.

Key themes of the disinfodemic have been suggested as follows:

- *Origin and spread of the disease:* Lack of clarity, transparency, and clear communication about the origin and spread of the pandemic fueled speculation, unease, and distrust.
- *False and misleading statistics:* False statistics can easily blend in with other legitimate findings or a singular study can be taken out of context and create confusion.
- *Economic impacts:* Social isolation directly impacted economic productivity with manufacturing shutdowns, supply chain bottlenecks, and loss of jobs and income.
- *Erosion in confidence in journalists and credible news outlets:* Politicized information regarding COVID-19 disseminated through news outlets undermined public trust and generated demand for alternative outlets which then could capitalize on audience potential.
- *Disinformation about treatment:* Disinformation about COVID-19 symptoms, diagnosis, treatment, immunity, prevention, and cure proliferated. Evidence-based practice embraces a triad of best available evidence, clinician experience, and patient preference. Lack of information combined with lockdown restrictions gave health care consumers time to search for information on the internet or seek it from their social network. Clinicians were faced with the challenge of public demand for experimental treatments, risky prevention strategies, and unproven cures and struggled to balance patient preference in the absence of evidence but fear of regulatory license oversight and potentially negative repercussions of prescribing these.
- *Impacts on society and the environment:* Lockdowns, stay-at-home orders, panic purchasing, absence of social gatherings, and loss of safety nets disrupted established prior practices of sharing information.
- *Politicization:* Partisan differences in public opinion emerged, with sharp divides over perceptions of governmental response to the pandemic

- *Content driven by fraudulent financial gain:* Through the age of internet access, content driven by fraudulent financial gain has risen, allowing users to become more susceptible to this type of disinformation through phishing and other forms of scamming. For example, some COVID-19 testing services were illegitimate with the intention of stealing sensitive information for financial gain (U.S. Department of Health and Human Services, 2023b).

Points of Care

Social Media

Over the past decade, social media has emerged as a dominant platform for information distribution, particularly consumer-generated information. Disinformation is often spread on social media platforms and can overpower legitimate information sources. In response, public health agencies increased their presence on key social media platforms, creating content and collaborating with social media influencers to curate and disseminate prevention messages (Basch et al., 2021; Cartwright et al., 2023). For example, in 2020, the state of Texas used a small portion of a $6 million campaign budget to pay influencers to promote mask use and social distancing on TikTok (Basch et al., 2021), prompting urgent need for further discussion on the ethics of paid public health messaging in rapidly evolving communication contexts. However, social media is also used to disseminate disinformation when either well-meaning but ill-informed persons or individuals with ignoble intent have disproportionate power to influence. One estimate suggested only 12 individual [so-called] superspreaders (including anti-vaccine advocates and alternative health entrepreneurs) were allegedly responsible for 65% of COVID-19-related information labeled as mis- or disinformation spread on popular social media platforms (Basch et al., 2021). Public outrage from some sectors over accusations of censorship and violation of First Amendment rights by social media companies unfairly moderating content or implementing bias in banning users led to highly publicized Congressional hearings and ongoing robust debate over free speech and the ethics of how information is categorized as mis- or disinformation, who or what entity gets to make that call, and the ethics of such censorship while balancing the right to free speech with protection of the public (Bond, 2021).

While there are challenges and causes for concern regarding unregulated sharing of COVID-19 content on social media, social media can play a vital role in disseminating accurate information rapidly. To the frustration of many and at times to the detriment of public good, content created by official public health agencies or credible health institutions and posted on their accounts often receives fewer views than communications posted by famous entertainers, influencers, or even ordinary consumer influencers (Basch et al., 2021). Younger generations and students use social media platforms to stay updated on daily news. Research shows 50% of adults get news at least sometimes from social media, and half or more of people ages 18–29 get their news primarily from Snapchat, TikTok, Reddit, and Facebook (Pew Research Center, 2024). Young people consider social media a primary source of credible information, and the majority share information posted without taking specific intentional steps to ensure the association of authenticity, including verifying the date of original publication to ensure the advice is current or verifying the information is generated by a credible source. Clickbait is content generated with the goal of attracting as many internet users as possible to click and navigate to a specific site, usually for financial gain of the poster (GFC Global, n.d.). Clickbait can amplify misinformation and disinformation with rapid spread. Partnerships between experienced content creators and credible health sources may help extend the reach of accurate health information on social media (Ali, 2020; Basch et al., 2021).

Education on evaluating credibility of information sources must be geared toward a heterogeneous population, with careful consideration of age, beliefs, culture, sociodemographics, literacy, and information-seeking sources. Gearing evidence-based content at the appropriate eHealth literacy level can allow for advancement in dissemination of credible COVID-19 information through social media avenues (Basch et al., 2021; Yammine, 2020). Digital media literacy curriculum in schools at all levels should empower children and young adults to be astute to the need to be savvy, well-informed consumers and recognize the spread of mis- and disinformation from uncredible sources on social media, while encouraging responsible sharing of information among their social communities.

Johns Hopkins offers the following advice for evaluating information credibility on social media sources:

1. The location of the poster—are they in the same location they are posting news about? Does the poster work in the field they are posting about?
2. The network—who is in the poster's network, and who follows them? Do you know this account? Is this an account you normally follow or is it being advertised in your feed or shared by someone else?
3. The content—can the information be corroborated from other credible sources?
4. Contextual updates—does the poster usually post about this topic? If so, what did the past or updated posts say? Do they fill in more details or give additional context or links to other sources of information to verify what they are saying?
5. Age—what is the age of the account in question? (Be wary of recently created accounts). What is the age of the content? Is this old news being recirculated?
6. Reliability—is the source of information reliable? (Johns Hopkins, 2023)

It is essential for parents to initiate discussion with children who have access to social media news sources and equip them to evaluate the credibility of information sources, with an invitation to bring any information in question to the parent or trusted adult for further scrutiny. Parents should talk with their children and have family discussions about what news sources will be considered credible, reliable, and trustworthy to guide family decision-making. A child or teen cannot only be personally harmed by mis- or disinformation, but they can harm others by distributing false information to their peers easily via social media and other digital information sharing. Children are active on social media and online settings and as users, they are not always prepared, continuously monitored, or cognitively capable of deciphering credible from uncredible. This can cause unnecessary fear and anxiety if children are exposed to and believe false information. Targeting children with disinformation is not uncommon because children use the internet to gain knowledge and are more likely to share it. The novelty and uniqueness of information are more appealing to young populations, creating an avenue for sharing disinformation. Although children in Generations Z and Alpha are born into a digital era as digital natives, they are not born as sophisticated, critical consumers of information. This is a skill that must be taught by parents and other adults who did not grow up in a digital world and often find it less intuitive and more difficult to navigate than their children do, creating opportunity for effective parent/child partnership to evaluate information together. Educating children on media literacy is crucial to empower them when navigating online activity (Howard et al., 2021).

Parents, pediatric health professionals, and educators can provide children with developmentally appropriate media literacy tools. Commitment to protecting children from disinformation acquired from the internet by improving media literacy is critical to successful interventions. Literacy skills applied to digital media are not the sole solution to prevent disinformation, but media literacy is a start. The minimum age set by federal policy governing responsibilities of digital data governance in the Childrens' Online Privacy Protection Rule is 13 years of age; however, this is very easy to get around by simply checking a box asserting the age of 13 and is often done with parental assent and subsequent parental confidence in their ability to be vigilant of their child's online activities and trust in personal responsibility of the child (Kohli, 2023). Parents are often caught off guard by the legal implications of violating an online platform's terms of use in regard to age requirement and don't realize it could void any legal protections available to qualified users should something nefarious happen to their child online. Investing in media and information literacy programs and training opportunities for educators and parents is helpful, and advocating for further research is needed to encourage policy decisions (Howard et al., 2021).

Lawmakers are approaching the issue of child social media use and safety from a legislative front. Utah recently signed the Social Media Regulation Act into law, which will limit minors' social media access between the hours of 10:30 pm and 6:30 am and require parental consent to access social media accounts such as Twitter, Instagram, and TikTok. The bill also allows Utah parents or guardians to access all their children's posts and prohibits social media companies from advertising to minors, collecting information about them, or targeting content to them. The law allowed for a year before implementation to seek public comment with consideration for technical logistics of implementing age verification. While other states proposed similar legislation in Utah's wake, Florida took Utah's law a step farther, introducing proposed legislation enacting an absolute ban on social media for all children in the state less than 16 years of age, requiring companies to delete pre-existing accounts (Bohannon, 2024). At the time of this writing, the United State Congress has pending legislation entitled the Kids Online Safety Act (KOSA), a bi-partisan proposal to enact sweeping reforms with a host of enhanced safety measures that social media companies would be required to enact that achieved support in the Senate with an affirmative vote of 91 with only 3 opposing (Blumenthal & Blackburn, 2024). Surrounding this is public debate over how to balance child safety with adult rights and expectations of privacy. These acts are generated in response to a wide variety of documented harms occurring through social media use and exposure to mis- and disinformation that could increase risk-taking behaviors is among them. Absolute prohibition of social media use by teens is likely unrealistic; however, educating young people on proper use of media platforms and empowering children to identify disinformation is essential. Creating opportunities for children to increase their media literacy and resilience allows critical thinking skills to expand (Howard et al., 2021).

While social media use can be problematic and have complexities of information sharing for adult populations, children have unique susceptibilities to mis- and disinformation. Children ages 7-to-12 think concretely, seeing things in terms of absolutes and in clearly demarcated categories such as "good" or "bad" and "right" or "wrong." At around 13 years of age, children start a cognitive development process of abstract thinking called formal operations. Younger teens are developmentally predisposed to mis- and disinformation because of limitations in cognitive development and an established neural framework of concrete thinking in which they are generally more trusting to accept things at face value. As formal operations begin to develop, older teens start to learn to carefully consider and discern messages they see on social media and are better able to consider complexities and nuances of such messaging. Providers can discuss with parents ways to determine if their teen is entering the formal operational thinking stage and becoming better able to navigate the nuances of evaluating information sources.

These characteristics of abstract thinking to consider can include:

- Actively considering new possibilities or exploring new ways of doing things
- Independently forming new ideas or asking questions about family beliefs or rules
- Considering many viewpoints and the feelings of others when thinking about a situation
- Sharing their thought process aloud when making decisions
- Asking questions about global concepts such as justice, history, and politics
- Talking about long-term plans and goals

Primary, Secondary, and Tertiary Prevention

Primary, secondary, and tertiary prevention can be used as a framework to prevent or debunk disinformation with relevant health messaging. Primary prevention includes messaging surrounding interventions to prevent COVID-19 infections with time-tested public health measures including effective handwashing, informed vaccine administration in recommended populations, advising proper-fitting mask-wearing in the presence of significant individual risk factors, social distancing in communities with increased transmission or for individuals with high-risk factors, and isolating when symptomatic with an active COVID-19 infection. Information about these interventions should be posted on well-established social media platforms by credible accounts and made easy to share. Secondary prevention includes messaging surrounding preventative measures leading to early diagnosis and prompt treatment. For example, social media platforms should direct users to reputable COVID-19 testing centers and provide real-time care management information with easy connections to escalate care access when needed. Tertiary prevention focuses messaging outreach on people who have already been affected by COVID-19 with a goal to prevent complications and reduce long-term side effects. Providers, governments, and both private and public health organizations can partner with social media influencers to post education on preventing infection, managing COVID-19 symptoms, and accessing high-quality care (Chikandiwa et al., 2022). Further information on developing an ethical framework for such partnerships is needed.

Another way to utilize social media for prevention of disinformation is the creation of a machine-learning tool utilizing artificial intelligence (AI) to assist social media platforms, online service providers, and government agencies in identifying and responding to misinformation or disinformation on social media (Alsmadi et al., 2024; Bontridder & Poullet, 2021; Cartwright et al., 2023) although many ethical and legal questions remain over implementation of such tools as concerns over censorship and suppression of free speech continue to grow. Debate over the boundaries in censorship of information is ongoing in litigation, legislative regulation, platform policies, and terms of use and other public communication forums. Public perception of lack of transparency in information sharing from governmental or other authoritative sources along with concurrent concerns over free speech suppression, biased censorship, arbitrary "fact checking," or banning of those who organically share information across social networks fuels mistrust and resentment (Grossman & Shapiro, 2023). The social and political complexities of this dynamic are beyond the scope of this chapter but it is important to consider in the context of the mindset of children and their families presenting for care and the need for transparency and respect in the patient–provider relationship.

Mistrust in Healthcare

Providers are responsible for maintaining their credentials and licensure and using their clinical expertise to ethically and responsibly guide patients on disease prevention, diagnosis and management, and available treatments. The disinfodemic accelerated the so-called death of expertise. In the early days of COVID-19, pediatric offices were empty as common childhood illnesses decreased because of lack of exposure resulting from social distancing while other families experienced fear in accessing their care environment with worries of COVID-19 exposure. In the absence of regular provider encounters and communication with families and with nationwide stay-at-home orders, parents increasingly sought information from their social networks and internet sources rather than their HCPs (Rivkees, 2023). Public trust in the healthcare system was declining even before the beginning of the pandemic, and the spread of misinformation regarding COVID-19 elevated this distrust.

Disinformation and lack of trust in healthcare are more common in marginalized populations who have experienced historical discrimination and who experience persistent health inequities including minoritized communities (Khullar et al., 2020). Perceptions of racism and inequality are inflamed by dissemination of disinformation. Xenophobia was evident at the onset of the COVID-19 pandemic, with reports of some public hostility demonstrated particularly toward persons of Asian ethnicity, occurring throughout the United States and around the world (Ali, 2020). The danger of mis- or disinformation is epitomized by its ability to incite violence and crime targeted at racial and ethnic minorities, including children (Ali et al., 2021).

When parents lose trust in their child's HCP, genuinely placed distrust can lead to well-intentioned but potentially harmful parental trial or adoption of treatments unsupported by research. General adherence to HCP recommendations and willingness to follow therapy modalities derives from a trusting foundation (Caronia & Ranzani, 2024). Trust between patient and HCP with a mutually respectful shared decision-making model is pivotal to optimal healthcare outcomes. Trust in a HCP decreases as parents increasingly become savvy healthcare consumers who first seek free information about a health issue from the internet and social networks before turning to the services of a HCP. Parents are increasingly turning to fragmented care environments such as urgent and emergent care or telehealth for convenience, diluting the frequency of interactions with a primary HCP in which there is opportunity to build trust for respectful, shared decision-making in which the expertise of the HCP in pediatric health is partnered with the primary influence of parental expertise based on lived experience with their own child. In addition, well-child care was severely disrupted and delayed, limiting opportunity for conversation and anticipatory guidance. This displaced continuity of care with primary care providers inflamed parental mistrust among conflicting provider recommendations on COVID-19 and negatively impacted child and family relationships with their HCP (Hong & Roy, 2023). There is a growing unease arising from parents toward pediatric HCPs as fears of subverting or usurping parental authority are inflamed by frightening, isolated reported cases of misplaced trust in a HCP. A recent high-profile case of what is being referred to as "medical kidnapping" captured the attention of the public in a highly publicized documentary and subsequent court case in which the family of a young girl was awarded $261 million in damages for false imprisonment after medical providers suspected maternal child abuse (Hauser, 2023). In addition, rising public conflict over issues like gender-based and reproductive rights allowing adolescents to seek care without parental consent contribute to growing unease or outright mistrust of clinician motivation to give a child access to care even if it is in clear opposition to parental preference. When clinician expertise is partnered respectfully with parental perspective and child voice, there is optimal opportunity for child health to flourish.

Off-Label Prescription Demand

Healthcare providers sometimes prescribe medications off-label based on best available evidence, which can cause an ethical dilemma, particularly for children. There is often a lack of research regarding dosing, efficacy, and safety of medication specifically for children and particularly for new or emerging therapies. This can be partially attributed to unfamiliarity with age-related developmental pharmacology in pediatric patients, ethical considerations limiting pharmaceutical research on children, and a lack of financial incentive for the pharmaceutical industry to do so (Allen et al., 2018). Parents may read about a prescriptive therapy online or hear an advertisement and expect HCPs to offer the medication or prescribe it upon request; however, pediatric HCPs are often understandably uncomfortable prescribing medications off-label. Medications approved for adult therapy are rarely simultaneously approved for children, meaning parents may get a prescription for themselves and then struggle to understand why they cannot get the same treatment for their children. Parents may then perceive HCPs as arbitrarily withholding prescriptions that seem to be safe in their estimation of information networks or according to personal experiences with themselves, friends or family.

Ivermectin is a medication that has been available for the last four decades with the initial purpose of treating roundworm parasites (https://pmc.ncbi.nlm.nih.gov/articles/PMC9135450/). Interest in ivermectin as a therapy soared after Australian researchers found it killed the COVID-19 virus in a laboratory setting, but at much higher doses than were recommended for prescribing. Based on current very low to low certainty, there is still a lack of professional scientific consensus regarding the safety and effectiveness of using ivermectin to treat COVID-19 (Popp et al., 2021). The overall reliable evidence does not support using ivermectin to treat or prevent COVID-19 outside of well-designed randomized controlled trials, and its use for such is not supported by the Federal Food and Drug Association (FDA, 2020), National Institute for Health (NIH) COVID Treatment Guidelines (discontinued and archived as of March 2024) (https://www.npr.org/sections/health-shots/2024/03/19/1239276507/nih-covid-treatment-guidelines) or the manufacturer at the time of this writing (U.S. Department of Health & Human Services, 2023a; Popp et al., 2021). Adverse reactions of ivermectin in children can include pruritus, skin rash, fever, fatigue, lymphadenopathy, arthralgia, tachycardia, hypotension (including orthostatic hypotension), edema, and abdominal pain (Campillo et al., 2021). Because ivermectin is used as a veterinary therapy for de-worming, concern ensued about human consumption of medication formulated for animals, leading the FDA to post on X (formerly known as Twitter) *"You are not a horse. You are not a cow. Seriously y'all. Stop it."* (Twitter, 2021), highlighting the problematic complexity of public interpretation of stodgy government agencies attempting to display relevance as contemporary influencers. However, many families perceived a therapy that had been on the market for 40 years without major incident to be a risk worth taking. This case study presents the serious dilemma of pediatric clinicians making prescribing decisions in real time in the best interests of children and their families when information is limited with a still-emerging scientific consensus. Providers are faced with risk assessment and risk assumption in prescribing with very real considerations of avoiding risk of endangering the status of their medical license if penalized for improper prescribing, a situation which emphasizes the need for established provider/patient relationships in which there is mutual trust and shared decision-making with informed consent and respect for both parental and provider boundaries.

Barriers and Breakthroughs

Provider Burnout

Healthcare providers are exhausted by the need to continually respond to disinformation regarding COVID-19 rather than focusing their efforts on providing credible information. At the beginning of the pandemic, a widely adopted public narrative espoused that children simply weren't impacted. While it is true, children were spared the burden of morbidity and mortality borne by adult populations, the pediatric care continuum was severely disrupted and pediatric HCPs were deeply impacted although often overlooked in the shadow of intensive care and emergency room HCPs. A 2021 survey of pediatric-focused APRNs distributed by the National Association of Pediatric Nurse Practitioners members ($n = 886$) found 34% of respondents expressed concern about moderate-to-extreme professional burnout, 25% reported feeling anxious or nervous, and 15% felt depressed or hopeless (Peck & Sonney, 2021). Responding to misinformation was the most common barrier reported by APRNs, with 55% reporting moderate-to-severe concern and another 29% reporting being somewhat concerned (Peck & Sonney, 2021). A follow-up 2023 study ($n = 1087$) alarmingly found that 87% of respondents now reported professional burnout and 80% reported concern for their own mental health. Responding to misinformation remained the number one clinical practice barrier with 64% of respondents now reporting moderate-to-severe concerns and another 25% reporting some level of concern (https://www.jpedhc.org/article/S0891-5245(23)00214-6/fulltext). Physicians face similar crises. In the United States, roughly 300–400 physicians die by suicide each year (American Foundation for Suicide Prevention, 2023). In a widely publicized tragic case, Dr. Lorna Breen died by suicide on April 26, 2020 after treating numerous confirmed COVID patients, contracting COVID-19 herself, and returning to an overwhelming number of sick patients, many of whom died in the emergency room waiting rooms and hallways (Dr. Lorna Breen Heroes Foundation, n.d.). In 2022, the American Medical Association found that 55% of pediatricians reported burnout and an astounding 48% did not feel valued. Pediatricians further revealed feeling alone, abandoned, and exhausted in their good-faith efforts to care for patients (American Medical Association, 2024).

Proposed solutions for both entities rely heavily on elevating clinician voice in professional decision-making forums as well as providing practical supports to alleviate stress and burnout. Physical protection and psychological support for HCPs during pandemic health crises should be a priority. Tools to help prevent provider burnout and fatigue include using resilience-based interventions, supporting HCPs to adopt health-seeking behaviors for mental health without fear of shame or stigma, and using online interventions. Adoption of coherence as resilience-enhancing technique can improve healthcare worker performance (Ali et al., 2021). However, it must be emphasized that interventions cannot be delivered with centralized messaging emphasizing solely the HCP's self-responsibility for developing resilience but must be matched by organizational structures and resources that promote work-life balance and healthy work cultures.

There are many ways HCPs can work to address mis- and disinformation with their patients and families. In general, best practices include:

- Avoid an argumentative stance with families. Rather than quickly dismissing their viewpoints or their fears as unfounded, be open to unfamiliar narratives and be respectful in hearing their specific concerns.
- Rather than engaging time and energy to disprove misinformation, respond proactively by providing families with credible facts, reputable sources, and scientifically sound evidence guiding your clinical practice.

eHealth Literacy

The American population often turns to the internet for current medical information. With immediate and unlimited access to both credible and noncredible health information, eHealth literacy is essential when looking for up-to-date and evidence-based information. Understanding the difference between credible and noncredible resources can help combat the spread of mis- and disinformation. Providers must work to understand each patient's knowledge, beliefs, and values to respond thoughtfully to fears of or resistance to accepting validated and scientifically based information (Polyzou et al., 2023). Kington et al. (2021) provided a flow diagram to guide conversations to help families identify credible online information. It is important for HCPs to convey an open invitation to respectfully discuss sources of information patients are using to seek health information, offering a collaborative approach to objectively evaluate source and subject credibility.

Partnerships with Media

Creating strategic partnerships to maintain accurate reporting can encourage truth in the presence of a disinfodemic. Newsrooms can partner with trusted researchers who can provide scientifically rigorous and reliable information because the media has a stronger influence on society's beliefs (Zviyita et al., 2022). In the pandemic, pre-print articles (preliminary drafts of scientific papers that are shared online prior to peer review and publication) proliferated. While this could potentially accelerate dissemination of life-saving medical breakthroughs, opportunity exists for rapid dissemination of so-called shoddy science when not properly vetted. Some discussion has been framed as comparing the pandemic with the "paperdemic," and calls out the risks of so-called "speed science" that could negatively influence the public trust (Dinis-Oliveira, 2020). With the contributing complexities of AI, it is clear there is a need for further discussion on professional standards for pre-prints (Chawla, 2024). In the meantime, partnerships between media and trusted researchers and scientists can help communicate data interpretation from such studies (Ratzan et al., 2020). Low-quality health information reinforcement loops on social media platforms can harm the general public (Kington et al., 2021). Information shared should be science-based, objective, and transparent/accountable. The US surgeon general encourages HCPs to proactively engage with patients and the public on health misinformation, use technology, and media platforms to share accurate health information with the public, and partner with community groups and other local organizations to prevent and address health misinformation (U.S. Surgeon General, 2021). However, this presents ethical considerations for use by pediatric clinicians who must have a confident grasp on the legal and ethical complexities and boundaries of professional use. Recommendations are included in the American Academy of Pediatrics clinical report entitled, *Ethical Considerations in Pediatricians' Use of Social Media,* which outlines the many benefits of social media as well as giving guidance on avoiding potential pitfalls. Positive elements include professional education and collaboration, patient education and advocacy, patient empowerment, increased patient access, clinical research and recruitment, identification of and counseling for high-risk behaviors, and nurturing compassion through narrative. Risks include inappropriate self-disclosure, blurring patient/provider boundaries, conflicts of interest, violation of confidentiality, and negative impacts on professional reputation emanating from disgruntled patients who voice their displeasure on social media (Macauley et al., 2021).

Cultural Responsiveness

Cultural responsiveness in healthcare is the ability to tailor care to meet patients' social, cultural, and linguistic needs and care for patients with diverse values, beliefs, and behaviors (American Hospital Association, 2023). All HCPs should receive regular training on culturally and linguistically appropriate healthcare, which can minimize the impact of mis- and disinformation in the context of a trusting and respectful patient/provider relationship. Providers should work to understand how social determinants of health, such as housing, income, and education, increase the risk of misunderstanding and believing mis- or disinformation regarding the pandemic. Providers can dispel mis-/disinformation by supporting people in different communities and cultures who may speak languages other than English.

Creating a task force of local leaders and community members to explain emergent issues and educate their community is also beneficial (Feinberg et al., 2021). Education provided by someone of the same culture and who speaks the same language is often better received because different cultures often receive and process information differently. For example, some cultures respond more favorably to storytelling or messaging from community leaders (Feinberg et al., 2021). Include other cultures' perspectives on risk, health, and wellness in the risk communication messages provided.

Suggestions for adopting a culturally responsive approach in a pandemic include:

- Cultivate partnerships between HCPs and trusted community organizations and leadership.
- Meet regularly with community leaders to share information, strategize, and collaborate on community-wide efforts to address the pandemic.
- Assess community needs and provide health information in relevant languages.
- Communicate through qualified interpreters. Utilize language lines instead of family members. Family members as interpreters can lead to reduced trust in HCPs, lower patient satisfaction, breaches of patient confidentiality, inaccurate communication, misdiagnosis, inadequate or inaccurate treatment, and reduced quality of care (Feinberg et al., 2021).

Lessons Learned

The importance of learning from current public health issues is crucial to move forward for the advancement of healthcare and future pandemic preparedness. Disinformation and misinformation are not new to healthcare, epidemics, or crisis; however, they appear to be more prevalent in a digital era. One of the most serious implications of mis- and disinformation within the professional healthcare arena is the intersection of regulatory and legal implications resulting in censure, revoking licensure (Baron et al., 2021) and even criminal implications and raises many complex questions for which there is continued ardent disagreement and lack of clarity (Farmer, 2022). What constitutes HCPs spreading mis- or disinformation and who gets to decide the definitions and thresholds? Where do individual rights intersect with professional restrictions or obligations? Is there a difference between HCPs spreading misinformation as opposed to disinformation? How does this intersect with individual rights of free speech? Can HCPs be held liable for not responding to mis- or disinformation? If so, how, by whom, and with what potential consequence? There are alarming reports of cases in which HCPs are grappling with these complex boundaries ranging from families suing providers who they say shared dangerous information that harmed a loved one to individual HCPs being sanctioned or threatened with losing their license by the overseeing regulatory body for spreading information deemed as false or misleading (AAMC News, 2023). The legal complexities of this issue are beyond the scope of this chapter but should generally be considered by regulatory and decision-making entities as well as employers in the overall picture of providers feeling pressured to rapidly navigate new and emerging complexities of information sharing with serious implications, which is likely contributing to feelings of anxiety and burnout (Peck & Sonney, 2021).

Providers are mentally and physically exhausted from interpreting and responding to mis- and disinformation regarding COVID-19. APRNs report feeling anxious, depressed, alone, and burnt out (Peck & Sonney, 2021). Healthcare providers benefit from administrative support, education, and access to mental health care when responding to a pandemic. Resilience-based interventions to support HCPs are essential during critical times of crisis. Strategies to mitigate fear are another lesson learned. The spread of mis- and disinformation on social media can appear faster than the spread of the disease itself (Ali et al., 2021). Educational campaigns and updates with daily releases from credible, trusted sources can help eliminate rising fear.

A proactive approach to effectively share credible information during the next crisis is ideal and can be managed with the collaborative efforts of media, healthcare professionals including nurses, political figures, and organizational leaders and should include representation from a diverse group of children and their families. Policy change and advocacy for health literacy resources within communities are powerful tools that HCPs can leverage to amplify credible messaging (Mistur et al., 2022). With the accountability of the community, advocacy for policy change can be accomplished with the goal of increased health literacy education for children, teens, and parents. Completely eliminating mis- and disinformation is unrealistic, but media health literacy goals for children are attainable.

Calls to Action
- Strength-based resilience supports are needed on an organizational and systems level to support pediatric HCPs to access mental health resources without shame or stigma and enact effective strategies to prevent provider burnout in the face of demands of responding to mis- and disinformation.
- Policy parameters need clarification with establishment of clear boundaries and legal frameworks to clarify obligations and restrictions of providers sharing information or not responding to mis- or disinformation to balance protection of professional autonomy and free speech with concerns for public safety.
- Advocacy is needed for policy support and resource allocation to provide health media literacy education for children and their families to teach them how to navigate information appraisal in online sources.

References

AAMC News. (2023). *Is spreading medical misinformation a physician's free speech right? It's complicated.* https://www.aamc.org/news/spreading-medical-misinformation-physician-s-free-speech-right-it-s-complicated

Ali, S. (2020). Combatting against covid-19 & misinformation: A systematic review. *Human Arenas, 5*(2), 337–352. https://doi.org/10.1007/s42087-020-00139-1

Ali, S., Khalid, A., & Zahid, E. (2021). Is covid-19 immune to misinformation? A brief overview. *Asian Bioethics Review, 13*(2), 255–277. https://doi.org/10.1007/s41649-020-00155-x

Allen, H. C., Garbe, M. C., Lees, J., Aziz, N., Chaaban, H., Miller, J. L., Johnson, P., & DeLeon, S. (2018). Off-label medication use in children, more common than we think: A systematic review of the literature. *The Journal of the Oklahoma State Medical Association, 111*(8), 776–783.

Alsmadi, I., Rice, N. M., & O'Brien, M. J. (2024). Fake or not? Automated detection of COVID-19 misinformation and disinformation in social networks and digital media. *Computational & Mathematical Organization Theory, 30*, 187–205. https://doi.org/10.1007/s10588-022-09369-w

American Foundation for Suicide Prevention. (2023). *Suicide prevention for healthcare professionals.* https://afsp.org/suicide-prevention-for-healthcare-professionals/#facts-about-mental-health-and-suicide

American Hospital Association. (2023). *Becoming a culturally competent healthcare organization.* https://www.aha.org/ahahret-guides/2013-06-18-becoming-culturally-competent-healthcare-organization#:~:text=Cultural%20competency%20in%20health%20care,social%2C%20cultural%20and%20linguistic%20needs

American Medical Association. (2024). *Most pediatricians have burnout. Here's what it takes to fix that.* https://www.ama-assn.org/practice-management/physician-health/most-pediatricians-have-burnout-here-s-what-it-takes-fix#:~:text=In%202022%2C%2055%25%20of%20pediatricians,the%20AMA's%20Organizational%20Biopsy%C2%AE

Baron, R., Nichols, D., & Newton, W. (2021). *Statement about dissemination of COVID-19 misinformation.* Statement about dissemination of COVID-19 misinformation | The American Board of Pediatrics. https://abp.org/news/press-releases/statement-about-dissemination-covid-19-misinformation

Basch, C. H., Meleo-Erwin, Z., Fera, J., Jaime, C., & Basch, C. E. (2021). A global pandemic in the time of viral memes: COVID-19 vaccine misinformation and disinformation on TikTok. *Human Vaccines & Immunotherapeutics, 17*(8), 2373–2377. https://doi.org/10.1080/21645515.2021.1894896

Blumenthal, R., & Blackburn, M. (2024). *The kids online safety act of 2022.* https://www.blumenthal.senate.gov/imo/media/doc/kids_online_safety_act_-_one_pager.pdf

Bohannon, M. (2024). *What to know about Florida's Social Media ban for kids under 16—Which DeSantis May Veto.* https://www.forbes.com/sites/mollybohannon/2024/02/23/what-to-know-about-floridas-social-media-ban-for-kids-under-16-which-desantis-may-veto/?sh=3d6a27707566

Bond, S. (2021). *Facebook, Twitter, Google CEOs testify before congress: 4 things to know.* https://www.npr.org/2021/03/25/980510388/facebook-twitter-google-ceos-testify-before-congress-4-things-to-know

Bontridder, N., & Poullet, Y. (2021, November 25). *The role of artificial intelligence in disinformation: Data & policy.* Cambridge Core. https://www.cambridge.org/core/journals/data-and-policy/article/role-of-artificial-intelligence-in-disinformation/7C4BF6CA35184F149143DE968FC4C3B6

Brennan, S., et al. (2020). *Types, sources, and claims of COVID-19 misinformation.* https://reutersinstitute.politics.ox.ac.uk/types-sources-and-claims-covid-19-misinformation

Campillo, J. T., Boussinesq, M., Bertout, S., Faillie, J. L., & Chesnais, C. B. (2021). Serious adverse reactions associated with ivermectin: A systematic pharmacovigilance study in sub-Saharan Africa and in the rest of the World. *PLoS Neglected Tropical Diseases, 15*(4), e0009354. https://doi.org/10.1371/journal.pntd.0009354

Caronia, L., & Ranzani, F. (2024). Epistemic trust as an interactional accomplishment in pediatric well-child visits: Parents' resistance to solicited advice as performing epistemic vigilance. *Health Communication, 39*, 838. https://doi.org/10.1080/10410236.2023.2189504

Cartwright, B., Frank, R., Weir, G., Padda, K., & Strange, S.-M. (2023). Deploying artificial intelligence to combat Covid-19 misinformation on social media: Technological and ethical considerations. https://doi.org/10.24251/HICSS.2023.266

Chawla, D. S. (2024). *COVID's preprint bump set to have lasting effect on research publishing.* https://www.nature.com/articles/d41586-024-00401-4

Chikandiwa, Zviyita, I., & Mapudzi, H. (2022). Social media and the COVID-19 disinfodemic in the digital space: Disempowering the public and threatening public health. *Acta Universitatis Danubius Communicatio, 16*(2).

Dinis-Oliveira, R. J. (2020). COVID-19 research: Pandemic versus "paperdemic", integrity, values and risks of the "speed science". *Forensic Sciences Research, 5*(2), 174–187.

Ekşi, A., Gümüşsoy, S., Utanır Altay, S., & Kirazlı, G. (2022). Effect of the COVID-19 pandemic on violence against pre-hospital emergency health workers. *Work, 73*(4), 1103–1108.

Farmer, B. (2022, February 22). *Medical Boards feel the pressure to let it go when doctors spread covid-19 misinformation.* Contemporary Pediatrics. https://www.contemporarypediatrics.com/view/medical-boards-feel-the-pressure-to-let-it-go-when-doctors-spread-covid-19-misinformation

Feinberg, R. Z., Owen-Smith, A., O'Connor, M. H., Ogrodnick, M. M., Rothenberg, R., & Eriksen, M. P. (2021). Strengthening culturally competent health communication. *Health Secure, 19*(S1), S41–S49. https://doi.org/10.1089/hs.2021.0048

GFC Global. (n.d.). *What is Clickbait?* https://edu.gcfglobal.org/en/thenow/what-is-clickbait/1/

Grossman, A. M., & Shapiro, K. A. (2023). *Shining a light on censorship: How transparency can curtail government social media censorship and more.* https://www.cato.org/briefing-paper/shining-light-censorship-how-transparency-can-curtail-government-social-media

Hauser, C. (2023). *Family in 'take care of maya' documentary is awarded $261 million.* https://www.nytimes.com/2023/11/10/us/take-care-of-maya-trial-damages-kowalski.html

Holcombe, M. (2022). *Homemade infant formula can be dangerous. Experts share how to feed your baby through the shortage.* https://www.cnn.com/2022/05/11/health/infant-formula-shortage-misinformation-wellness/index.html

Hong, Y., & Roy, R. (2023). Communication in the time of uncertainty and misinformation. *Journal of Creative Communications, 18*(2), 131–132.

Johns Hopkins (2023). https://guides.library.jhu.edu/evaluate/internet-resources

Howard, P. N., Neudert L.-M., & Prakash, N. (2021, August). *Rapid analysis digital misinformation/disinformation.* UICEF Global Insite. https://www.unicef.org/globalinsight/media/2096/file/UNICEF-Global-Insight-DigitalMis-Disinformation-and-Children-2021.pdf

Khullar, D., Darien, G., & Ness, D. L. (2020). Patient consumerism, healing relationships, and rebuilding trust in health care. *JAMA, 324*(23), 2359–2360. https://doi.org/10.1001/jama.2020.1293

Kington, R. S., Arnesen, S., Chou, W. S., Curry, S. J., Lazer, D., & Villarruel, A. M. (2021). Identifying credible sources of health information in social media: Principles and attributes. *NAM Perspectives.* https://doi.org/10.31478/202107a

Kohli, A. (2023, March 25). Utah's new law restricting social media use for minors isn't clear on enforcement. *Time.* https://time.com/6266100/utah_teens_social_media_laws/

Lorna Breen Heroes Foundation (n.d.). https://drlornabreen.org/about-lorna/

Macauley, R., Elster, N., Fanaroff, J. M., & the Committee on Bioethics, Committee on Medical Liability and Risk Management. (2021). Ethical considerations in pediatricians' use of social media. *Pediatrics, 147*(3), e20200496852021.

Mistur, E. M., Givens, J. W., & Matisoff, D. C. (2022). Contagious covid-19 policies: Policy diffusion during times of crisis. *Review of Policy Research, 40*(1), 36–62. https://doi.org/10.1111/ropr.12487

Oswald, S., Lewinski, M., Greco, S., & VIllata, S. (2022). *The pandemic of argumentation* (Vol. 43). Springer Nature. https://doi.org/10.1007/978-3-030-91017-4

Peck, J. L., & Sonney, J. (2021). Exhausted and burned out: COVID-19 emerging impacts threaten the health of the pediatric advanced practice registered nursing workforce. *Journal of Pediatric Health Care, 35*(4), 414–424. https://doi.org/10.1016/j.pedhc.2021.04.012

Pew Research Center. (2024). *Social Media and News Fact Sheet.* https://www.pewresearch.org/journalism/fact-sheet/social-media-and-news-fact-sheet/

Polyzou, M., Kiefer, D., Baraliakos, X., & Sewerin, P. (2023). Addressing the spread of health-related misinformation on social networks: An opinion article. *Frontiers in Medicine, 10*, 1167033. https://doi.org/10.3389/fmed.2023.1167033

Popp, M., Stegemann, M., Metzendorf, M.-I., Gould, S., Kranke, P., Meybohm, P., Skoetz, N., & Weibel, S. (2021). Ivermectin for preventing and treating COVID-19. *Cochrane Database of Systematic Reviews, 2021*(7), CD015017. https://doi.org/10.1002/14651858.CD015017.pub2

Posetti, J., & Bontcheva, K. (2020a, April 23). *Key themes and formats of the COVID-19 disinfodemic, according to UN-ICFJ research.* https://ijnet.org/en/story/key-themes-and-formats-covid-19-disinfodemic-according-un-icfj-research

Posetti, J., & Bontcheva, K. (2020b). *Disinfodemic: Deciphering COVID-19 disinformation.* Policy brief. https://unesdoc.unesco.org/ark:/48223/pf0000374416

Ratzan, S., Sommariva, S., & Rauh, L. (2020). Enhancing global health communication during a crisis: Lessons from the covid-19 pandemic. *Public Health Research and Practice, 30*(2), e3022010. https://doi.org/10.17061/phrp3022010

Rivkees, S. A. (2023, February 22). A war on pediatric care is putting children at risk. *Time.* https://time.com/6257272/pediatric-care-political-war/

Twitter. (2021). https://twitter.com/US_FDA/status/1429050070243192839?lang=en

U.S. Department of Health and Human Services. (2023a). *Ivermectin.* National Institutes of Health. https://www.covid19treatmentguidelines.nih.gov/therapies/miscellaneous-drugs/ivermectin/

U.S. Department of Health and Human Services. (2023b). *Fraud alert: COVID-19 scams.* https://oig.hhs.gov/fraud/consumer-alerts/fraud-alert-covid-19-scams/

U.S. Food and Drug Administration. (2020, July 15). *FDA cautions against use of hydroxychloroquine or chloroquine for COVID-19 outside of the hospital setting or a clinical trial due to risk of heart rhythm problems.* https://www.fda.gov/drugs/drug-safety-and-availability/fda-cautions-against-use-of-hydroxychloroquine-or-chloroquine-covid-19-outside-hospital-setting-or

US Surgeon General (2021) *Confronting health misinformation: The U.S. surgeon general's advisory on building a healthy information environment*

World Health Organization. (2023). *Coronavirus disease (COVID-19): Hydroxychloroquine.* https://www.who.int/news-room/questions-and-answers/item/coronavirus-disease-(covid-19)-hydroxychloroquine

Yammine, S. (2020). Going viral: How to boost the spread of coronavirus science on social media. *Nature, 581*, 345.

Zhang, S., Zhao, Z., Zhang, H., Zhu, Y., Xi, Z., & Xiang, K. (2023). Workplace violence against healthcare workers during the COVID-19 pandemic: A systematic review and meta-analysis. *Environmental Science and Pollution Research International, 30*(30), 74838–74852.

Zviyita, I., Mapudzi, H., & Chikandiwa, C. T. (2022). Social media and the COVID-19 disinfodemic in the digital space: Disempowering the public and threatening public health. *Acta Universitatis Danubius Communicatio, 16*(2).

Implications for Health Care System Leaders: Organizational Policies Impacting Care Delivery

Aaron Carpenter, Andrea Kline-Tilford, and Rajashree Koppolu

> *The way we've been thinking has gotten us to where we are, but where we are going requires a new way of thinking.*
>
> —Brenda Bence, Executive Leadership Coach

Introduction and Background

There are more than 250 children's hospitals in the United States providing care for acutely ill children requiring subspecialty and critical care services (Casimir, 2019). The impact of the COVID-19 pandemic, especially in its first surge, was largely concentrated in adult healthcare. While the experience of children's health systems (CHS) was different in timing and impact, severity was no less significant. In February of 2020, the Centers for Disease Control and Prevention (CDC) announced efforts to mitigate transmission of the novel virus, followed soon after in March 2020 by state government shutdowns affecting nearly every aspect of the economy, including CHS (Centers for Disease Control and Prevention, 2023). This chapter will discuss the multifactorial impact of COVID-19 on pediatric healthcare systems and pediatric-specific obstacles navigated by healthcare system leaders.

A. Carpenter
Nemours Children's Health, Delaware Valley, Wilmington, DE, USA
e-mail: aaron.carpenter@nemours.org

A. Kline-Tilford (✉)
University of Michigan Health, Ann Arbor, MI, USA

R. Koppolu
Stanford Medicine Children's Health, Palo Alto, CA, USA
e-mail: rkoppolu@stanfordchildrens.org

© The Author(s), under exclusive license to Springer Nature Switzerland AG 2025
J. L. Peck (ed.), *COVID-19 Impacts on Child Health*,
https://doi.org/10.1007/978-3-031-80369-7_18

Operational Impacts

In the early stages of the pandemic, many CHS experienced an almost immediate cessation of elective procedures, closure of ambulatory clinics, and a significant drop in average daily inpatient census (Ferry et al., 2022; Gill et al., 2021). In comparison to prior years, pediatric inpatient admissions decreased by 45.4% in April of 2020, resulting in revenue losses that directly impact CHS ability to deliver on their mission and provide needed care to children (Pelletier et al., 2021). Children's hospitals saw a decrease in healthcare encounters, charges, emergency room visits, and surgery encounters (Synhorst et al., 2021). Generally, revenue declines represented anywhere from 5% to 20% and were not unique to any specific region or market. Furthermore, 90% of children's hospitals experienced some kind of negative financial impact in 2020 and are continuing to recover (Children's Hospital Association, 2021). These early shutdowns were a harbinger that would lead to exceptional workforce challenges for CHS. As a result of the economic impact of reduced volumes and revenues in addition to other factors, employment for nurses in ambulatory care, hospitals, home health, and nursing homes in the United States (U.S.) dropped significantly from March to April 2020 (Beurhaus et al., 2022). Revenue losses for some CHS in the early months of the pandemic led to furloughs or reductions in force (Beurhaus et al., 2022).

In early 2021, the Children's Hospital Association (CHA) published a report highlighting the challenges specific to pediatric hospitals and health systems. CHA utilized data from 33 children's hospitals across the U.S. and identified six unique challenges to pediatric healthcare: (Children's Hospital Association, 2021).

- Large volume and revenue losses.
- Slow recovery with estimates of $7 billion dollar losses between 2020 and 2021
- Ninety percent of children's hospitals experienced negative financial impact
- Children admitted to children's hospitals were sicker due to deferral of care during early months of the pandemic
- Untreated behavioral and mental health problems led to an acute exacerbation of these health concerns culminating in crisis
- Children's hospitals did not have the same level of federal relief provided to all U.S. hospitals

In response to a concern for suboptimal federal funding, the CHA advocated on behalf of CHS in a letter to the U.S. Senate and House of Representatives, recognizing the possibility of a pullback in emergency funding for children and emphasizing the need for continued funding in children's health, specifically around children's mental health interventions, bolstering of the pediatric workforce, and strengthening health coverage for children (Wietecha, 2022).

A common misunderstanding that children were not as affected by COVID-19 as adults is misleading. Although there was greater mortality associated with COVID-19 in the adult population, COVID-19 was not a benign virus for children. In a study that assessed COVID-19 as the underlying cause of death in children and young people aged 0–19, investigators determined COVID-19 ranked eighth among all causes of death in this age-group and fifth in disease-related causes of death (Flaxman et al., 2023). Importantly, COVID-19 disproportionately affected children in low socioeconomic classes, and Black, multicultural, and urban families (Barioja et al., 2023). Children's hospitals did not see the same level of surge volumes in intensive care units (ICUs) and acute care units as adult hospitals. This did not, however, protect children or CHS from other devastating effects in the aftermath of the pandemic. In 2021, the American Association of Pediatrics (AAP), American Academy of Child and Adolescent Psychiatry (AACAP), and the Children's Hospital Association (CHA) collectively declared a national state of emergency of children's mental health (Children's Hospital Association, n.d.).

Health System Response

CHS saw an initial decrease in patient activity and inpatient volumes in the wake of government shutdown (Children's Hospital Association, 2021). Leaders in CHS responded to decreasing patient volumes and revenue with varied operational plans, including temporary furloughs and reductions in workforce (Children's Hospital Association, 2021) As patient volumes returned, community exposure to the virus further impacted the healthcare workforce. This, in combination with operational challenges such as supply chain disruption, concerns about adequate personal protective equipment (PPE), and fear of exposure to a novel virus led to initiation of hospital incident command system (HICS) activation (Westley et al., 2023).

In the 1980s, HICS was established by the Orange County Emergency Medical Service to foster a standardized emergency management approach for significant emergency response (EMSA, 2023). The framework has evolved over time, most recently updated in 2014. The HICS provides a standardized and structured approach to leading a response to large scale impact on health systems in the event of an emergency requiring considerable resource (EMSA, 2023). Incident command (IC) is a clearly defined transparent structure with an identified leader (incident commander), and a structure that identifies accountable leaders (section chiefs) for standard incident management responsibilities, such as operations, planning, logistics, finance, and others.

Activation of the IC structure in CHS allowed leaders and teams to rapidly address threats to patients, families, and staff, increasing timeliness and activation of decisions. Implicit in the activation of IC is a centralized location for the gathering of the response team identified above. Innovation was the hallmark of pandemic incident response from the earliest stages of activation as gathering in a room was contrary to the infection prevention protocols hospitals employed during the early stages of the pandemic. Unique to CHS was the extension of screening protocols to caregivers. Interdisciplinary taskforces contributed to the development of protocols by regular assessment of regional and local disease burden, case rate positivity, and their impacts on operations. This was particularly critical in CHS where limitations on caregivers' ability to be at bedside with their child had significant impact on the patient's recovery and support. One large children's hospital in the Northwest U.S. reported their incident command structure allowed for rapid decision-making and process improvements throughout the pandemic response (Parikh et al., 2020). Leaders transitioned IC structures to the virtual format and flexed from standardized approach to adapt processes to the new environment. The IC structure allowed CHS leaders to rapidly respond to ongoing threats to the delivery of care and create immediately responsive countermeasures to maintain operations.

As the pandemic progressed, the IC structure was employed by some CHS for focused incident management. One children's hospital described their experience in utilizing the IC structure in managing the surge in patients presenting for mental and behavioral health crises. The institution of the IC structure as a focused response to behavioral healthcare promoted rapid decision-making and allowed the system to, "quickly advance short—and long-term solutions to this unprecedented challenge" (Westley et al., 2023). The IC response to the COVID-19 pandemic provides a framework for agile decision-making. CHS can learn from the experience of pandemic IC structures and novel approaches developed through the pandemic to significant operational challenges in CHS, such as viral and behavioral health patient surges in the future.

Financial Implications

Children's hospitals, which provide a critical safety net for the pediatric population, were not spared from significant economic challenges during the COVID-19 pandemic. While the total volume of pediatric patients requiring hospital-based care was not as numerous as adult patients, children with chronic illness and those with co-morbidities were at higher risk for COVID-19-related hospitalizations, particularly among Black and Hispanic children (Koppolu, 2021). Furthermore, children admitted to the hospital for care related to COVID-19 required multidisciplinary services and potentially long hospital stays. One in three children admitted with COVID-19 was admitted to an intensive care unit (Kim et al., 2020) and the case mix index (CMI) as a measure of clinical complexity increased by 11% from January to December 2020 (Children's Hospital Association, 2021). Many hospitals had to cancel non-essential procedures, increase capacity to accommodate pediatric patients with COVID-19, and invest in capital costs of newly established testing and vaccination sites. In 2018, elective and ambulatory procedures accounted for approximately 63% of an average hospital's revenue (Khullar et al., 2020). Hospitals reallocated resources for additional personal protective equipment, employee wellness, and drug shortages. In many cases, infrastructures including space and staff within children's hospitals were used to admit adult patients. Lastly, children's hospitals saw a dramatic increase in emergency room visits related to behavioral and mental health crisis (Children's Hospital Association, n.d.). As a result of all these dynamic, abrupt, and complex changes, children's hospitals were operating under tight financial margins.

Children's health insurance coverage saw important shifts during the pandemic. Unfortunately, one in five children in the United States experienced the job loss of an adult in the household in the first few months of the COVID-19 pandemic (Bokun et al., 2020). The majority of children in the United States are covered as dependents on a parent's employer-based health insurance plan with 52% as of 2015 (Currie & Chorniy, 2021; Murphey, 2017). Furthermore, increasing unemployment rates and economic instability, driven by the pandemic, threatened the ability of children to have stable housing, food security, and child and family well-being (Coley, 2020). This abrupt change was intensified by the increasing number of uninsured children in the United States prior to the pandemic. The number of uninsured children increased from 4.7% in 2016 to 5.7% in 2019 and the number for Hispanic children increased to 9.2%, largely thought to be due to declines in public insurance (Berchick & Mykyta, 2019). Possessing health insurance coverage is generally associated with improved access to care for children and adults (Office of Disease Prevention and Health Promotion, Office of the Assistant Secretary for Health, Office of the Secretary, U.S. Department of Health and Human Services, 2022). Children with health insurance are more likely than those who lack insurance coverage to receive early care and are at lower risk for hospitalization (Murphey, 2017). Expansion in public health insurance programs has led to not only short-term declines in infant mortality and preventable hospitalization but have also been associated with long-term effects such as higher educational attainment, earnings, self-reported health, and lower mortality compared to those who did not benefit from expansions (Currie & Chorniy, 2021).

Public insurance programs, such as Medicaid, have historically served as an option for children during prior economic downturns (Dorn et al., 2008). Medicaid and the Children's Health Insurance (CHIP) programs are administered by states, but the cost is shared with the federal government. To administer the program, states absorb over 15% of its total budget on average (Currie & Duque, 2019). Given this robust financial investment, Medicaid is vulnerable to cuts during budget shortfalls (Currie & Chorniy, 2021). Many states struggled to balance their state budgets and their Medicaid program in the setting of competing public health demands. In states like California where Medi-Cal (state's Medicaid program) expansions of the Affordable Care Act were implemented, Medi-Cal was noted to be the most important payer in stabilizing the financial status of many California hospitals during the pandemic (Melnick & Maerki, 2021). Therefore, there was variability in the ability for states to maintain their Medicaid budgets in the setting of many children needing access to affordable and accessible health insurance coverage.

Children's hospitals experienced a shift in payor mix during the pandemic. Medicaid is the primary payer for children's hospitals covering more than 50% of patients (Children's Hospital Association, 2021). As such, children's hospitals are the highest Medicaid provider hospitals in the United States (Children's Hospital Association, 2021). The U.S. Department of Health and Human Services distributed nearly 72.4 billion to healthcare providers (HCPs) in the Coronavirus Aid, Relief, and Economic Security (CARES) Act and the Paycheck Protection Program and Health Care Enhancement Act (Schwartz & Damino, 2020). Programs such as the

Provider Relief Fund targeted various healthcare systems including children's hospitals that diagnosed, tested, and cared for individuals with suspected or actual COVID-19 and had healthcare expenses and lost revenues related to COVID-19 (Kleinpell et al., 2021). While this federal relief funding helped address some of these direct costs, high-Medicaid providers were largely left out of receiving these funds made available through the Medicare program (Children's Hospital Association, 2021). One analysis demonstrated that HCPs and hospitals with the highest share of private insurance revenue received a disproportionately high share of total funds (Schwartz & Damino, 2020). Therefore, it seems that hospitals with a low share of private insurance received less than half as much funding (Schwartz & Damino, 2020). Based on the nature of children's hospitals general payor mix, they experienced a disproportionate amount of relief funding.

Public health infrastructure has been largely underfunded in the last 20 years yet is necessary to promote disease prevention and health promotion (Isasi et al., 2021). Therefore, more attention has been placed on seeking care within hospital-based settings instead of investing resources in areas such as emergency preparedness. There is an opportunity to strategically think about the needed financial investment in future public health initiatives and how to coordinate those with children's healthcare systems. CHS worked hard to maintain financial solvency with the many changing dynamics of the pandemic. Existing hospital resources and federal assistance from the Coronavirus Aid, Relief and Economic Security Act helped mitigate some of the needed revenue but were not sufficient to provide all the resources needed for these healthcare systems to operate. Given the unique needs of pediatric patients, the difference in payor mix, and the insurance programs which support children's access to care, there are many lessons to be gained from the COVID-19 pandemic. Through our collective experience, there is a tremendous opportunity to think about how we can create sustainable programs, receive consistent funding, and predictive care models to help us provide the critical care which children need during another public health emergency.

Federal and State Policy Impacts

During the height of the COVID-19 pandemic, many U.S. states with reduced or restricted advanced practice registered nurses (APRN) practice, suspended practice restrictions on an emergency basis. Suspension of practice restrictions facilitated patient care, allowing full scope practice for APRNs in 21 states with reduced or restricted practice through promulgation of governor-implemented executive orders (Kleinpell et al., 2021). Five states implemented a temporary suspension of all practice restrictions, while 16 states invoked a temporary waiver of select practice restrictions and 7 states took no action on temporarily expanding APRN practice (Kleinpell et al., 2021). Time during the pandemic with expanded practice was an unanticipated opportunity to examine the impact of the cost-effective and more accessible care provided by APRNs. Pediatric healthcare leaders and APRNs must employ this information to continue to inform legislators and to advance health policy agendas on reducing barriers to APRN practice (Kleinpell et al., 2021).

Regulatory bodies required U.S. health systems to implement systems to control disease transmission during this pandemic (Maung et al., 2022). Self-reported COVID-19 screening and temperature assessment for healthcare workers entering healthcare facilities during the COVID-19 pandemic were commonly adopted by health systems as part of this plan (Chowdhury et al., 2020; Maung et al., 2022; Zhang et al., 2020) A study at one large academic health system described the development and implementation of a web-based mobile COVID-19 employee screening attestation for daily use prior to entering the healthcare facility (Zhang et al., 2020). This tool was developed to be the primary mode of daily symptom screening for this large health system with >25,000 employees screening daily, while paper and kiosk screening options were offered for employees unable or preferring not to use mobile application. A "glanceable" indicator was displayed on the mobile digital screen, demonstrating the employee passed the screening without symptoms concerning for COVID-19, which was then shown to screening staff upon entering the health facility. Screenings suggestive of possible COVID-19 (e.g., fever, cough, sore throat, shortness breath) did not generate the glanceable indicator of passing screening and provided guidance on next steps for the employee related to their symptoms (Zhang et al., 2020). After 3 months of implementation, 2,169,406 screenings were complete, identifying 1865 employee with symptoms, 91% of the positive screenings were identified on the mobile app and the remainder were identified via manual or kiosk symptom reporting (Zhang et al., 2020). This mobile application was quickly adopted by employees and was important in identifying employees with symptoms who may have otherwise reported to work, potentially infecting other employees or patients/families (Zhang et al., 2020). Adopting this mobile application reduced the need for manual reporting and reduced lines to kiosks at health system entrance.

Additional screening strategies included routine employee temperature assessment upon entrance to health care facilities in conjunction with symptom screening questionnaires for patients and families (Chowdhury et al., 2020). In a study from March 2020 to March 2021, only 1 screening of 6000 employee temperature screenings at a health system in California identified a healthcare worker fever without other reported symptoms (Maung et al., 2022). Upon re-take of the temperature, it was documented to be normal (Maung et al., 2022). Use of daily temperature assessment, when used in conjunction with an online symptom screening, failed to identify additional cases suspicious for COVID-19 (Maung et al., 2022). Screening strategies were common during the height of the pandemic and were slowly reduced after vaccination was widely available, though, varied by health system. These mechanisms for screening were important in keeping staff, patients, and families safe during the pandemic, however, undoubtedly added a new operational burden. The lessons learned from these approaches can operationalize optimal disease screening in future pandemic planning.

The Centers for Medicare and Medicaid Services (CMS) implemented a regulatory requirement for COVID-19 vaccination policies and procedures for health care staff on November 5, 2021 with the "Omnibus COVID-19 Health Care Staff

Vaccination." Providers and suppliers (e.g., hospitals, ambulatory surgical centers, hospice services, home health services) participating in Medicare and Medicaid programs, were required to implement these changes or face risk of penalty up to termination of provider agreement with Medicare and Medicaid (Department of Health and Human Services, 2023). With the high proportion of children receiving services with the support of Medicaid, fund streams could be severely impacted, if not fully adopted. On May 31, 2023, CMS released regulatory changes removing the requirement for COVID-19 vaccination policies for staff effective August 4, 2023 (Department of Health and Human Services, 2023). While requirements for COVID-19 vaccination were lifted, quality measure requirements for evaluating the proportion of healthcare workers who are vaccinated against COVID-19 remained in place (American Hospital Association, n.d.; Department of Health and Human Services, 2023). Pediatric health system leaders continue to evaluate policies and procedures around COVID-19 vaccination requirements for healthcare personnel in considering safe and optimal care for patients and families.

Workforce Vaccine Hesitancy Implications

In December of 2020, when the U.S. Food and Drug Administration (FDA) granted emergency use authorization of the COVID-19 vaccine, many pediatric healthcare systems offered and encouraged vaccination of healthcare workers (Food and Drug Administration, n.d.). When the FDA approved, the first COVID-19 vaccine in August 2021 (Food and Drug Administration, n.d.), increasing numbers of children's hospitals began mandating vaccination as part of employment, providing nurses the ability to protect themselves, their families, and the fragile children they care for in the healthcare setting (Toth-Manikowski et al., 2022). Not all healthcare workers, including nurses, embraced the mandate to be vaccinated. A December 2020 survey study of over 4000 children's hospital clinical and non-clinical staff at a free-standing children's hospital evaluated vaccine hesitancy among staff (Kociolek et al., 2021). Nearly 60% reported that would definitely receive the vaccine and 8.6% had already received the vaccine. Vaccine hesitancy, defined as have not decided, probably will not or definitely will not receive the vaccine, was noted in nearly 20% of the children's hospital staff (Kociolek et al., 2021). Notably, respondents identifying as having a high-risk medical condition were three times more likely to respond as vaccine hesitant. Concerns reported by vaccine-hesitant individuals included vaccine safety associated with speed of novel vaccine development (Kociolek et al., 2021).

Leaders and healthcare organizations were positioned to support patient safety through healthcare workforce health and wellness while minimizing absences related to illness. Vaccine requirements for pediatric healthcare workers were not a new concept, as most have been required to have influenza, hepatitis B, and tetanus vaccines at the start of employment (Emanuel & Skorton, 2021) for many years to reduce risk of disease transmission to children in their care. Ultimately, many institutions upheld vaccine requirements and enforced separation from employees not willing to be vaccinated while acknowledging the risk that mandates could result in backlash and further mistrust (Toth-Manikowski et al., 2022). Study findings suggest targeting efforts in relationship building to increase employee confidence in vaccination and targeted educational and advocacy programs to address and overcome concerns with the COVID-19 vaccine (Kociolek et al., 2021). Frequently, individuals cite HCPs, and local and national experts as trusted sources influence their decisions, providing an opportunity for pediatric APRNs to provide evidence-based vaccine education to patients and families (Kociolek et al., 2021). Further dialogue is needed to guide policy and ethical implications of vaccination mandates for HCPs.

Impacts on Daily Operations

CHS navigated maintaining patient operations while managing staff absences for COVID-19 infection in themselves or family members. At the onset of the pandemic, it was recommended that staff infected with COVID-19 remain out of the workforce for a minimum of 2 weeks, resulting in increased workload burden for the healthy workforce. As more was learned about COVID-19 infection, return to work after COVID-19 infection guidelines resulted in reduced time for work return clearance. Like the constant changes in patient care guidelines with COVID-19, there were frequent changes to quarantine guidelines for infected individuals, requiring hospital leaders to manage constant outpouring of new information, adapting staffing plans appropriately (Nelson & Hylton Rushton, 2021). Amid staffing challenges during the pandemic, some nursing staff struggled with guilt when experiencing their own illness during the COVID-19 pandemic, knowing their absence would result in greater impacts on their co-workers during a time of an already meager staffing situation. This resulted in higher rates of presenteeism among nursing staff, though unable to work to full potential due to illness symptoms (Nelson & Hylton Rushton, 2021). Not only were staff not feeling well themselves, but they also placed others are risk of contracting a contagious disease (Nelson & Hylton Rushton, 2021). Frequently, nurses reported to work during the pandemic, knowing their contributions to patient care were needed, especially as the workforce contracted, leaving less staff available to care for patients and families (Nelson & Hylton Rushton, 2021). Children's healthcare leaders can support staff in making supported and informed decisions through adhering to published public health standards and offering accessible rapid testing (Nelson & Hylton Rushton, 2021).

It became necessary to adopt new operations/processes to mitigate staffing infectious risk and to disseminate information swiftly and widely during the pandemic. To protect staff from exposure to infected patients, new methods of patient care delivery were temporarily adopted to maintain high standards to care for patients. Some teams performed daily rounds with a portion of team members on videoconferencing or other virtual platforms away from patients to reduce the risk of COVID-19 disease transmission (Bavare et al., 2021; Temsah et al., 2021).

Information on COVID-19 was shared across systems at an astounding pace, requiring constant adjustments to policies, procedures, and protocols. The rapidity of new information increased strain and stress on the daily care delivery. Leadership teams were instrumental in assuring appropriate digital platforms were available to disseminate information quickly and efficiently to team members delivering care during the pandemic. For example, in the pediatric population, a novel inflammatory disease was identified associated with COVID-19, multi-system inflammatory syndrome in children (Centers for Disease Control and Prevention, n.d.). This newly identified syndrome resulted in pediatric critical illness and several iterations of diagnostic criteria and management necessitating real-time information dissemination of latest guidelines. Renke et al. describe methods for keeping up-to-date with the updates associated with COVID-19 that were happening at a lightning pace during the pandemic including shared online documents and protocols, in-person education and webinars (Renke et al., 2020). Leaders ensured that staff had access to the latest information using platforms that were most appropriate for their CHS.

Impacts on Children and Their Families

In effort to reduce the risk of spreading COVID-19 to both patients and staff, and in some cases, to reduce the utilization of personal protective equipment, most children's hospitals adopted new visitor policies during the pandemic (Moss et al., 2021; Vance et al., 2021). A systematic review of publicly available children's hospital visitor policies during the COVID-19 pandemic demonstrated varying policies, the most stringent restricting all visitors (Vance et al., 2021). Others specified visitor policy changes including allowing one adult visitor at a time, reducing visiting duration, elimination of visitation by children <18 years of age, or eliminated overnight visiting (Vance et al., 2021). Not only were patients and families impacted, nurses and HCPs reported anguish from stringent visitor restrictions as family members are crucial in delivery of family-centered care and supporting hospitalized children (Andrist et al., 2020; Vance et al., 2021). Separation of children from their family is distressing for children, families, and HCPs (Andrist et al., 2020). Opportunities for future pandemic response should prioritize strategies to balance disease transmission risk reduction efforts and maintaining visitor policies that maximize child wellness and promote family-centered care while maintaining adjustments for patient conditions (Andrist et al., 2020; Vance et al., 2021).

Impacts on Clinician Work and Workflow

The COVID-19 pandemic took a significant toll on pediatric nurses and HCPs, both professionally and personally. Nurses and other HCPs were repeatedly asked to do more with less and were often fearful of their own safety, particularly as supply chain issues plagued all areas of life including healthcare systems (Wahlster &

Hartog, 2022). This included basic supplies such as personal protective equipment (PPE), which were often used beyond manufactured recommended recommendations or decontaminated for reuse, particularly at the onset of the pandemic (Tabah et al., 2020; Zorko et al., 2020). Face masks, particularly N-95 masks, were commonly worn for those providing direct patient care during the COVID-19 pandemic. Protection from disease transmission with prolonged N-95 mask use has been associated with facial rashes, acne, skin breakdown, and headaches (Rosner, 2020). Leaders can help advocate for mask breaks, hydration, and adequate skin care to help alleviate these challenges.

With stay-at-home orders and a reduction in surgical procedures, children's hospital census plummeted, providing capacity for pediatric registered nurses (RN) and advanced practice registered nurse (APRN) workforce to temporarily adapt their practice to new roles or areas. Nurses were often called upon to fill alternate roles, modulate care delivery and float to new units with unfamiliar staff (Brown et al., 2021; Endacott et al., 2022; Pountney et al., 2023; Renke et al., 2020). Renke et al. (2020) described pediatric nurse practitioners (NPs) from one academic children's hospital who voluntarily deployed to the adult COVID ICU to serve as front line providers among a multidisciplinary team (Renke et al., 2020). This short-term care model adjustment was only possible during the state governor's executive order that expanded APRN ability to practice without the restriction of outdated supervision requirements during the COVID-19 pandemic in concert with implementation of health system emergency privileging. Lessons learned from this model of pediatric NP deployment to an adult COVID ICU include the need for a more robust orientation, clustering days on service to allow for greater time away from the mental and psychological toll of the clinical environment and partnerships with the medical staff services department to facilitate emergency privileging (Renke et al., 2020).

Ambulatory pediatric care delivery was also modulated during the pandemic. One example highlighting pivotal ambulatory pediatric healthcare delivery during COVID-19 included administration of routinely recommended vaccinations using a "drive-through/drive-up" method in effort to combat the dwindling childhood vaccination rates, which threaten outbreaks of vaccine-preventable disease (Center for Disease Control and Prevention, n.d.). These experiences help equip CHS leaders prepare for future pandemic planning and modulation of staffing and care delivery models to meet the needs of rapidly changing care in crisis state. Leaders must adopt strategies to address these challenges to promote the success of the pediatric workforce through developing psychologically safe environments for staff to process distress, advanced planning for supply chain challenges, and early and flexible staffing models to meet the needs of patient care.

Impacts on Clinician Well-Being

The American Nurses Association (ANA) conducted a survey in March through April of 2020 to assess nurses' concerns about the pandemic (American Nurses Association, n.d.). The survey provides a snapshot of the experience of 32,000 nurses in the U.S., 68% of whom reported concerns about being short-staffed (American Nurses Association, n.d.). Factors contributing to the concern for a national nursing workforce shortage predate the COVID-19 pandemic. In a cross-sectional study of hospitals before and during the COVID-19 pandemic, data suggests that nursing burnout and intent to leave the profession worsened only slightly during the pandemic in hospitals that have historically poor working environments and suboptimal nurse staffing (Aiken et al., 2022). This was additive to a profession already identified as at higher risk for mental health challenges, anxiety, depression, and suicide in pre-pandemic state (Davis et al., 2021). A study reviewing data from 2007 to 2018 demonstrated that nurses, particularly female, have a significantly increased risk of suicide when compared to the general population (Davis et al., 2021).

The American Association of Critical Care Nurses (AACN) compiled responses from more than 6500 United States (U.S.) critical care nurses with devastating findings. Nearly 92% of respondents reported that they believe the pandemic was professionally depleting and will cut their careers short and 66% reported considering leaving the nursing profession after their experience with the pandemic (American Association of Critical Care Nurses, 2021). COVID-19 resulted in significant retention challenges of RN staff across all healthcare settings with spikes in moral distress, emotional exhaustion, and anxiety, yielding a ballooning challenge for healthcare leaders (American Association of Critical Care Nurses, 2021). In a meta-analysis examining nurses' motivations to leave the profession, reasons did not all point to experiences during COVID-19. Nurses commonly cited poor working conditions, bullying, lack of career advancement opportunities, lack of support from managers, and stress as rationale for separation from the nursing profession (Bahlman-van Ooijen et al., 2023). These factors, coupled with an aging workforce have amplified staffing challenges (McKenna et al., 2023). In fact, the International Council of Nurses projects the need for an additional 10.6 million nurses globally by 2030 to address the workforce shortfall (Anon, 2022).

Staffing challenges in healthcare systems led to struggles to properly staff units and keep beds open for patients in need of care. In ambulatory settings, reduced staffing led to strain in providing ambulatory access for primary and subspeciality care clinics. Staffing challenges led to further economic strain in healthcare systems as the demand for staffing began to propel reliance on staffing agencies to meet the needs of frontline staff in some healthcare settings and systems. Significant increases in opportunities for travel RNs and other healthcare professionals flourished during the pandemic, often accompanied by attractive sign-on bonuses. These staffing solutions were necessary in some children's hospitals to maintain operations, though, are less desirable than permanent staff due to the amplified hourly wage and lack of continuity of care (Chervoni, 2022). Other short-term solutions included recruiting RNs who had recently retired or expanding contingent/per diem staff and implementing incentive hourly payments for staff deployed to high-risk units, such as COVID-19 units where pediatric nurses sometimes cared for adult patients (Buccione et al., 2022).

Evidence has indicated higher incidence of moral distress, burnout, and post-traumatic stress disorder among pediatric critical care nurses prior to the pandemic when compared with other HCPs in pediatric critical care (Pountney et al., 2023). Pandemic-associated PPE shortages, re-purposing of pediatric critical care work, and inability to achieve work-life balance were accentuated during the pandemic, resulting in new challenges with pediatric critical care well-being (Pountney et al., 2023). In a study of pediatric ICU nurses, female nurses were more likely to experience post-traumatic stress disorder and sleep disturbances (Buccione et al., 2022). These results highlight the critical state of pediatric nurse well-being and implore pediatric nursing leaders to strategize efforts to address these issues.

Moral distress was heightened during the pandemic in both ambulatory and inpatient APRNs with ambulatory APRNs reporting more isolation and inpatient APRNs reporting more post-traumatic stress from traumatic experiences; however, both groups experienced mental and physical exhaustion (Wood et al., 2022). In the only study of its kind surveying COVID-19 impacts on pediatric-focused APRNs in 2021 (Peck & Sonney, 2021), more than one-third of the APRN workforce felt professionally burned out and 25% reported feeling anxious or nervous. Additionally, 15% of respondents reported feeling hopeless or depressed (Peck & Sonney, 2021). These findings support what had already been reported in other nursing populations and indicate severity of risk to the workforce and additional action needed by healthcare leaders to address this challenge.

It is clear that the continued suggestion of promoting individual resilience in nurses is not sufficient to address the crisis surrounding RNs and APRNs. Individual pediatric nursing professionals need the help of their leaders and organizations to promote organizational resilience and transform environments into supportive havens promoting psychological safety (Udod et al., 2021). Reducing non-clinical activities, such as meetings, promoting self-care including physical activity, building staffing schedules to promote sleep hygiene, and access to workplace counselling and resilience support can be used in providing support for nursing staff during pandemic response and beyond (Holthof & Luedi, 2021).

Impacts on Health Leaders

Leaders themselves experienced many personal and professional challenges while working hard to support their teams, units, and their employees. Leaders needed to remain committed to the mission of their respective organizations, ensuring quality, safety, service, research, and education were not compromised while trying to develop the skills of effective leadership during times of crisis. In addition, leaders were challenged with making high-impact decisions during times of uncertainty, complexity, and ambiguity (Kaul et al., 2020). Shingler-Nace (2020) notes that emergency management is a skill and not all leaders are equipped to navigate with ease through these unique challenges (Shingler-Nace, 2020). She identifies five elements to successful leadership during crisis: staying calm, communicating, collaborating, coordinating, and supporting teams through these times. Exemplary leadership has also been studied and resulted in a variety of traits and actions capable of an effective response (Nicola et al., 2020). These include open communication, acting early and decisively, not ignoring any sections of the community, and leading by example (Nicola et al., 2020). Additional principles which have been identified for effective leaders during crisis are communication, decision making, humanism, innovation, realism, and core values (Kaul et al., 2020). Critical care leaders speak to principles of presence, transparency, and empathy to ensure we emerge from this pandemic with better outcomes for our teams and ourselves (Hayes & Cocchi, 2022). Leaders need to have presence in a time of social isolation, offer praise and recognition to staff while potentially not receiving any themselves, increase transparency regarding organization decisions while data and context may not have been readily available, and keep constant organizational and community awareness while worrying about the health and well-being of themselves and their families.

The long-term impacts of the pandemic on advanced practice leaders have yet to be realized. There will be ongoing challenges related to vaccinations, masking policies, new variants, supply chain, and workforce shortages. And yet the resilience and adaptive change with which leaders responded cannot be underscored enough. An important priority of leaders is to complete an assessment of the landscape at all levels and practice the humility and wisdom to recognize lessons learned (Kaul et al., 2020). While we reflect and learn many lessons of leadership from the pandemic, let's not forget the direct impact that leading through this public health emergency had on pediatric leaders themselves. Future research directed toward the unique needs of pediatric-focused leaders and training for leaders to best respond during crisis is essential to not only having a resilient leader, but also an effective response for our teams.

Impacts on Pediatric Nursing Recruitment

In the years following the COVID-19 pandemic, pediatric nurses faced unique challenges that require support and investment from health system leaders. NCLEX-RN pass rates dropped in the years surrounding the pandemic, taking several years to recover (Larsen et al., 2003). The fourth quarter (October–December) of 2022 marked the nadir in NCLEX-RN pass rates since the initiation of the COVID-19 pandemic, with the lowest pass rates for more than a decade, 50.48%. This pass rate included first and repeat test takers from the United States and abroad (National Council of State Boards of Nursing, n.d.-a). The pass rate decline has been attributed to decreases in clinical hours, particularly in-person experiences during nursing school and the worsening mental well-being of nursing students related to pandemic stressors. Additionally, early in the pandemic, it was necessary to conserve PPE and distance staff, limiting resources, and space to accommodate in-person student learners. The NCLEX-RN pass rates began to rebound in 2023, with improved rates of 81.6% for the second quarter of 2023. Throughout the pandemic, the National Council of State Boards of Nursing did not waive from its established standards for pass rates, upholding established test-taking standards.

In parallel, Pediatric Nursing Certification Board (PNCB) Pediatric Nurse Practitioner pass rates were also impacted during the pandemic. In a 5-year span, between 2017 and 2022, Pediatric Nurse Practitioner—Primary Care (PNP-PC) pass rates fell from 92% to 80.44% and Pediatric Nurse Practitioner—Acute Care (PNP-AC) pass rates fell from 80% to 72.83% (Pediatric Nurse Practitioner Certification Board, n.d.). Certification standards are necessary to ensure clinicians have achieved minimum requirement for entry to practice; however, lower pass rates also reduced qualified candidate pools of RN and APRN staff when workforce pipeline is critical for CHS. Pediatric healthcare leaders must partner with nursing schools to maximize opportunities for accommodating student placement requests and invest in the experience of the preceptors and students to ensure rich and meaningful experiences for students.

Recruitment of individuals interested in becoming nursing professionals is essential to keeping hospital doors and clinics open to serve the health needs of children is a paramount issue for nursing leaders to address in conjunction with other key stakeholders. A study of U.S. nursing students identified experience of illness or hospitalization or that of a loved one or self, a family member or friend with a career in nursing, or previous healthcare setting work experience as leading factors in their decision to pursue the nursing profession (Larsen et al., 2003). The same study explored characteristics of the nursing professional that influenced career decisions and identified concern for others, variety of career paths, and job security ranked most highly (Larsen et al., 2003). An Indonesian study identified several factors influencing decisions entering the nursing profession. These include a desire to serve others and God, a personal calling to join the profession, and influence from family members and others to join the nursing profession (Cilar et al., 2020). These findings demonstrate influences that CHS leaders can commission in nursing workforce pipeline challenges, including highlighting the endless opportunities of the profession and the exquisite impact nurses have on individuals and societies.

Understanding the current landscape of the nursing profession must be leveraged to attract potential candidates to sustain the current and future nursing workforce. The 2022 National Workforce study showed that 80% of the U.S. nursing workforce identified as White/Caucasian, severely mismatched to the nation's current and future demographics and impeding universal delivery of culturally responsive care (National Council of State Boards of Nursing, n.d.-b). The study also revealed 11.2% of survey respondents identified as male, which further highlights opportunities for expanded efforts to recruit males to the profession to increase the workforce and to mirror the population (National Council of State Boards of Nursing, n.d.-b; Linden et al., 2022) more appropriately. Post-pandemic efforts are critically needed for CHS leaders to partner with nursing educators in attracting a diverse, culturally responsive supply line of students to the nursing and APRN profession through advocating for increased nursing workforce development funding, partnering with professional organizations, establishing strong supportive transition-to-practice programs, and fostering supportive, safe, and enriching environments to nursing students and early career staff (American Association of Colleges of Nursing, n.d.).

Barriers and Breakthroughs

Financial Impact Barrier

- Access to children's health insurance coverage is key to having access to health-care coverage. However, barriers such as out-of-pocket expenses, time, lost wages, food or housing insecurity, and a robust pediatric healthcare workforce are all key barriers which need to be addressed.
- Worsening health disparities in the number of children without health insurance covered were brought to the forefront during the pandemic.

Financial Impact Breakthrough

- The COVID-19 pandemic underscored the importance of legislative and administrative actions toward children's hospitals to support key initiatives such as telehealth expansion, HCP well-being, pediatric emergency preparedness, behavioral and mental health care services, and research.
- Continued support for programs such as Medicaid, Children's Health Insurance Program (CHIP), and the Affordable Care Act have brought the rate of uninsured children significantly down, and advocacy to improve outreach and enrollment efforts needs to continue after the public health emergency ended.

State and Federal Barrier

- Lack of universal adoption of full practice authority for APRNs.

State and Federal Breakthrough

- State-based emergency executive orders allowed APRNs in some states to practice to the full extent of their training, certification, and licensure and APRNs answered the call.

Clinician Impact Barrier

- Clinicians were operating in dynamic healthcare environments where they were had to adjust to new PPE requirements, potential deployment to new clinical areas, and strict COVID-19 testing guidelines.
- Clinicians experienced significant moral distress, burnout, and staffing challenges.

- Healthcare leaders were pushed to be transparent and manage complex operational systems with abruptly changing guidelines.

Clinician Breakthrough

- CHS pivoted to developing robust mental health and resilience support and resources for staff.
- As a result of the pandemic, CHS further examined staffing models and emergency preparedness workflows to be best prepared for future public health emergencies.
- New and novel strategies for recruitment of nursing professionals are increasing with opportunities to build a diverse pipeline of pediatric-focused HCPs.

Lessons Learned

The COVID-19 pandemic had widespread and lasting impacts challenging CHS leaders to stretch in all aspects of their role. The pediatric COVID-19 experience resulted in barriers including fast-paced influx of massive amounts of information and uncertainties, revenue stream and expense changes, staffing model adjustments, and mitigation strategies to keep patients, families, and staff safe and new vaccination requirements. Overarching breakthroughs from the pandemic include rapid deployment of ICS, showcasing APRN success at top of license practice, telehealth expansion, and identification of the many opportunities for supporting pediatric RN and APRN workforce well-being. The collective response of CHS and their leaders was essential to navigating the multifaceted impacts of pediatric COVID-19 and its impact on the workplace.

Calls to Action
- Expand the investment in public health infrastructure and promote increased coordination with children's healthcare systems to better holistically prepare for public health emergencies.
- Invest in the pediatric advanced practice profession by supporting efforts which focus on HCP well-being, resilience, and burnout avoidance.
- Promote strategies for pediatric workforce recruitment and retention to support future children's health system operations, acute and critical care access, and optimal patient care delivery.
- Advocate for full practice authority for all pediatric-focused APRNs in all states to optimize access to high-quality, affordable, and safe patient care.
- Continued advocacy for robust state and federal funds to support children's hospitals during a public health emergency, irrespective of payer mix.

References

Aiken, L., Sloane, D., McHugh, M., Pogue, C., & Lasater, K. (2022). A repeated cross-sectional study of nurses immediately before and during the COVID-19 pandemic: Implications for action. *Nursing Outlook, 71*, 101903. https://doi.org/10.1016/j.outlook.2022.11.007

American Association of Colleges of Nursing. (n.d.). *Fact sheet: Enhancing diversity in the nursing workforce*. https://www.aacnnursing.org/Portals/0/PDFs/Fact-Sheets/Enhancing-Diversity-Factsheet.pdf. Accessed 8 Oct 2023.

American Association of Critical Care Nurses. (2021). *Hear us out campaign*. https://www.hearusout.com/. Accessed 14 July 2023.

American Hospital Association. (n.d.). *CMS eliminates COVID-19 vaccination requirements for health care workers*. https://www.aha.org/news/headline/2023-05-31-cms-eliminates-covid-19-vaccination-requirements-health-care-workers. Accessed 1 Oct 2023.

American Nurses Association. (n.d.). *Initial COVID-19 survey*. www.nursingworld.org. https://www.nursingworld.org/practice-policy/work-environment/health-safety/disaster-preparedness/coronavirus/what-you-need-to-know/covid-19-survey-results/urvey. Accessed 5 July 2023.

Andrist, E., Clarke, R. G., & Harding, M. (2020). Paved with good intentions: Hospital visitation restrictions in the age of coronavirus disease 2019. *Pediatric Critical Care Medicine, 21*(10), e924–e926.

Anon. (2022). The NCSBN 2022 environmental scan: Resiliency, achievement, and public protection. *Journal of Nursing Regulation, 12*(4), S1–S56. https://doi.org/10.1016/S2155-8256(22)00015-1. Epub 2022 Jan 18. PMID: 35070487; PMCID: PMC8764909.

Bahlman-van Ooijen, W., Malfait, S., Huisman-de Waal, G., & Hafsteinsdóttir, T. B. (2023). Nurses' motivations to leave the nursing profession: A qualitative meta-aggregation. *Journal of Advanced Nursing, 00*, 1–17. https://doi.org/10.1111/jan.15696

Barioja, K., Elenwo, C., & Hartwell, M. (2023). Disparities in pediatric medical and childcare disruption due to COVID-19. *JAMA Pediatrics, 177*(4), 1–3.

Bavare, A. C., Goldman, J. R., Musick, M. A., Sembera, K. A., Sardual, A. A., Lam, A. K., Tume, S. C., Thammasitboon, S. X., & Williams, E. A. (2021). Virtual communication embedded bedside ICU rounds: A hybrid rounds practice adapted to the coronavirus pandemic. *Pediatric Critical Care Medicine, 22*(8), e427–e436. https://doi.org/10.1097/PCC.0000000000002704

Berchick, E. R., & Mykyta, L. (2019). *Children's public health insurance coverage lower than in 2017*. https://www.census.gov/library/stories/2019/09/uninsured-rate-for-children-in-2018.html

Beurhaus, P., Staiger, D., Auerbach, D., Yates, M., & Donelan, K. (2022). Nurse employment during the first fifteen months of the COVID-19 pandemic. *Health Affairs, 1*(1), 79–85. https://doi.org/10.1377/hithaff.2021.01289

Bokun, A., Himmelstern, J., Jeong, W., Meier, A., Musick, K., & Warren, R. (2020). *The unequal impact of COVID-19 on children's economic vulnerability*. https://econofact.org/the-unequal-impact-of-covid-19-on-childrens-economic-vulnerability

Brown, H., Carrera, B., & Stanley, L. (2021). Optimizing nurse staffing during a pandemic. *Journal of Continuing Education in Nursing, 52*(3), 109–111.

Buccione, E., Santella, B., Fiani, M. E., Maffeo, M., Tedesco, B., D'Errico, A., Della Pelle, C., Bambi, S., & Rasero, L. (2022). Quality of life of pediatric nurses during the COVID-19 pandemic: A cross-sectional study. *Dimensions of Critical Care Nursing, 41*(5), 246–255. https://doi.org/10.1097/DCC.0000000000000537. PMID: 35905426.

Casimir, G. (2019). Why children's hospitals are unique and so essential. *Frontiers in Pediatrics, 7*, 305. https://doi.org/10.3389/fped.2019.00305

Center for Disease Control and Prevention. (n.d.). *Considerations for planning curbside/drive-through vaccination clinics*. https://www.cdc.gov/vaccines/hcp/admin/mass-clinic-activities/curbside-vaccination-clinics.html. Accessed 19 July 2023.

Centers for Disease Control and Prevention. (2023, July 10). *CDC Museum COVID-19 timeline*. www.cdc.gov/museum/timeline/covid19.html. Accessed 7 July 2023.

Centers for Disease Control and Prevention. (n.d.). *Information for healthcare providers about multisystem inflammatory syndrome in children (MIS-C)*. https://www.cdc.gov/mis/mis-c/hcp_cstecdc/index.html. Accessed 28 July 2023.

Chervoni, T. (2022). The staffing shortage pandemic. *Journal of Radiology Nursing, 41*, 74–75.

Children's Hospital Association. (2021). *The financial impact of the Covid-19 pandemic on children's hospitals*. https://www.childrenshospitals.org/-/media/files/migration/cor_covid_financial_impact_report_2020.pdf. Accessed 27 July 2023.

Children's Hospital Association. (n.d.). *Declaration of a National Emergency in Child and Adolescent Mental Health*. https://www.childrenshospitals.org/news/newsroom/2021/11/declaration-of-a-national-emergency-in-child-and-adolescent-mental-health. Accessed 29 July 2023.

Chowdhury, J. M., Patel, M., Zheng, M., Abramian, O., & Criner, G. J. (2020). Mobilization and preparation of a large urban academic center during the COVID-19 pandemic. *Annals of the American Thoracic Society, 17*(8), 922–925. https://doi.org/10.1513/AnnalsATS.202003-259PS

Cilar, L., Spevan, M., Čuček Trifkovič, K., & Štiglic, G. (2020). What motivates students to enter nursing? Findings from a cross-sectional study. *Nurse Education Today, 90*, 104463. https://doi.org/10.1016/j.nedt.2020.104463

Coley, R. L. (2020). *COVID-19 job and income loss jeopardize child well-being: Income support policies can help*. https://www.srcd.org/research/covid-19-job-and-income-loss-jeopardize-child-well-being-income-support-policies-can-help

Currie, J., & Chorniy, A. (2021). Medicaid and child health insurance program improve child health and reduce poverty but face threats. *Academic Pediatrics, 21*(8S), S146–S153. https://doi.org/10.1016/j.acap.2021.01.009

Currie, J., & Duque, V. (2019). Medicaid: What does it do, and can we do it better? *The Annals of the American Academy of Political and Social Science, 686*(1), 148–179. https://doi.org/10.1177/0002716219874772

Davis, M., Cher, B., Friese, C., & Bynum, J. (2021). Association of US nurse and physician occupation with risk of suicide. *JAMA Psychiatry, 78*, 651. https://doi.org/10.1001/jamapsychiatry.2021.0154

Department of Health and Human Services. (2023). *Medicare and Medicaid Programs; Policy and Regulatory Changes to the Omnibus COVID-19 Health Care Staff Vaccination Requirements; Additional Policy and Regulatory Changes to the Requirements for Long-Term Care (LTC) Facilities and Intermediate Care Facilities for Individuals With Intellectual Disabilities (ICFs-IID) To Provide COVID-19 Vaccine Education and Offer Vaccinations to Residents, Clients, and Staff; Policy and Regulatory Changes to the Long Term Care Facility COVID-19 Testing Requirements*. https://public-inspection.federalregister.gov/2023-11449.pdf?utm_source=federalregister.gov&utm_medium=email&utm_campaign=pi+subscription+mailing+list. Accessed 20 July 2023.

Dorn, S., Garrett, B., Holahan, J., & Williams, A. (2008). *Medicaid, SCHIP and economic downturn: Policy challenges and policy responses*. Executive summary. Kaiser Commission on Medicaid and the Uninsured. https://www.kff.org/wp-content/uploads/2013/01/7770es.pdf

Emanuel, E. J., & Skorton, D. J. (2021). Mandating COVID-19 vaccination for health care workers. *Annals of Internal Medicine, 174*, 1308. https://doi.org/10.7326/M21-3150

EMSA. (2023, July 20). *HICS history and background*. https://emsa.ca.gov/hics-history-and-background/

Endacott, R., Pearce, S., Rae, P., Richardson, A., Bench, S., Pattison, N., & the SEISMIC Study Team. (2022). How COVID-19 has affected staffing models in intensive care: A qualitative study examining alternative staffing models (SEISMIC). *Journal of Advanced Nursing, 78*, 1075–1088. https://doi.org/10.1111/jan.15081

Ferry, A. M., Dibbs, R. P., Ward, A., Velez, V., Ringold, S. L., Archer, N. M., Winebar, J. M., Andropoulos, D. B., & Hollier, L. H., Jr. (2022). Operational effect of COVID-19 on surgical care at a tertiary pediatric hospital. *AORN Journal, 115*(2), 147–155. https://doi.org/10.1002/aorn.13604. PMID: 35084769; PMCID: PMC9011624.

Flaxman, S., Whittaker, C., Semenova, E., Rashid, T., Parks, R., Blenkinsop, A., Unwin, J., Mishra, S., Bhatt, S., Gurdasani, D., & Ratmann, O. (2023). Assessment of COVID-19 as the underlying cause of death among children and young people aged 0 to 19 years in the US. *JAMA Network Open, 6*(1), e2253590. https://doi.org/10.1001/jamanetworkopen.2022.53590

Food and Drug Administration. (n.d.). *Emergency use authorization.* Retrieved July 21, 2023, from https://www.fda.gov/emergency-preparedness-and-response/mcm-legal-regulatory-and-policy-framework/emergency-use-authorization. Accessed 21 July 2023.

Gill, P. J., Mahant, S., Hall, M., & Berry, J. G. (2021). Reasons for admissions to US children's hospitals during the COVID-19 pandemic. *JAMA, 325*(16), 1676–1679. https://doi.org/10.1001/jama.2021.4382. Erratum in: JAMA. 2021 Jul 13;326(2):190. PMID: 33904877; PMCID: PMC8080216.

Hayes, M. M., & Cocchi, M. N. (2022). Critical care leadership during the COVID-19 pandemic. *Journal of Critical Care, 67*, 186–188. https://doi.org/10.1016/j.jcrc.2021.09.015

Holthof, N., & Luedi, M. M. (2021). Considerations for acute care staffing during a pandemic. *Best Practice & Research. Clinical Anaesthesiology, 35*(3), 389–404. https://doi.org/10.1016/j.bpa.2020.12.008. Epub 2020 Dec 10. PMID: 34511227; PMCID: PMC7726522.

Isasi, F., Naylor, M., Skorton, D., Grbowski, D., Hernandez, S., & Rice, V. (2021). *Patients, families, and communicated COVID-19 impact assessment: Lessons learned and compelling needs.* National Academy of Medicine. https://nam.edu/patients-families-and-communities-covid-19-impact-assessment-lessons-learned-and-compelling-needs/

Kaul, V., Shah, V. H., & El-Serag, H. (2020). Leadership during crisis: Lessons and applications from the COVID-19 pandemic. *Gastroenterology, 159*(3), 809–812. https://doi.org/10.1053/j.gastro.2020.04.076

Khullar, D., Bond, A., & Schpero, W. (2020). COVID-19 and the financial health of US hospitals. *JAMA, 323*(21), 2127–2128. https://doi.org/10.1001/jama.2020.6269

Kim, L., Whitaker, M., O'Halloran, A., et al. (2020). Hospitalization rates and characteristics of children aged < 18 years hospitalization with laboratory-confirmed COVID-10—COVID-NET, 14 states. *MMWR Morbidity and Mortality Weekly Report, 69*, 1081–1088. https://doi.org/10.15585/mmwr.mm6932e3

Kleinpell, R., Myers, C., Schorn, M., & Likes, W. (2021). Impact of COVID-19 pandemic on APRN practice: Results from a national survey. *Nursing Outlook, 69*(5), 783–792. https://doi.org/10.1016/j.outlook.2021.05.002

Kociolek, L. K., Elhadary, J., Jhaveri, R., Patel, A. B., Stahulak, B., & Cartland, J. (2021). Coronavirus disease 2019 vaccine hesitancy among children's hospital staff: A single-center survey. *Infection Control and Hospital Epidemiology, 42*(6), 775–777. https://doi.org/10.1017/ice.2021.58. Epub 2021 Feb 9. PMID: 33557977; PMCID: PMC7925985.

Koppolu, R. (2021). Children's hospitals and impact of COVID-19. *Journal of Pediatric Health Care, 35*(2), 239–241. https://doi.org/10.1016/j.pedhc.2020.12.001

Larsen, P. D., McGill, J. S., & Palmer, S. J. (2003). Factors influencing career decisions: Perspectives of nursing students in three types of programs. *The Journal of Nursing Education, 42*(4), 168–173. https://doi.org/10.3928/0148-4834-20030401-07

Linden, M. A., Mitchell, G., Carlisle, S., Rainey, D., Mulvenna, C., & Monaghan, C. (2022). Recruiting males to the nursing profession: Acceptability testing of the 'make a difference with nursing' intervention for post-primary school students. *BMC Nursing, 21*(1), 173. https://doi.org/10.1186/s12912-022-00956-5

Maung, Z., Kristensen, M., Hoffman, B., & Jacobson, M. (2022). Temperature screening of healthcare personnel is ineffective in controlling COVID-19. *Journal of Occupational and Environmental Medicine, 64*(5), 382–384. https://doi.org/10.1097/JOM.0000000000002518

McKenna, L., Mambu, I., Sommers, C., Reisenhofer, S., & McCaughan, J. (2023). Nurses' and nursing students' reasons for entering the profession: Content analysis of open-ended questions. *BMC Nursing, 22*(1), 152. https://doi.org/10.1186/s12912-023-01307-8

Melnick, G., & Maerki, S. (2021, August 27). *The financial impact of COVID-19 on California hospitals: January 2020 through June 2021.* California Healthcare Foundation. https://www.chcf.org/wp-content/uploads/2021

Moss, S. J., Krewulak, K. D., Stelfox, H. T., Ahmed, S. B., Anglin, M. C., Bagshaw, S. M., Burns, K. E. A., Cook, D. J., Doig, C. J., Fox-Robichaud, A., Fowler, R., Hernández, L., Kho, M. E., Kredentser, M., Makuk, K., Murthy, S., Niven, D. J., Olafson, K., Parhar, K. K. S., Patten, S. B., Rewa, O. G., Rochwerg, B., Sept, B., Soo, A., Spence, K., Spence, S., Straus, S., West, A., Parsons Leigh, J., & Fiest, K. M. (2021). Restricted visitation policies in acute care settings during the COVID-19 pandemic: A scoping review. *Critical Care, 25*(1), 347. https://doi.org/10.1186/s13054-021-03763-7. PMID: 34563234; PMCID: PMC8465762.

Murphey, D. (2017). *Health insurance coverage improves well-being.* Child Trends Research Brief. https://cms.childtrends.org/wp-content/uploads/2017/05/2017-22HealthInsurance_finalupdate.pdf

National Council of State Boards of Nursing. (n.d.-a). *NCLEX_Stats_2022-Q4-PassRates.* https://www.ncsbn.org/public-files/NCLEX_Stats_2022-Q4-PassRates.pdf. Accessed 28 Sept 2023.

National Council of State Boards of Nursing. (n.d.-b). *National nursing workforce study.* Retrieved October 8, 2023, from https://www.ncsbn.org/research/recent-research/workforce.page. Accessed 8 Oct 2023.

Nelson, K., & Hylton Rushton, C. (2021). Working while ill during COVID-19: Ethics, guilt, and moral community. *AACN Advanced Critical Care, 32*(3), 356–361. https://doi.org/10.4037/aacnacc2021342

Nicola, M., Sohrabi, C., Mathew, G., Kerwan, A., Al-Jabir, A., Griffin, M., Agha, M., & Agha, R. (2020). Health policy and leadership models during the COVID-19 pandemic: A review. *International Journal of Surgery, 81*, 122–129. https://doi.org/10.1016/j.ijsu.2020.07.026

Office of Disease Prevention and Health Promotion, Office of the Assistant Secretary for Health, Office of the Secretary, U.S. Department of Health and Human Services. (2022). *Healthy People 2030: Health care access and quality.* https://health.gov/healthypeople/objectives-and-data/browse-objectives/health-careaccess-and-quality

Parikh, S., Avansino, J., Dick, A., Enriquez, B., Geiduschek, J., Martin, L., McDonald, R., Yandow, S., Zerr, D., & Ojemann, J. (2020). Collaborative multidisciplinary incident command at Seattle children's hospital for raid preparatory pediatric surgery countermeasures to the COVID-19 pandemic. *Journal of the American College of Surgeons, 231*(2), 269–274. https://doi.org/10.1016/j.jamcollsurg.2020.04.012

Peck, J., & Sonney, J. (2021). Exhausted and burned out: COVID-19 emerging impacts threaten the health of pediatric advanced practice registered nursing workforce. *Journal of Pediatric Health Care, 35*(4), 414–424.

Pediatric Nurse Practitioner Certification Board. (n.d.). *PNCB exams—Exam types, accreditation, and statistics.* https://pncb.org/pncb-exams. Accessed 28 Sept 2023.

Pelletier, J., Rakkar, J., Au, A., Fuhrman, D., Clark, R., & Horvat, C. M. (2021). Trends in US pediatric hospital admissions in 2020 compared with the decade before the COVID-19 pandemic. *JAMA Open Network, 4*(2), e2037227. https://doi.org/10.1001/jamanetworkopen.2020.37227

Pountney, J., Butcher, I., Donnelly, P., Morrison, R., & Shaw, R. L. (2023). How the COVID-19 crisis affected the well-being of nurses working in paediatric critical care: A qualitative study. *British Journal of Health Psychology, 00*, 1–16. https://doi.org/10.1111/bjhp.12661

Renke, C., Callow, L., Egnor, T., Honstain, C., Kellogg, K., Pollack, B., Reske, J., et al. (2020). Utilization of pediatric nurse practitioners as adult critical care providers during the COVID-19 pandemic: A novel approach. *Journal of Pediatric Health Care, 34*(5), 490–494.

Rosner, R. (2020). Adverse effects of prolonged mask use among healthcare professionals during COVID-19. *Journal of Infectious Diseases and Epidemiology, 6*, 130. https://doi.org/10.23937/2472-3658/151013

Schwartz, K., & Damino, A. (2020, May 13). *Distribution of CARES act funding among hospitals*. Kaiser Family Foundation. https://www.kff.org/coronavirus-covid-19/issue-brief/distribution-of-cares-act-funding-among-hospitals/

Shingler-Nace, A. (2020). COVID-19: When leadership calls. *Nurse Leader, 18*(3), 202–203. https://doi.org/10.1016/j.mnl.2020.03.017

Synhorst, D. C., Bettenhausen, J. L., Hall, M., Thurm, C., Shah, S. S., Auger, K. A., Williams, D. J., Morse, R., & Berry, J. G. (2021). Healthcare encounter and financial impact of COVID-19 on children's hospitals. *Journal of Hospital Medicine, 16*(4), 223–226. https://doi.org/10.12788/jhm.3572

Tabah, A., Ramanan, M., Laupland, K. B., Buetti, N., Cortegiani, A., Mellinghoff, J., Conway, A., Morris, L., Camporota, L., Zappella, N., Elhadi, M., Povoa, P., Amrein, K., Vidalz, G., Derde, L., Bassetti, M., Francois, G., Ssi yan kai, N., & De Waele, J. J. (2020). Personal protective equipment and intensive care unit healthcare worker safety in the COVID-19 era (PPE-SAFE): An international survey. *Journal of Critical Care, 59*, 70–75.

Temsah, M. H., Alhboob, A., Abouammoh, N., Al-Eyadhy, A., Aljamaan, F., Alsohime, F., Alabdulhafid, M., Ashry, A., Bukhari, A., ElTahir, O., Jamal, A., Halwani, R., Alhasan, K., Alherbish, A., Temsah, R., Al-Tawfiq, J. A., & Barry, M. (2021). Pediatric intensive care hybrid-style clinical round during COVID-19 pandemic: A pilot study. *Frontiers in Pediatrics, 9*, 720203. https://doi.org/10.3389/fped.2021.720203. PMID: 34490169; PMCID: PMC8417365.

Toth-Manikowski, S., Swirsky, E., Gandhi, R., & Piscitello, G. (2022). COVID-19 vaccination hesitancy among health care workers, communication, and policy-making. *American Journal of Infection Control, 50*, 20–25.

Udod, S., MacPhee, M., & Baxter, P. (2021). Rethinking resilience. Nurses and nurse leaders emerging from the post-COVID-19. *Environment, 51*(11), 537–540.

Vance, A. J., Duy, J., Laventhal, N., Iwashyna, T. J., & Costa, D. K. (2021). Visitor guidelines in US children's hospitals during COVID-19. *Hospital Pediatrics, 11*(6), e83–e89. https://doi.org/10.1542/hpeds.2020-005772

Wahlster, S., & Hartog, C. (2022). Coronavirus disease 2019 aftermath: Psychological trauma in ICU healthcare workers. *Current Opinion in Critical Care, 28*(6), 686–694. https://doi.org/10.1097/MCC.0000000000000994. Epub 2022 Oct 18. PMID: 36302198.

Westley, L., Manworren, R., Griffith, D., Hoffman, J., Janssen, A., Routburg, S., & Richey, K. (2023). Using hospital incident command systems to respond to the pediatric mental and behavioral health crisis of the COVID-19 pandemic. *The Journal of Nursing Administration, 53*(2), 96–103. https://doi.org/10.1097/NNA.0000000000001254

Wietecha, M. (2022). *End of year priorities congress letter*. Children's Hospital Association. https://www.childrenshospitals.org/-/media/files/public-policy/mental_health/letters/2022/110222_end_of_year_priorities_congress_letter.pdf

Wood, E., King, R., Robertson, S., Senek, M., & Tod, A. (2022). Moral distress in advanced practice nurses during the COVID-19 pandemic. *Nursing Standard, 37*, 44. https://doi.org/10.7748/ns.2022e11885

Zhang, H., Dimitrov, D., Simpson, L., Plaks, N., Singh, B., Penney, S., Charles, J., Sheehan, R., Flammini, S., Murphy, S., & Landman, A. (2020). A web-based, mobile-responsive application to screen health care workers for COVID-19 symptoms: Rapid design, deployment, and usage. *JMIR Formative Research, 4*(10), e19533. https://doi.org/10.2196/19533. PMID: 32877348; PMCID: PMC7546861.

Zorko, D., Gertsman, S., O'Hearn, K., Timmerman, N., Ambu-Ali, N., Dinh, T., Sampson, M., Sikora, L., McNally, J. D., & Choong, K. (2020). Decontamination interventions for the reuse of surgical mask personal protective equipment: A systematic review. *The Journal of Hospital Infection, 106*(2), 283–294.

Concluding Thoughts

Moira Szilagyi

The COVID-19 pandemic came upon us seemingly out of nowhere disrupting our safety as it created fear, anxiety, and upheaval across the entire world, including in the United States. The underpinnings of our lives (our daily routines and rituals, our social connections, and our expectations for what our life was and could be) were suddenly no more. The pandemic quickly became a pan-disruptor.

Despite long-standing fears that a pandemic, likely influenza, was on the horizon, our country, with its immense wealth and infrastructure, was woefully unprepared. Our public health infrastructure had been largely decimated following 9/11, and pediatric healthcare had been undervalued and underfunded for decades. Vaccines that have protected people from debilitating and potentially deadly diseases are still regarded as the crowning public health achievement of all time, but vaccine misinformation and disinformation had fueled hesitancy and refusal. When the pandemic hit, the hesitancy and refusal escalated and led to questioning other public health recommendations such as masking, distancing, and isolating. At the time, our country was also mired in conflict and disagreement fueled by social media opportunists. It was in this context that we were brought to a literal standstill in 2020 by a virus about which we understood little.

This comprehensive book on the pandemic reminds us of those frightening times early on when people, especially the elderly, were hospitalized and dying in droves. It reminds us of the almost paralyzing uncertainty we felt because solid information was sparse and the disinformation machine filled the data void with fiction. In this book, expert authors revisit the breadth and depth of the upheaval we endured, across systems, socioeconomic levels, and ages. They detail the effects on the pediatric workforce as our practices and clinics closed, elective surgery was suspended, our pediatric units were converted to adult care, and our emergency departments witnessed a dramatic increase in child and youth visits for mental health problems

M. Szilagyi
UCLA Geffen School of Medicine, Los Angeles, CA, USA

© The Author(s), under exclusive license to Springer Nature
Switzerland AG 2025
J. L. Peck (ed.), *COVID-19 Impacts on Child Health*,
https://doi.org/10.1007/978-3-031-80369-7

and suicidality. They recall that pediatric training shifted overnight to a virtual model, compromising education of our future healthcare professionals. They review the impacts on pregnant women and newborns, minoritized populations and immigrants, children in foster care and juvenile justice settings, and those with special health care needs. The authors reviewed the literature and remind us that no one was left untouched, and some of us fared worse than others. A harsh light was shone on the inequities in healthcare access that were deeply embedded into our systems and structures, especially for marginalized populations, such as those of color, immigrants, and the poor.

In pediatrics, children initially had lower rates of infection and their health appeared less harmed, so it is easy to forget that children and families suffered in other critical ways as schools, childcare, recreation sites, and libraries are closed. Because there was no vaccine and limited understanding of how the virus spread, isolation replaced social connection. Family stress increased as supply chains for food and daily essentials became depleted, and many families experienced a significant drop in income as employers reduced the size of their workforce.

Some of our most marginalized populations were on the front lines of health care and by mid-2021, over 140,000 US children, mostly Black, Latino, and Native American, had lost a primary caregiver to the virus, and many other children were separated from caregivers and other family members who were hospitalized. While some parents were able to home-school and some children could access school on-line, learning was compromised for children with poor internet access. Children with disabilities and special health care needs lost vital school services (special education, school-based health, and mental health). And, then, in 2021, Multi-system Inflammatory Syndrome (MIS-C) was diagnosed in children and toddlers. In 2022, as schools and childcare re-opened, the tripledemic of influenza, COVID-19, and RSV, led to a surge in pediatric hospitalizations, including intensive care admission, for infants and toddlers. The major impact on children though was the loss of relational experiences and social-emotional learning. Societal conflict and anger streamed into their lives by social media continue to feed the anxiety, depression, grief, loss, and loneliness as the world has opened back up. And, our pediatric workforce has not fully recovered from its losses.

We were fortunate in the US—fortunate that we were well-resourced and our government could invest in vaccine development; fortunate that research on mRNA and its potential had been ongoing for decades; fortunate that antivirals and immunoglobulin treatments were available and new ones came to market; fortunate that we have a vaccine reporting system to quickly monitor for "signals" that might indicate potential side effects; and fortunate that the safety profiles of the recommended COVID-19 vaccines have been excellent. We were also fortunate that the American Academy of Pediatrics became the repository for data about children and developed 30 different scientifically grounded guidance tools to help pediatricians, other pediatric healthcare professionals, parents, and government leaders respond to protect children. Science often evolves slowly, but "COVID science" grew rapidly. Sadly, the science was often drowned out by the misinformation and purposeful disinformation that fed hesitancy and distrust.

Another pandemic will happen. We don't know which organism will cause it or when it might happen—the experts worry about influenza and measles. The authors of this book go beyond describing what happened over 3 years of a global pandemic. They advocate for the United States to take the lessons learned that are described in each chapter and make recommendations about how our country could and should invest in preparing for another pandemic. They suggest rebuilding our infrastructure in public health and investing in our pediatric health system and workforce, increasing the size of the mental health workforce, and making sure that all pediatric healthcare professionals understand and use trauma-informed principles in caring for children. They have ample suggestions and we can hope that our leaders not only read this book but use the recommendations to make wise decisions and investments, to communicate the science that saved hundreds of thousands of lives, and to prevent the chaos that added to the disruptions caused by the COVID-19 pandemic.